Steering against Superbugs

Steering against Superbugs

The Global Governance of Antimicrobial Resistance

Edited by

OLIVIER RUBIN

Professor in Global Studies, Roskilde University, Roskilde, Denmark

ERIK BAEKKESKOV

Senior Lecturer in Public Policy, University of Melbourne, Melbourne, Australia

AND

LOUISE MUNKHOLM

Consultant, PhD in sociology of law, Roskilde University, Roskilde, Denmark

Cover image: Earth encircled by the genome of MRSA strain SO-1977 from Sudan.
The circular map of the chromosome is reproduced from Ali, M.S., Isa, N.M., Abedelrhman, F.M. et al.
Genomic analysis of methicillin-resistant Staphylococcus aureus strain SO-1977 from Sudan.
BMC Microbiol 19, 126 (2019). https://doi.org/10.1186/s12866-019-1470-2. The globe is reproduced from
Johan Swanepoel/Shutterstock.com

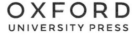

OXFORD
UNIVERSITY PRESS

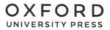
OXFORD
UNIVERSITY PRESS

Great Clarendon Street, Oxford, OX2 6DP,
United Kingdom

Oxford University Press is a department of the University of Oxford.
It furthers the University's objective of excellence in research, scholarship,
and education by publishing worldwide. Oxford is a registered trade mark of
Oxford University Press in the UK and in certain other countries

© Oxford University Press 2023

The moral rights of the authors have been asserted

First Edition published in 2023

Published in the United States of America by Oxford University Press
198 Madison Avenue, New York, NY 10016, United States of America

British Library Cataloguing in Publication Data

Data available

Library of Congress Control Number: 2022952180

ISBN 978–0–19–289947–7

DOI: 10.1093/oso/9780192899477.001.0001

Printed and bound in the UK by
TJ Books Limited

This volume collects together key insights from across social sciences on AMR governance. AMR is now the third-leading underlying cause of death globally, which is why a global approach and global governance is necessary. Through a global perspective, the case studies in this volume highlight both successes and challenges of local, regional, and global governance for AMR. As we work together across the world to tackle the 'silent' AMR pandemic, I strongly recommend this book for all in the global and public health and policy sphere to help galvanise action to address the insidious and complex health emergency of AMR.

Professor Dame Sally Davies
UK Special Envoy on Antimicrobial Resistance (AMR)

Steering against Superbugs comprehensively unpacks the root social drivers of antimicrobial resistance and masterfully situates these drivers in their cultural, historical and political contexts. Rubin, Baekkeskov, and Munkholm have brought together some of the world's leading thinkers in this field and have provided us with some of the best ideas yet to tackle this intensifying global health challenge that already kills more than 1.2 million people each year.

Professor Steven J. Hoffman, Director of the Global Strategy Lab and
the WHO Collaborating Centre on Global Governance of Antimicrobial
Resistance, York University, Canada

This exciting volume achieves what many have been waiting for: a compendium of social science approaches to antimicrobial resistance. With a focus on governance, the authors demonstrate the strengths of different disciplines by providing evidence at multiple scales of the ways in which antibiotics, and drug resistance, is—and can be—governed. From clinics, to bednets, to global policy spaces, the book introduces the reader to detailed case studies that enlighten and awaken interest in the multiple dimensions that make up the complex challenge of antimicrobial resistance globally.

Professor Clare Chandler, Anthropology of Antimicrobial Resistance
lead and founding Director, AMR Centre, London School of
Hygiene & Tropical Medicine.

Microbes, humans, One Health, and the interplay between them through AMR. This book introduces the reader to the conceptual issues of AMR, and then steers her through governance challenges, One Health aspects, global awareness, advocacy and regulatory matters. This is essential reading, not just for those working in this critical field but also for policy-makers, healthcare leaders, One Health professionals, and the wider community—providing an armament of knowledge, insight, and perspectives in the fight against AMR.

Professor & Head Sujith J Chandy, Department of Pharmacology & Clinical Pharmacology, Christian Medical College Vellore, India

Preface

'Superbugs' is not entirely new as a term referring to drug-resistant microbes and their threat to medicine and society. In October of 1966, amidst articles on fashion and football, *Look* magazine offered a two-page commentary, entitled 'Are Germs Winning the War Against People?' (Osmundsen, 1966). As John Osmundsen began his piece, in the wake of the discovery of the horizontal transmission of resistance across bacteria: 'Recent reports in medical journals and the press warn that the problem of controlling infectious disease caused by bacteria may be getting out of hand.' Describing multi-drug-resistant 'superbugs' that 'might get loose and create an epidemic of invulnerability to drugs among germs throughout the world', Osmundsen warned that unless antimicrobials were used more rationally, 'we may find ourselves no better off than we were in the 1930s, before the advent of sulfa drugs and penicillin, when cleanliness was about the only weapon we had against bacterial infections'.

The notion of rational antibiotic use that Osmundsen implied was itself in transition by the time he wrote his article. Starting in the 1950s, reformers focused on the seemingly irrational nature of particular antibiotic combinations and their pervasive (and persuasive) advertising, culminating in the passage in the United States in 1962 of the Kefauver–Harris amendments, mandating proof of drug efficacy through controlled clinical trials before permitting new drugs on the market. With seemingly inappropriate drugs off the market, from the late 1960s onward, reformist physicians, pharmacists, public health workers, and politicians increasingly discussed the 'rational' or 'irrational' prescribing of *appropriate* antibiotics, considering the relative impacts of clinician education versus regulation in ensuring the individual prescription of the right drug for the right bug for the right patient at the right time at the right cost (Podolsky, 2015). More recently still, scholars in disciplines like anthropology, sociology, and history have turned to examining the larger structural forces (in both the Global North and South) shaping and often constraining the practice of such would-be 'rational' prescribing.

This shift in the notion of 'rational' prescribing has taken place amidst larger shifts with respect to antibiotic development, prescribing, and reform. First, the heady technological optimism of the 1950s and 1960s—when antibiotics remained a leading sector for pharmaceutical profitability, and when even Osmundsen could conclude his article with the reassurance that 'meanwhile, the pharmaceutical industry is working harder than ever to develop new antibiotics so that we can at least stay even in the war against our bacterial enemies'—has been replaced by concern (if not panic) about the inability of industry to 'stay even' with resistant superbugs, and by consideration of the necessary means to incentivize industry to re-engage in such antimicrobial development in the first place (Morel et al., 2020). Second, and starting in the 1980s (and escalating in recent decades), the attention of antibiotic reformers has extended from local, and even national, to global concerns and actions, at least as conceptualized by would-be reformers invoking antimicrobial resistance as a shared moral and pragmatic concern regarding microbes that respect neither species nor national boundaries (Overton et al., 2021). Such 'global' reframing would eventually entail more nuanced considerations of various tensions: between global and local (as well as regional) needs, opportunities, and implementation; concerning the evolving relationship between the Global North and South in the production, consumption, and regulation of antimicrobials; and among the forces shaping both antimicrobial excess and access in different parts of the globe (Kirchhelle et al., 2020). Third, antimicrobial usage and its consequences have since the 2000s been reframed as a 'One Health' concern, mandating considerations across multiple sectors of usage (humans, animals, agriculture), and the alignment of supranational entities like the World Health Organization (WHO), the World Organization for Animal Health (OIE), and the Food and Agriculture Organization (FAO), as well as their parallels within nations and regions (Khan, 2016). And fourth, and still more recently, we have seen social scientists increasingly and productively engage with the political, economic, social, cultural, legal, and moral contexts in which antibiotics are developed, regulated, prescribed (or not), and taken, and in which resistance develops and is encountered (Chandler et al., 2016). In the hands of such social scientists, simple equations of supply and demand have given way to more nuanced considerations of the global, regional, and local forces shaping antimicrobial usage and resistance.

Against this background, *Steering against Superbugs* appears at a propitious moment. In 2015, with antimicrobial resistance having been surfaced (at least momentarily) as a global public health and economic concern on par with climate change, the WHO released its Global Action Plan on Antimicrobial Resistance, followed a year later by the United Nations' first-ever High Level Meeting on Antimicrobial Resistance (Davies, 2013; O'Neill, 2016; WHO, 2015). By 2023, well over 100 countries have developed National Action Plans (WHO, 2022). And yet, while such initiatives represent a significant shift in mobilization around antimicrobial usage and resistance, the responses to date have exposed important limitations, not the least the gap between the paper aspirations of the plans and the necessary funding and structural capacities to implement change (IACG, 2018).

And this is where this volume's contributors—from across a range of social sciences—play such a valuable role in framing and examining such apparent mobilization, its successes and limitations to date, and the prospects for (and potential nature of) global governance concerning antimicrobial usage and resistance moving forward. They examine collaborations and tensions across animal, human, and agricultural sectors, often across a second axis concerning local, regional, and global needs and actors. They underscore the historical path-dependency of how such efforts have unfolded to date in locations ranging from Bangladesh and India to Switzerland and the European Union. And while revealing the similarities between antimicrobial resistance and climate change, they demonstrate the degree to which antimicrobial resistance has to this point lacked the degree of consistent advocacy and activism applied to climate change.

This last comparison merits its own consideration. After all, antimicrobial resistance is not only a rich topic through which social scientists can thoughtfully examine interactions among germs, people, and the structures and societies in which they are embedded. It is a critical public health and social justice concern whose evolving 'solutions' should merit the continuing input of social scientists moving forward. As we reconsider the very nature of 'winning' a 'war' against germs, we can be thoughtful in how we collectively and productively live with them, and with each other.

Scott Harris Podolsky, MD

Professor of Global Health and Social Medicine

Department of Global Health and Social Medicine, Harvard Medical School,

USA Director, Center for the History of Medicine, Countway Medical Library

References

Chandler, C., Hutchinson, E., and Hutchison, C. (2016). *Addressing Antimicrobial Resistance Through Social Theory: An Anthropologically Oriented Report*. London School of Hygiene & Tropical Medicine. http://www.lshtm.ac.uk/php/ghd/research/app/anthropologyofantimicrobial resistance.html;. see also https://antimicrobialsinsociety.org/

Davies, S. C. (2013). *Annual Report of the Chief Medical Officer. Volume Two, 2011: Infections and the Rise of Antimicrobial Resistance* (London: Department of Health).

Interagency Coordination Group on Antimicrobial Resistance (IACG). (2018). *Antimicrobial Resistance: National Action Plans*. https://cdn.who.int/media/docs/default-source/antimicrobial-resistance/iacg-amr-national-action-plans-110618.pdf?sfvrsn=53e4eb22_4

Kahn, L. (2016). *One Health and the Politics of Antimicrobial Resistance* (Baltimore, MD: Johns Hopkins University Press).

Kirchhelle, C., Atkinson, P., Broom, A., Chuengsatiansup, K., Ferreira, J. P., Fortané, N., et al. (2020). 'Setting the Standard: Multidisciplinary Hallmarks for Structural, Equitable and Tracked Antibiotic Policy', *BMJ Global Health*, 5/9, e003091.

Morel, C. M., Lindahl, O., Harbarth, S., de Kraker, M. E. A., Edwards, S., and Hollis, A. (2020) 'Industry Incentives and Antibiotic Resistance: An Introduction to the Antibiotic Susceptibility Bonus', *Journal of Antibiotics*, 73: 421–28.

O'Neill, J. (2016). *Tackling Drug-Resistant Infections Globally: Final Report and Recommendations* (London: The Review on Antimicrobial Resistance). https://amr-review.org/sites/default/files/160518_Final%20paper_with%20cover.pdf

Osmundsen, J. A. (1966). 'Are Germs Winning the War Against People?', *Look* (18 October 1966), 140–41.

Overton, K., Fortané, N., Broom, A., Raymond, S., Gradmann, C., Orubu, E. S., et al. (2021). 'Waves of Attention: Patterns and Themes of International Antimicrobial Resistance Reports, 1945–2000', *BMJ Global Health*, 6, e006909. doi:10.1136/bmjgh-2021-006909.

Podolsky, S. H. (2015). *The Antibiotic Era: Reform, Resistance, and the Pursuit of a Rational Therapeutics* (Baltimore, MD: Johns Hopkins University Press).

World Health Organization. (2015). *Global Action Plan on Antimicrobial Resistance* (Geneva: World Health Organization).

World Health Organization. (2022). *Library of AMR National Action Plans*. https://www.who.int/teams/surveillance-prevention-control-AMR/national-action-plan-monitoring-evaluation/library-of-national-action-plans.

Contents

Contributors

Erik Baekkeskov is Senior Lecturer in the School of Social and Political Sciences at the University of Melbourne, Melbourne, Australia.

Daniel Carelli is a Phd-candidate in the Department of Political Science at the University of Gothenburg, Gothenburg, Sweden.

Raphael Chanda is Senior Policy Officer in the Action on Antibiotic Resistance (ReAct), Africa.

Ipshita Chaturvedi is a Partner at Dentons Rodyk LLP, Singapore.

Francesca Chiara is Director of Antimicrobial Stewardship Project, Center for Infectious Disease Research and Policy (CIDRAP) at University of Minnesota, Minneapolis, USA.

Jessica Craig is Senior Research Analyst at the Center for Disease Dynamics, Economics & Policy, Nairobi, Kenya.

Mark D. M. Davis is Associate Professor in the Centre to Impact Antimicrobial Resistance at Monash University, Melbourne, Australia.

Chris Degeling is Associate Professor in the Australian Centre for Engagement, Evidence and Values at the University of Wollongong, Wollongong, Australia.

Bernadette Dunham is Professorial Lecturer in the Milken Institute School of Public Health at George Washington University, Washington, DC, USA.

Alina Engström is a Analyst at Swedish Defence Research Agency, Kista, Sweden.

Isabel Frost is a Consultant to the WHO in Geneva.

Sebastián Andres Frugone Cádiz is a Risk Analysis and Governance Graduate at the University of Stavanger, Norway.

Christoph Gradmann is Professor in the Department of Community Medicine and Global Health at the University of Oslo Institute of Health and Society, Oslo, Norway.

Tabitha Hrynick is Researcher in the Institute of Development Studies at the University of Sussex, Brighton, United Kingdom.

Sarah Humboldt-Dachroeden is a PhD candidate in the Department of Social Sciences and Business at Roskilde University, Roskilde, Denmark.

Carsten Strøby Jensen is Associate Professor in the Department of Sociology at the University of Copenhagen, Copenhagen, Denmark.

Jyoti Joshi is Antimicrobial Resistance (AMR) Advisor at the International Centre for AMR Solutions (ICARS), Copenhagen, Denmark.

Natasha Kavalakkat is Counsel at Singularity Legal in Mumbai, India.

Claas Kirchhelle is Assistant Professor in the School of History at the University College Dublin, Dublin, Ireland.

Hayley MacGregor is Professor in the Institute of Development Studies at the University of Sussex, Brighton, United Kingdom.

Philip Mathew is Advisor at the International Centre for Antimicrobial Resistance Solutions, Copenhagen, Denmark.

Louise Munkholm is Consultant, PhD in sociology of law, at Roskilde University, Roskilde, Denmark.

Katerina Mitkidis is Associate Professor in the Department of Law at Aarhus University, Aarhus, Denmark.

Mirfin Mpundu is Director of ReAct Africa, Partnership & Engagement Lead Africa at the International Centre for Antimicrobial Resistance Solution (ICARS), Copenhagen, Denmark.

Jon Pierre is Professor in the Department of Political Science at the University of Gothenburg, Gothenburg, Sweden.

Arjun Rajkhowa is project officer at the National Centre for Antimicrobial Stewardship, in the Department of Infectious Diseases at the Melbourne Medical School, Melbourne, Australia.

Kabir Rajkhowa is Professor at the Gauhati Medical College and Hospital, Guwahati, Assam, India.

Susan Rogers Van Katwyk is Managing Director of the WHO Collaborating Centre on Global Governance of Antimicrobial Resistance at York University, Canada.

Björn Rönnerstrand is a PhD and researcher at the SOM Institute of the University of Gothenburg, Gothenburg, Sweden.

Oliver Rubin is Professor in Global Studies, Roskilde University, Roskilde, Denmark.

Syed Shahid Abbas is a Researcher at the Institute of Development Studies, University of Sussex, Brighton, United Kingdom.

Reidar Staupe-Delgado is Associate Professor at UiT, the Arctic University of Norway, Norway.

Nancy Leys Stepan is Professor Emerita of History of Medicine at Colombia University, New York, USA.

Muriel Surdez is Professor in the Department of Social Sciences at the University of Fribourg, Switzerland.

Karin Thursky is Professor at the National Centre for Antimicrobial Stewardship, in the Department of Infectious Diseases at the Melbourne Medical School, Melbourne, Australia.

Ahmad Wesal Zaman is a Postdoc in the Department of Social Sciences and Business at Roskilde University, Roskilde, Denmark.

1

Steering against Superbugs

Research Agenda and Four Perspectives for Global Governance

Erik Baekkeskov, Louise Munkholm, and Olivier Rubin

Introduction

Many people correctly understand that superbugs can threaten health. Superbugs are microbial organisms, including bacteria, viruses, parasites, or fungi, that resist one or more antibiotic or other antimicrobial treatments. What may be less widely understood is that the threat is global, growing, and encompasses human systems surrounding healthcare, agriculture, and the environment. In 2019, 1.3 million people around the world are estimated to have died from resistant microbes (Murray et al., 2022). This is similar to how many succumb annually to HIV/AIDS and malaria combined (Laxminarayan 2022). The recent coronavirus pandemic may have further exacerbated the global health challenge posed by superbugs (Adebisi et al., 2021; Rizvi and Ahammad, 2022; Rodríguez-Baño et al., 2021). By 2050, worst-case projections include annual superbug fatalities of 10 million people (O'Neil, 2016). Some experts have started to refer to the increase and spread of superbugs as the overlooked or silent pandemic (Laxminarayan, 2022; Mahoney et al., 2021; UN, 2020). Other experts warn that we might be heading towards a 'post-antibiotic' era where minor infections become increasingly severe or even impossible to treat (Kwon and Powderly, 2021; Reardon, 2014). Annual economic losses related to superbugs are already estimated in the tens of billion U.S. dollars (Hall et al., 2018). As a response to these global challenges, this book analyses and discusses ways to reduce barriers to and create opportunities for global governance of antimicrobial resistance. Or more briefly, steering against superbugs.

Antimicrobial resistance (AMR) is the more generally used term for the superbug challenge. Microbes can mutate to develop resistance either spontaneously or through selective pressure from being exposed to antimicrobials (Halpern, 2009). Antimicrobials—such as antibiotics—are an essential component of modern medical and veterinary practice. But when humans use antimicrobials, microbes that by chance have greater resistance to particular antimicrobials will survive and proliferate, while more vulnerable microbes die off. Hence, using antimicrobials undermines their long-term effectiveness because of evolutionary pressures they exert on affected microbial species. Antimicrobials used to combat harmful microbes become increasingly ineffective. Such diminishing efficacy has affected each new antimicrobial used since the

Erik Baekkeskov, Louise Munkholm, and Olivier Rubin, *Steering against Superbugs* In: *Steering against Superbugs*. Edited by: Olivier Rubin, Erik Baekkeskov, and Louise Munkholm, Oxford University Press. © Oxford University Press 2023. DOI: 10.1093/oso/9780192899477.003.0001

discovery of penicillin in the 1940s (Podolsky, 2018). At the same time, antimicrobials have been used increasingly around the world to enhance health and agricultural production (see Chapters 2 and 3). For some decades, research and pharmaceutical development supplied new antimicrobials to supplement those losing their efficacy. Since the 1990s, however, microbial evolution of AMR has outstripped development of new antimicrobial treatments. As a result, many resistant microbes have emerged that threaten human and animal health, health sectors, food systems, and the environment.

How can human societies steer against superbugs? Like many other issues that are collectively governed, governance directed against AMR is an ongoing process. It includes two general goals: developing new treatments against microbial diseases (increasing supply), and improving stewardship of current antimicrobials so that they remain effective for longer (lowering demand). Both goals necessitate coordination globally and domestically. The increasingly interconnected world means that health and food systems are vulnerable to resistant pathogens that spread across national borders. Likewise, antimicrobials are produced in many countries and used in all societies, making emergence of AMR possible everywhere.

Achieving policy coordination between countries is non-trivial, however. International relations scholarship often characterizes the international system as anarchical, in the sense that it lacks a government able to monitor and enforce legal compliance. This means that global governance of AMR is likely to suffer from collective action problems common to international relations. Benefits from using antimicrobials are local, whereas the costs of AMR are global, making it a tragedy of the commons observed in other global challenges such as climate change, overfishing, and pollution. Thus, antimicrobial resources are depleted through overuse as they become less effective due to increasing AMR.

Such depletion also means that antimicrobial resources are not as accessible to present generations as they were to generations in the past. In this way, there is a tension between inter-generational and intra-generational justice in relation to AMR. Ensuring that there is equal access for all to effective treatments of microbial infections now *and* in the future arguably requires that all countries accept constraints on current use (intergenerational perspective). However, there are substantial distributional inequalities between nations—and indeed within nations—when it comes to antibiotic use (intra-generational perspective). Almost 6 million deaths annually in the Global South can be attributed not to AMR but to the *lack of access* to antibiotics (Rochford et al., 2018).

These distributional considerations between the Global North and South have direct repercussions for the prospect of setting up an effective system of global governance: distributional consequences (in terms of responsibility, impacts, and costs) need to be addressed to ensure that many countries take actions against AMR. Achieving global solidarity relies on global settlements over how to pursue just distributions of existing and new antimicrobials and how to develop just burden-sharing mechanisms. Such a burden-sharing governance regime is complicated by an international system with limited capacity for oversight and enforcement. These issues mean that autonomous actors and sovereign countries pursuing their own interests have weak incentives to act against AMR, even though they collectively stand to gain from maintaining effective antimicrobials. Thus, although the need for global coordination to fight AMR might seem obvious, AMR is difficult to address at the global level because of these complex and multifaceted dynamics.

The current solution is to create action plans and guidelines that member states of the World Health Organization (WHO) and other global bodies endorse to regulate antimicrobial usage. A Global Action Plan on AMR was endorsed in 2015 with the WHO member states committing to implementing national action plans based on the global guidelines. Around 150 member states reported having finalized their national action plans by 2021. However, although most national action plans are well aligned with the global guidelines on paper, the actual implementation of the guidelines is lagging, particularly in low and middle-income countries (LMICs) (Munkholm and Rubin, 2020). One explanation for asymmetry in efforts against AMR is that national governments do not have the same resources, capabilities, and mandates to govern their societies. Another explanation is divergence in national interests when it comes to mitigating AMR. For instance, the problem of resistant microbes may be relatively less important in countries that struggle to provide any access at all to antimicrobials for many citizens. Hence, the complexity and multidimensionality of AMR requires a multisectoral and multinational approach based on global coordination and actions (see Chapters 11 and 13).

As mentioned at the outset, this book analyses and discusses ways to reduce barriers to and create opportunities for global governance of AMR. Its chapters bring a specific and original focus that links to global AMR governance. While contemporary AMR research tends to be medical, biological, clinical, or epidemiological, this book draws heavily on contributions from the social sciences. We have previously argued that seeing AMR through a socio-political prism results in identifying different challenges than those emphasized by medical science alone (Baekkeskov et al., 2020; Frid-Nielsen et al., 2019). This book expands this perspective. Numerous factors beyond biology contribute to the production and propagation of AMR, including behavioural, economic, environmental, political, and social forces. Discussing opportunities and caveats of different global governance regimes of any transboundary threat, be it climate change, cyber terrorism, pandemics, or as in this case AMR, benefits greatly from insights and perspective from social science disciplines. Drawing on perspectives from public health, legal studies, public administration, history, political science, and sociology, the book brings to the fore perspectives and approaches to complement those of natural and medical sciences.

Importantly, the book should be understood as a pitch of ideas rather than consolidated and thoroughly tested solutions. Our aim is to establish a new research agenda based on the need to complement technical solutions with social science research that offers new perspectives. The book characterizes the AMR challenge as a complex of changing, transboundary, and creeping crises (Chapter 4). It helps to define the roles for top-down and bottom-up governance. It discusses dichotomies such as binding and non-binding agreements, global and local initiatives, and technical and social responses. We argue that the social sciences provide vital information and insights for any debates about how to steer against superbugs. The next section presents cross-cutting themes and opportunities for global AMR governance based on the book's chapters and the final section provides a thematic summary of the chapters.

Four perspectives on global AMR governance

A key question at the global level of AMR governance is how international organizations, national governments, and local actors collectively should articulate and pursue principles that govern factors contributing to AMR. To an extent, answers to this question depend on what works. International action plans and guidelines, such as those created by the WHO, the Food and Agriculture Organization of the United Nations (FAO), and the World Organisation for Animal Health (OIE), arguably have epistemic and moral authority. Indeed, most countries adopted the goals of the Global Action Plan on AMR (2015) in their own AMR national action plans (Munkholm and Rubin, 2020). Yet there is a long distance from a strategic document to policies and programmes that really steer how antimicrobials are developed, produced, sold, and used (Rubin and Munkholm, 2021). The disconnect between policy formulation and implementation is a persistent challenge in governance. Solving it calls for multiple social science perspectives. Indeed, enactment and implementation problems explain why many chapters in this volume look beyond global and even national strategies for AMR governance. Based on the insights gained from these rich and original accounts of contemporary political and regulatory responses to AMR, we draw out four perspectives for how to globally steer against superbugs:

1. Approach global AMR governance as polycentric.
2. Build new cross-sectoral coalitions.
3. Target actions rather than adopting grand strategies.
4. Shift the intervention focus from individuals to structures.

In the following, we elaborate on each of these perspectives in turn.

1. Approach global AMR governance as polycentric

One central theme emerging from the book's chapters is to problematize the current push for global coordination of efforts against AMR. Rather than broadly assuming that coordination at the global level will resolve AMR issues, most chapters in the book pinpoint challenges and opportunities on multiple levels that shape governance initiatives directed against AMR and examine their effectiveness. Governing AMR surely depends on global coordination and leadership. The WHO and many other health agencies, joined by organizations for agriculture and animal health, have successfully mounted worldwide initiatives against AMR since 2010 (Chapter 2). Yet the effectiveness of those initiatives depends crucially on how countries, localities, private organizations, and individuals act to mitigate AMR. Such agents need to align themselves globally while acting according to how problems and solutions exist in their specific local contexts. Hence, governing AMR goes far beyond forums that only include international organizations and national governments.

As previously described, local social conditions vary with respect to how they contribute to AMR. Local or national initiatives have sometimes worked to mitigate AMR very effectively inside their specific settings. That is, while resistant organisms spread, they do not necessarily do so, and resistance can be locally halted if selection pressures from uses of antimicrobials are sufficiently reduced. These distinct biological AMR characteristics combined with diverse socio-economic settings mean that AMR phenomena and their intrinsic challenges can vary considerably by location. In some locations, the most effective solution may be to provide incentives for patients, doctors, and farmers to reduce their use of antibiotics. In other locations, access to clean drinking water or fast diagnostics matter more than adjustments in antibiotic consumers' behaviour. In turn, this suggests that mitigating AMR is a global concern but strategies to do so depend very much on how AMR appears in specific regions, countries, and even specific localities. Hence, governing AMR calls for polycentric and 'glocal' governance approaches, rather than one uniform global approach alone. Ostrom (2010) argues that a single governance unit is poorly suited to solving global collective-action problems in situations where—as is the case with AMR—global governance relies heavily on national, regional, and local efforts. Instead, Ostrom recommends polycentric governance where a system of multiple governing authorities at differing scales (rather than a monocentric global unit) draws on local knowledge, mutual monitoring, and network learning. Polycentric governance is easier to implement as both the initiative and implementing capacity originate from a bottom-up network of stakeholders.

A move towards understanding global governance as the term 'polycentric' begs the question of what productive roles international organizations, such as WHO, FAO, OIE, or the United Nations Environment Programme (UNEP), may play. The chapters in this book suggest several roles for international actors. Concretely, the book highlights the opportunity to shift thinking about how AMR governance should be organized globally, from uniform top-down action plans towards polycentric and 'glocal' models adapted to social and biological variations in how AMR is induced. Global actors have soft tools related to information that are already deployed against AMR in various ways. They can push AMR onto political agendas through international forums and meetings, facilitate dialogue among national governments and with private actors, and pool and analyse data from AMR surveillance activities. Likewise, global actors, such as the WHO, FAO, OIE, or UNEP, can continue to play normative or moral roles by presenting goals (such as limiting antimicrobial use (AMU), increasing Infection Prevention Control (IPC), etc.) and general means and standards (the One Health

(OH) approach, individual behavioural interventions) against which regional, national, and local efforts can be measured. In addition, global AMR surveillance initiatives can create transparency. These actions could potentially represent soft power that
nudges national governments towards deeper commitments (e.g., through 'naming
and shaming') (Nye, 1990; Rothman, 2011). At the regional level, the European Union
runs several AMR initiatives that due to the EU's supranational characteristics have
stronger mandates than those of global actors (see Chapters 5 and 6). On this basis,
stronger collaborations among global and regional institutions may also be seen as the
way forward.

2. Build new cross-sectoral coalitions

Understanding global governance of AMR as polycentric also pushes us to consider
and boost the advocacy ecology of AMR (Chapter 14). One opportunity highlighted
in this book is to exploit how technical insights and approaches to AMR can enable
political solutions. The OH approach recognizes interdependencies between human,
animal, and environmental health. AMR health problems traverse realms that are usually separated in how governments and societies organize activity, including jurisdictions, sectors, policy areas, and entities. Yet, when a problem in one realm spills into
another, entrepreneurial political actors can frame and use shared aspects of these challenges to align interests between the realms.

However, as chapters in this book demonstrate, this alignment rarely happens.
Bureaucracies and practitioners that matter to AMR still work in separate silos
(Chapters 7, 10, 12, and 13). Recognizing common problems can potentially be used
politically to engineer common fronts against AMR. A key political challenge is to
build upon mobilizations of common attention to the AMR problem (cf. Hannah
and Baekkeskov, 2020). Further common ground should be sought where similar solutions are possible in different realms. For instance, limiting antibiotic prescriptions
has been possible across much of Europe, as has outlawing antibiotics in animal feed.
Europe has the advantage of established regional actors able to mediate common solutions, primarily the European Commission (Chapter 6). Yet the example demonstrates
that active political entrepreneurship can combine technical knowledge of AMR and
negotiating skills to identify effective solutions that many sovereign actors can agree
to enact within their own areas. Hence, it suggests a pragmatic front line for future regional or cross-sectoral efforts.

Relatedly, AMR is currently outside the focus of potentially important supporters,
such as activists and non-governmental organizations (NGOs) with interests in areas
in which AMR is entangled, such as developmental and environmental problems
(Chapters 14 and 15). Thus, mobilizing civil society and grassroots is critical to raising
and sustaining political attention to AMR in national and local contexts. AMR's cross-
cutting character—across sectors, borders, and policy areas—can potentially be a key

to political success. The political front line here is to demonstrate the interdependencies to established activists, NGOs, businesses, and more. Such demonstrations—or targeted awareness raising—should aim to mobilize cross-issue support, for instance between developmental or environmental advocates and AMR response efforts. Of course, such alliances are mutual. Actors leading AMR initiatives could be called upon to support developmental or environmental agendas in return. Relatedly, international donors, such as the Bill Gates Foundation, need to acknowledge and integrate the adverse dynamics of AMR in their eradication campaigns as means to fight infectious disease (Chapter 3).

3. Target actions rather than adopting grand strategies

The chapters in this volume also recommend pursuing targeted and pragmatic actions rather than grand strategies against AMR. This entails identifying and picking 'low-hanging fruit' rather than general abstract goals. A key example presented from different perspectives in two chapters is supply chain management targeting effluents from production of antimicrobial medicines (Chapters 17 and 18). Much of the production capacity for antimicrobials is located in LMIC contexts, such as in India and Bangladesh. Regulating effluents at these sites of production has proven difficult. Targeting purchasers is a different matter, however, particularly in highly developed contexts such as some EU Member States. By targeting end-product standards for purchasers, policy actors can use markets to affect what happens 'upstream' at the production site. Also, targeting actions provide an avenue for introducing hard law tools to ensure progress in AMR mitigation, such as binding agreements inspired by international trade law which oblige all parties to perform in accordance with agreed upon rules (Chapter 19). Chapters in the book that analyse AMR governance issues in LMIC settings also suggest several targeted actions that would foster immediate progress. These include implementing infection prevention control (IPC) and water, sanitation, and hygiene programmes, and interventions at community level co-designed and implemented by all relevant local stakeholders in a combined effort to strengthen AMR response (Chapters 7 and 9).

4. Shift intervention focus from individuals to structures

Finally, polycentric global governance with new types of coalitions and based on targeted actions would benefit from shifting focus away from how individuals behave to the structures that direct them. Current action plans place great emphasis on individual choices, particularly around awareness of AMR and use of antimicrobials (Chapter 8). Yet mobilizing politically is important because many—and perhaps most—choices that people face are structured by laws, programmes, norms, beliefs, incentives, and other constraints and opportunities that come from society, markets, and government. Political action and regulation are crucial because they structure individuals' choices.

Shifting global governance focus from individual choices in isolation towards how choices depend on structures is likely to highlight problems and solutions that will prove far more efficacious because they address deeper and more enduring contributors to AMR. The book's chapters show this in various ways. Some show that AMR governance depends on contextual organizations, rules, and norms, leaving individuals unable to control how they use antimicrobials (Chapters 8, 10, and 16). Others highlight the importance of economic development (Chapters 2, 7, and 9). Governing AMR in LMICs is interlinked with issues such as supplying clean water, stable food sources, functioning hospitals, and adequate and equitable access to high-quality pharmaceuticals. All such issues strongly constrain how individuals can behave towards antimicrobials. Finally, several chapters in this book highlight the need to see AMR as a sustainable developmental issue, arguing that we will never be able to mitigate AMR if we do not achieve sustainability in development as well as AMU (Chapters 5 and 7).

Structure and content of the book

The book is structured in six parts that cover different aspects of global AMR governance. Its eighteen chapters represent distinct takes on global steering against superbugs.

Part I: Framing and conceptualizing AMR

The three chapters in this section apply different social science perspectives to address the current framing and conceptualization of AMR. An argument common across the chapters is the need to complement the current dominant technical framing of AMR with a broader, social perspective. Such an encompassing perspective would be better equipped than a monodisciplinary perspective to overcome the socio-economic cleavages between the Global North and South, produce social and behavioural insights about AMR and AMU, and investigate AMR vulnerabilities and resilience that cut across countries and social groups.

Claas Kirchhelle and Christoph Gradmann (Chapter 2) trace the global history of AMR from the 1940s, where it was seen as an isolated failure of treatment, to today, where AMR is acknowledged as a global challenge across multiple sectors. The chapter illuminates long-term path dependencies that shape current initiatives and understandings of AMR. Historically, solutions to AMR have been impeded by fluctuating global attention spanning from indifference to moral panic. The authors argue that the current push to address AMR is shaped by large-scale movements in pharmaceutical markets and supply chains from the Global North to the Global South. The chapter notes how in the 'triangle' of pills, markets, and policies, the Global North now only controls policy. The current global governance regime, therefore, is characterized by a tension between pills (produced in Global South) and policy (pushed by the Global North).

Nancy Stepan (Chapter 3) also questions the global focus on AMR as primarily a biotechnical challenge. Through an analysis of the global eradication campaign of malaria from the 1950s onwards, the chapter problematizes the tension between recognizing the challenge of AMR on the one hand and the pursuit of disease eradication based on the large-scale use of antimicrobial drugs and insecticides on the other. The perspective of *eradicationism* has endured in public health strategies despite the accepted knowledge that using antimicrobials and insecticides generates endless cycles of resistant strains of microorganisms and insects. The author suggests that eradicationism based on biological innovations should be but one part of a broader set of global governance solutions. As the chapter notes with respect to malaria, housing with insect screens appears to provide better protection than biocides. The author thus identifies a need to reintegrate the biosocial with the biotechnical in a broader ecological OH approach.

Reidar Staupe-Delgado, Alina Engström, and Sebastián Frugone (Chapter 4) explicitly link the fluctuating global attention to AMR to the creeping and elusive nature of AMR. As an umbrella term for a number of individual health emergencies, AMR lacks clearly definable temporal and spatial boundaries. As such, it constitutes an endemic condition that continually evolves. Occasional outbreak episodes invite attention and concern, only for the challenge of AMR to subside again from the public view. AMR is thus an inevitable outcome in the sense that resistance is a fact of biology while at the same time being a societally constructed disaster risk. The authors recommend a disaster theory lens with its focus on vulnerability and resilience to offer a fresh perspective to the global governance of the AMR crisis.

Part II: Coordination and leadership in AMR governance

In the absence of a hegemonic power at the international level, coordination and leadership of global AMR governance is left to dedicated international organizations, regional actors, and national governments. In this part, two chapters focus on EU leadership in improving regional and global AMR responses, while one chapter discusses how to bridge the important divide between the Global North and South when it comes to global coordination. At the regional level, the EU has proven to be an effective arbiter of AMR response both through binding legislation and as a normative power spurring the implementation of key AMR initiatives. However, coordination at the global level is still hampered by a lack of accountability mechanisms in the Global North and inadequate capacities and competing health concerns in the Global South.

Carsten Strøby Jensen (Chapter 5) analyses the EU's recent track record in combating AMR. By comparing antimicrobial consumption in human and livestock sectors across EU Member States, Jensen identifies a strong trend of convergence across Member

States towards lower levels of antimicrobial consumption. The EU has enacted several agricultural policies, most notably the ban on the use of antimicrobials as growth promoters in 2006. Human health policies continue to be an area of national competence, yet here the EU pursues softer measures rooted in guidelines, surveillance, and transparency. Jensen shows how normative arbiters such as the EU can effectively encourage more sustainable antimicrobial use without relying on binding forms of legislation.

Daniel Carelli, Jon Pierre, and Björn Rönnerstrand (Chapter 6) also focus on the EU but they analyse how COVID-19 has presented a window of opportunity for closer coordination on human health challenges across EU Member States. They show how health experts point to the global and national levels as the most effective venues in tackling AMR. Yet at the same time, experts highlight the role of the EU when asked which actor would be best suited to lead coordination of AMR policies. Hence, although AMR is recognized as a transnational problem in need of global coordination, EU health experts prefer a regional agency with some decision-making power over a global agency with limited influence. The authors argue that the 'EU4Health' programme, launched in the wake of the COVID-19 pandemic, is enacting this preference and could prove to be a game-changer in European AMR governance. The initiative reinforces the important role that regional coordination agencies can play in AMR mitigation.

Mirfin Mpundu, Philip Mathew, Raphael Chanda, and Francesca Chiara (Chapter 7) consider the steps needed to move the AMR agenda forward in the Global South. Their chapter identifies three governance challenges that limit progression in LMIC settings: (i) confusion regarding responsibilities for implementation (lack of leadership); (ii) limited knowledge about the scope and relevance of AMR (lack of mobilization); and (iii) capability traps (lack of resources). These factors impede implementation of AMR national action plans (NAPs). As a way forward, the authors suggest integration between AMR response and the Sustainable Development Goals (SDGs). At country level, this would mean that experts working with the SDGs at head of state's offices engage also in AMR policy implementation. This could spur resource mobilization and understanding of AMR as not only a health challenge but also a sustainable developmental issue.

Part III: AMR governance from below

The three chapters in this part share a focus on the agency of social actors and individuals. Each analysis recognizes that the struggle against AMR will be shaped by how organizations, social groups, or individuals act. Mitigating AMR depends on individuals and organizations collectively adhering to principles of sustainable AMU, yet such adherence is difficult to manufacture by handing down public policies from on high. The contributions in this part illustrate interdependencies between contexts and individual or organizational choices. Global AMR governance should not misdiagnose the AMU problem as merely one of individual choice but instead recognize that such choices are influenced by contextual specifics, most notably the extent to which actors at community or local levels can be engaged and involved.

Mark Davis (Chapter 8) uses a Foucauldian governmentality perspective (with a focus on how the exercise of power that constrain behaviour through surveillance, legal or administrative structures) to show how AMR governance in a high-income country (Australia) can over-emphasize individual choices and awareness and ignore systems that constrain and direct these. In numerous ways, Australia's AMR policies place individual commitment and information as central to mitigating AMR. Davis argues that individuals are merely 'one element of the biological–social–economic systems that circulate antimicrobials across species and in the environment'. How individual actions affect AMR is biologically complex rather than linear or clear. In addition, social science research shows that individual demand has limited power to explain antimicrobial use and is itself contingent on how care systems are organized and regulated. Finally, several years of AMR awareness raising and communication in Australia and elsewhere have failed to make most citizens understand AMR, challenging the assumption that more information will alter behaviours. In consequence, Davis argues, AMR governance would benefit from improved and nuanced reckoning with what individuals need to help them play their part in antimicrobial stewardship.

Tabitha Hrynick, Syed Shahid Abbas, and Hayley MacGregor (Chapter 9) analyse cases from a lower income country (Bangladesh) to illustrate how effective AMR governance can depend on context-specific solutions developed by local stakeholders. The analysis provides a critical corrective to discourse that frames inappropriate drug usage as the primary global AMR governance challenge, and qualifies the role of associated one-size-fits-all, 'top-down' solutions. Bangladesh enjoys relatively low-cost antibiotics produced domestically, but the government is unable to regulate sales. In addition, its relatively unregulated healthcare system offers highly uneven access and quality of care for citizens. Bangladesh is also home to high-density populations and much farming, creating significant burdens of infection and high demand for antimicrobials. In the absence of government capability to regulate uses of antimicrobials for humans and animals, pilot projects in Bangladesh have demonstrated that mitigating AMR is possible through 'bottom-up' initiatives and dialogue within local communities and agricultural sectors.

Muriel Surdez (Chapter 10) uses the sociology of professions to analyse the case of AMR policy implementation in a high-income but decentralized country (Switzerland). Surdez argues that implementing Switzerland's 2015 NAP has been bound by pre-existing divisions between human and animal health professions and between national (federal) and local (cantonal) authority. In particular, changing antimicrobial uses and surveillance in the Swiss food production sector depends on whether cantonal departments and professionals in private practice choose to accept and act. Hence, when the federal food safety agency sought to implement the NAP, it had to negotiate with cantonal departments and the professional organization of veterinarians. As a consequence, global initiatives against AMR were dependent on how such established veto players adopted, adapted, or resisted the measures.

Part IV: A One Health (OH) perspective on AMR

The three chapters in this part share a focus on AMR as a multi-sectoral challenge demanding cross-sectoral solutions. OH approaches build upon recognition of interdependencies between the health of humans, animals, and environments. The OH term indicates the unity of health in all sectors, problematizing the sectoral separations and independence suggested by how fields of research and policy are organized. OH has been widely accepted in global and national action plans as the general principle for mitigating AMR, because resistant organisms can spread across species barriers and in natural environments. However, questions remain about opportunities and limitations of OH approaches to AMR governance, and the chapters help to highlight these.

Laura H. Kahn and Bernadette Dunham (Chapter 11) describe the OH approach to mitigating AMR, and its applications. Their chapter also offers an OH three-dimensional matrix as a tool to examine complex issues such as AMR. Exemplary national cases are drawn from the United States and Denmark, where OH has been applied with some success in the struggle to limit AMR. OH has also been applied in several global AMR initiatives, showing global reach. The chapter argues, however, that four general barriers limit implementation of OH against AMR: (i) the OH concept is ill-defined; (ii) international organizations across food safety and human and animal health have very different resources; (iii) AMR action plans are poorly enforced; and (iv) AMR is a complex problem.

Jessica Craig, Isabel Frost, and Jyoti Joshi (Chapter 12) consider challenges of implementing the OH approach against AMR in LMIC countries. NAPs tend to prescribe OH. Yet several factors have made moving NAPs 'from paper to practice' particularly difficult in many LMICs. Among these are shortages of funding for NAP-related programmes, competing health and development priorities, difficulties in sustaining inter-sectoral collaborations, and lack of legal mandates. The chapter illustrates such challenges through in-depth reviews of AMR surveillance and infection prevention and control.

Sarah Humboldt-Dachroeden and Chris Degeling (Chapter 13) report on a survey of European experts involved in multiple sectors that contribute to AMR to describe OH practices. The survey includes responses from 104 experts in twenty-three countries involved in regulating human or animal health, food safety, or the environment. The chapter indicates the extent of multi-sectoral governance in the field of AMR surveillance and suggests how well the OH approach is realized in practice. For instance, agency and department portfolios sometimes overlap, suggesting redundancy, and AMR-related initiatives often fail to include representatives from the environmental and social science sectors that would enable more comprehensive perspectives when implementing OH initiatives.

Part V: Global advocacy and awareness of AMR

The three chapters in this part analyse different cases of awareness raising and mobilization activities. They share the concern that scientific communities appear to face difficulties when turning AMR into an issue with broad public appeal. The chapters highlight different obstacles for advocacy by discussing the role of different actors and structures in shaping AMR awareness and mobilizing political recognition These obstacles relate to the relationship between experts and politicians, the ability to frame and translate scientific information, and the (social) media coverage of AMR.

Olivier Rubin and Erik Baekkeskov (Chapter 14) take a global perspective on AMR policy advocacy. They seek to explain why recent increases in global attention and agenda-setting do not appear to have produced an equivalent increase in implementation of AMR policy initiatives. The authors argue that this lack of implementation is linked to an 'advocacy ecology' that relies almost exclusively on problem brokers among committed public health experts across national and international agencies. While these health experts successfully placed the threat of AMR on the global agenda, this attention has often failed to yield implemented policies in national and local contexts. The main political challenge for progressing AMR policy, according to the authors, is not further awareness raising activities aimed at popularizing scientific knowledge but rather mobilizing potential policy entrepreneurs among non-health stakeholders, such as invested bureaucrats, powerful activist organizations, and relevant private companies.

Ahmad Wesal Zaman (Chapter 15) investigates and compares social media attention to AMR and climate change (CC). Based on a large-N analysis of Twitter data, the author finds that CC receives much more attention than AMR and explains the difference by discussing the role of digital policy entrepreneurs in shaping agendas and public debates. Digital policy entrepreneurs for CC have been successful in attracting public attention through aesthetic and dramatic presentation of the CC problem. In contrast, AMR digital policy entrepreneurs have been scientifically oriented, dispassionate, and uncontroversial. On that basis, the author concludes that in order to increase attention to AMR and keep AMR on the agenda, there is a need for transforming the language of communication from scientifically oriented language to more emotional language. Such communication can be achieved through simplified and symbolic communication strategies that would attract public and political attention, without compromising scientific facts.

Arjun Rajkhowa, Karin Thursky, and Kabir Rajkhowa (Chapter 16) analyse AMR mitigation in India with focus on the role of medical experts in AMR policy-making. Awareness and recognition among politicians about AMR have increased due to the engagement of the medical expert community in the policy formulation process, yet local (state) implementation lags behind national (federal) enactment of AMR policies. The authors propose that local ownership of AMR mitigation efforts is crucial.

Over half of India's states did not participate in a federally led consultation in 2017 on state-level implementation actions. The authors discuss initiatives that are informed by awareness and experiences of stakeholders on the ground, which could change such lack of state-level engagement and effort against AMR.

Part VI: Regulatory responses to AMR

The three chapters in this part analyse and discuss existing national, supranational, and international opportunities for regulating antimicrobial production and consumption. The chapters draw inspiration from both public and private international law. Two chapters look at pharmaceutical waste management and suggest supply chain regulation modelled over EU law as a promising avenue for combatting one of the drivers of AMR. A third chapter investigates lessons learnt from fifteen years of implementing the International Health Regulations (IHR) to inform a broader discussion of the pros and cons of international legal agreements on AMR.

Ipshita Chaturvedi and Natasha Kavalakkat (Chapter 17) recommend using a supply chain-based regulatory framework to mitigate AMR. Addressing supply chains for antimicrobial sales, they argue, will overcome gaps in regulation of effluents that can increase AMR. To illustrate their point, the authors analyse the case of the Patancheru region, home to the biggest cluster of pharmaceutical manufacturing companies in India. For more than twenty years, improper disposal of pharmaceutical waste has contributed to an increase in AMR in the surrounding environment, yet attempts to regulate manufacturing waste have suffered from lack of accountability and liability measures, including no mechanisms for determining compliance at production sites. The authors suggest a supply chain approach that imposes due diligence obligations on end-product companies marketing pharmaceuticals. This would force such companies to avoid sourcing drugs with adverse environmental impacts, which in turn will pressure drug manufacturers that supply them to invest in proper waste treatment systems.

Katerina Mitkidis (Chapter 18) also directs attention to pharmaceutical industries and the need for stimulating change in ways antimicrobials are manufactured. The author advocates for introducing 'governance by contract' in the global governance regime of AMR. One example could be EU public procurement law, which encourages public buyers of pharmaceuticals to include sustainability criteria in their tenders. The author proposes integrating public procurement with corporate procurement practices from the private sector. While public procurement focuses on articulating sustainability requirements primarily in the initial phases of the procurement process (pre-tender and tender), private procurement does the opposite and focuses on contract language and contract execution. This would oblige vendors to clean up their own production and source only from minimally polluting suppliers.

Louise Munkholm and Susan Rogers Van Katwyk (Chapter 19) discuss the potential of applying already existing binding agreements for the global governance of AMR, exemplified by the IHR. The authors analyse the extent to which the IHR incentivize action, institutionalizes accountability, and activate interest groups relevant to AMR mitigation. Their analysis shows that IHR implementation suffers from: (i) lack of sustained action, particularly in LMICs that struggle with developing and maintaining the core capacities required under the IHR; (ii) a soft approach to accountability with no enforcement mechanisms in place (e.g., there are no legal consequences if member states do not comply with their obligations); and (iii) a lack of activation of all interested groups when it comes to IHR implementation. Instead of using the IHR as an overall framework, the authors conclude that a global AMR governance regime could be built around a new standalone AMR treaty developed and monitored either by the UN or a new multisectoral body.

References

Adebisi, Y. A., Alaran, A. J., Okereke, M., Oke, G. I., Amos, O. A., Olaoye, O. C., et al. (2021). 'COVID-19 and Antimicrobial Resistance: A Review', *Infectious Diseases: Research and Treatment*, 14, 11786337211033870.

Baekkeskov, E., Rubin, O., Munkholm, L., and Zaman, W. (2020). 'Antimicrobial Resistance as a Global Health Crisis', in E. Stern, ed., *Oxford Encyclopaedia of Politics* (Oxford, Oxford University Press). Retrieved 27 January 2023, from https://oxfordre.com/politics/view/10.1093/acrefore/9780190228637.001.0001/acrefore-9780190228637-e-1626

Frid-Nielsen, S. S., Rubin, O., and Baekkeskov, E. (2019). 'The State of Social Science Research on Antimicrobial Resistance', *Social Science & Medicine*, 242, 112596.

Hall, W., McDonell, A., and O'Neil, J. (2018). *Superbugs: An Arms Race against Bacteria.* (Cambridge, MA: Harvard University Press).

Halpern, N. E. (2009). 'Antibiotics in Food Animals: The Convergence of Animal and Public Health, Science, Policy, Politics and the Law', *Drake Journal of Agricultural Law*, 14(3), 401–36.

Hannah, A., and Baekkeskov, E. (2020) 'The Promises and Pitfalls of Polysemic Ideas: "One Health" and Antimicrobial Resistance Policy in Australia and the UK', *Policy Sciences*, 53, 437–52,

Kwon, J. H., and Powderly, W. G. (2021). 'The Post-antibiotic Era Is Here', *Science*, 373(6554), 471.

Laxminarayan, R. (2022). 'The Overlooked Pandemic of Antimicrobial Resistance', *The Lancet*, 399(10325), 606–7.

Mahoney, A. R., Safaee, M. M., Wuest, W. M., and Furst, A. L. (2021). 'The Silent Pandemic: Emergent Antibiotic Resistances Following the Global Response to SARS-CoV-2', *Iscience*, 24(4), 102304.

Munkholm, L., and Rubin, O. (2020). 'The Global Governance of Antimicrobial Resistance: A Cross-Country Study of Alignment between the Global Action Plan and National Action Plans', *Globalization and Health*, 16/1, 109.

Murray, C. J., Ikuta, K. S., Sharara, F., Swetschinski, L., Aguilar, G. R., Gray, A., et al. (2022). 'Global Burden of Bacterial Antimicrobial Resistance in 2019: A Systematic Analysis', *The Lancet*, 399/10325, 605–94.

Nye, J. S. (1990). 'Soft Power', *Foreign Policy*, 80, 153–72.

Ostrom, E. (2010) 'Beyond Markets and States: Polycentric Governance of Complex Economic Systems', *American Economic Review*, 100, 641–72.

Podolsky, S. H. (2018). 'The Evolving Response to Antibiotic Resistance (1945–2018)', *Palgrave Communications*, 4, 124.

Reardon, S. (2014). 'WHO Warns against "Post-antibiotic" Era', *Nature*, https://doi.org/10.1038/nature.2014.15135, accessed 27 January 2023.

Rizvi, S. G., and Ahammad, S. Z. (2022). 'COVID-19 and Antimicrobial Resistance: A Cross-Study', *Science of the Total Environment*, 807, 150873.

Rochford, C., Sridhar, D., Woods, N., Saleh, Z., Hartenstein, L., Ahlawat, H., et al. (2018). 'Global Governance of Antimicrobial Resistance', *The Lancet*, 391/10134, 1976–78.

Rodríguez-Baño, J., Rossolini, G. M., Schultsz, C., Tacconelli, E., Murthy, S., Ohmagari, N., et al. (2021). 'Key considerations on the potential impacts of the COVID-19 pandemic on antimicrobial resistance research and surveillance', *Transactions of the Royal Society of Tropical Medicine and Hygiene*, 115(10), 1122–29.

Rothman, S. (2011). 'Revising the soft power concept: What are the means and mechanisms of soft power?', *Journal of Political Power*, 4(1), 49–64.

Rubin, O., and Munkholm, L. (2021). 'Isomorphic dynamics in national action plans on antimicrobial resistance', *Public Administration and Development*. https://doi.org/10.1002/pad.1966.

UN. (2020). 'Silent Pandemic: Overuse renders antimicrobials less effective—UN agriculture agency', https://news.un.org/en/story/2020/11/1077972.

PART I

FRAMING AND CONCEPTUALIZING AMR

2

Pills and Politics

A Historical Analysis of International Antibiotic Regulation since 1945

Christoph Gradmann and Claas Kirchhelle

Introduction

The history of international antibiotic regulation and policy is one of unrelenting dynamism and unforeseen challenges. In contrast to successful action against other planetary challenges like ozone depletion or pathogenic threats like rinderpest, international attempts to regulate antibiotics and curb antimicrobial resistance (AMR) have trailed behind evolving targets, new scientific knowledge, and changing forms of use. They have also been undermined by fragmented political action, different priorities, and the failure to address underlying structural inequalities simultaneously (Kirchhelle et al., 2020).

In this chapter, we draw on the growing number of historical and social sciences reviews of antibiotic use and AMR as well as select primary sources to discuss the emerging long lines of the history of international antibiotic regulation that by now covers over seventy-five years. We will first explain why the post-war period saw both new antibiotic classes and new forms of antibiotic use proliferate in the presence of only minimal national or international regulation. Secondly, we will look at the 1960s and 1970s when early attempts at policing were suggested but either failed to find their way to implementation or failed to solve identified problems. In a third step, we will look at the years around 1990, when discussions about antibiotic policy changed in intensity, tone, and scale. This shift happened against the background of a stalling research and development pipeline for new antibiotics, proliferating antimicrobial resistance (AMR), and concerns by countries of the Global North about biosecurity hazards arising from the Global South. In a fourth step, we will look at the new millennium when discussions surrounding antibiotic policy began to recognize and explicitly target LMICs and the One Health nexus of human, animal, and environmental health.

From proliferation to international concern (1950–1970)

In 1935, the arrival of Prontosil marked the beginning of a golden era of antimicrobial research and development. As a result of systematized screening and biochemical

Christoph Gradmann and Claas Kirchhelle, *Pills and Politics* In: *Steering against Superbugs.* Edited by:
Olivier Rubin, Erik Baekkeskov, and Louise Munkholm, Oxford University Press. © Oxford University Press 2023.
DOI: 10.1093/oso/9780192899477.003.0002

modification, the decades between 1935 and the 1970s saw a stream of targeted treatments for microbial infections enter global markets (Lesch, 2007). Initially, neither the synthetic sulfonamides nor the biological antibiotics discovered from the 1940s onwards seemed in need of international policing. As 'wonder drugs' and objects of wartime propaganda, the scope of their beneficial application seemed almost unlimited. As a consequence, international discussions primarily focused on standardizing and boosting production rather than controlling antimicrobial access (Bud, 2007).

What policing existed was national or even local at the hospital or clinical level. In Western countries, early regulations focused on protecting supplies of a still scarce resource as well as human and non-human antibiotic users from toxic side effects and residues in food and milk (Kirchhelle, 2020). Although knowledge of evolving 'drug fastness'—the ability of microbes to resist antimicrobials—had existed since the 1910s (Gradmann, 2011), concerns about AMR remained isolated. As a biological phenomenon, AMR was still very much tied to its previous history as a biologically interesting phenomenon and a laboratory tool in molecular biology and medical genetics (Gradmann, 2011). Outside the laboratory, drug resistance was deemed controllable via 'rational' prescription and by combining and switching drugs (Landecker, 2019; Podolsky, 2018).

For our history, this benign view of AMR had the consequence that the skyrocketing production, marketing, and use of antibiotics in the 1950s went mostly unregulated. Driven by industry's attempts to find new market outlets and economic pressure for enhanced productivity in health and food production systems, two new forms of usage in particular would soon emerge as major regulatory challenges: in agriculture, the licensing of often low-dosed antibiotic applications to enhance animal and plant productivity and combat disease led to the mass proliferation of mostly unsupervised antibiotic use (Kirchhelle, 2020); in human medicine, the introduction of oral antibiotics opened the door for antibiotics' widespread use in general practice and indiscriminate application against respiratory tract infections (MacFarlane and Worboys, 2008). Although individual researchers warned about side effects including AMR selection, antibiotics' status as symbols of technological progress and cost- and labour-saving impact made concerns about access rather than restriction the order of the day (Podolsky, 2015; Smith-Howard, 2017).

Hospitals, which were traditionally supposed to serve as lighthouses of therapeutic progress, became the first places where drug resistance resulting from increased antibiotic use emerged as a prominent challenge. As an author noted in 1955, 'clinicians may properly start treating an infection due to a susceptible strain or strains … [and] end treating a new bacterial infection in the patient as a result of penicillin therapy' (Spink, 1955: 586). During the late 1940s, AMR had already surfaced as a problem in the treatment of burns victims and of persistent infections like typhoid (Bud, 2007; Colquhoun and Weetch, 1950). In agriculture, veterinarians had similarly reported emerging problems surrounding the treatment of drug resistant mastitis in cows (Woods, 2014).

However, it was the pandemic spread of drug resistant *Staphylococcus aureus* phage-type 80/81 from 1953 onwards that transformed perceptions of AMR from a local into an international problem. Explosive outbreaks of drug resistant mastitis, conjunctivitis, and pyoderma among patients and carers in neonatal wards triggered calls for international diagnostic standards in medicine (Hillier, 2006). The pandemic also highlighted worrying early signs that problems of antibiotic overuse in human and animal medicine might be interlinked. From the mid-1950s onwards, Western European and North American research on abattoir workers, in prison dairies, and on rural military recruits began highlighted rising levels of resistant organisms in animal production while use of bacteriophage-typing indicated potential connections of infection and AMR selection across species boundaries (Kirchhelle, 2020; McKenna, 2018).

Contemporaries responded to the identified challenges in line with prevailing post-war optimism in technological solutions: most commonly, treatment failure resulted in higher doses of the same drug, supplementation with other antibiotics, and increasing reliance on newer antibiotics (Podolsky, 2015). While this response overcame treatment failures in the short term, it did little to address the underlying drivers of AMR and increasing antibiotic dependence in health systems and food production. Famously, after methicillin was marketed in 1959 as the ultimate answer for penicillin resistant Staphylococcal infections, it took only two years for Methicillin-resistant *Staphylococcus aureus* (MRSA) to be isolated in the United Kingdom (McKenna, 2010).

Another response to the perceived overuse of antibiotics was to call for more 'rational drug use' in medicine and agriculture. This usually entailed a certain clinical and economic restraint with regards to the quantity of drugs used, insistence on proper diagnosis of a disease, calls to improve infection control in health and agricultural settings, and a revival of public health epidemiology in clinical settings (Kirchhelle, 2020; Podolsky, 2015).

With new categories of prescription-only drugs only recently introduced in many countries, the implied universal common-sense nature of appeals for 'rational drug use' belied underlying conflicts over antibiotic control, professional rivalries, and economic interests. In hospital settings, calls for AMR control often took the form of moralizing appeals to a past in which hygienic standards had allegedly been practised with more vigour—and controlled by clinical microbiologists. Thus British bacteriologist Mary Barber remarked in 1960 that 'the principles for preventing hospital cross-infection enunciated long before the introduction of antibiotics remain the same to-day, but the ubiquity of the staphylococcus makes their strict application difficult in relation to this microbe' (Barber et al., 1960: 11) While medical lobbies in most countries managed to resist government efforts to regulate prescription practices, the 1962 US Kefauver–Harris Bill combatted 'irrational' industry marketing practices by introducing regulatory requirements for new antibiotics to show efficacy in clinical trials (Podolsky, 2015). In agriculture, transatlantic calls for antibiotic reform and enhanced consumer protection from residues triggered power struggles between veterinarians, regulators, feed and pharmaceutical producers, and farmers' unions over the degree of veterinary supervision and government control of on-farm antibiotic access and marketing (Smith-Howard, 2010, 2017). Medical calls for antibiotic restraint in animal medicine triggered swift and aggressive rebuttals from the veterinary profession (Kirchhelle, 2020).

It was in this situation of a growing awareness of problems that the World Health Organization (WHO) initiated a first attempt to create an international system of diagnostic standards for AMR and a network of public health inspired reference laboratories (Gradmann, 2013). So far, diagnostic equipment had been locally produced and—with some exceptions like centralized microbiological surveillance in England and Wales and regional solutions in Scandinavia—resulting epidemiologies of AMR had been local too. It was hoped that standardized diagnostic technology would facilitate the creation of comparable epidemiological statistics that would serve as a basis for policing antibiotics application in human medicine. The prevailing situation in 1960 was, as the WHO committee deemed, one of chaos and low-quality data (Gradmann, 2013: 563).

Hans Ericsson and John Sherris, who were leading the WHO study, envisioned a future in which clinical antibiotic use would be guided by laboratory science—a vision inspired by Ericson's position as head of a Swedish public health laboratory that executed such an authority over clinicians in the country. Alas, what worked in Scandinavia proved unpalatable to countries that were big producers of antibiotics. In the course of a decade, the comprehensive standardization of diagnostic standards that the International Collaborative Study had envisioned was reduced to the standardization of the paper discs used in clinical laboratories. The proliferation of the so-called Kirby–Bauer high content disc test, of which Sherris had been one of the co-inventors, was the one thing that remained of the work. The other was a landmark manual of diagnostic work with regards to AMR (Ericsson and Sherris, 1971).

In contrast to the relative stagnation of national and international reform efforts in human medicine, agricultural antibiotics emerged as the first successful target of transnational regulation in Western Europe. Profiting from an integrated system of public health surveillance and influenced by Japanese research on transferable AMR, British microbiologists had begun to campaign for restrictions of therapeutically relevant antibiotics in agriculture from around 1960 onwards. As a result of their campaigning, real-world data on transferable resistance on farms, and national scares involving deadly typhoid and gastroenteritis outbreaks, the British government agreed to enact the first precautionary antibiotic restrictions in 1969. Proposed by the so-called Swann Report, the restrictions centred on prohibiting the use of low-dosed feeds containing medically important antibiotics like penicillin and the tetracyclines in animal production. It was hoped that reserving these antibiotics for therapeutic use and providing ongoing access to feeds containing non-therapeutic antibiotics that were not used in human medicine would protect medically relevant drugs without jeopardizing agricultural productivity. During the 1970s, successful British promotion of the 'Swann gospel' within the European Economic Community (EEC) led to the adoption of similar bans on the continent and repeated—though ultimately futile—ban attempts by the American Food and Drugs Administration (FDA). Unfortunately, the bans' limited nature, emerging cross-resistance between therapeutic and non-therapeutic antibiotics, and surging antibiotic demand meant that the Swann reforms were unable to stop rising agricultural antibiotic usage or AMR (Kirchhelle, 2020,2016; Thoms, 2014, 2017).

Superbugs and super committees (1970–2010)

Despite the Swann report's lasting influence on regulatory thinking (Kirchhelle, 2018), the 1970s thus continued to be characterized by slow-moving and fragmented reform efforts at the national and transnational levels. With the exception of expert workshops on AMR surveillance and resistance hazards in agriculture, action also ground to a halt at the international level. The International Collaborative Study was stopped in its tracks by the US Centers for Disease Control and Prevention (CDC) and Food and Drug Administration (FDA) in the early 1970s, defending what they saw as intellectual and material property of antibiotics producers against the onslaught of Nordic public health extremists. Similarly, the domestic defeat of FDA attempts to ban low-dosed antibiotic feeds led to US opposition to international attempts to condemn antibiotic growth promotion via WHO or the Codex Alimentarius (Gradmann, 2013).

And for the time being, it did seem that there was an alternative to ever stricter regulation: to solve the problems of AMR with drug innovation. Since the 1950s, the pharmaceutical industry had seen AMR not just as a challenge to existing antibiotics but as a chance to market new antibiotics. In medicine and agriculture, professional magazines regularly praised the properties of new AMR-busters (Gradmann, 2016; Kirchhelle, 2020). Meanwhile, crises that might have tilted the regulatory balance in favour of restrictions like the emergence of multiple drug-resistant (MDR) typhoid in Asia and South America around 1970 occurred just before the marketing of multiple new classes of effective antibiotics (Kirchhelle et al., 2019). In this sense, the AMR problems created by the mass adoption of first-generation antibiotics in the 1950s paved the way for the commercial success of later broad-spectrum antibiotics from ampicillin to ciprofloxacin (Podolsky, 2015). Meanwhile, the structural factors driving increasing antibiotic use—and growing infrastructural antibiotic dependency (Chandler et al., 2016)—in both human medicine and food production remained unaddressed.

It was only from around 1990, in an atmosphere of crisis, that international antibiotic policy began to make meaningful steps forward. Several factors created this window of opportunity: in popular culture, the notion of a post-antibiotic age that had occasionally popped up since the late 1960s gained increasing traction. Feeding off anxieties about HIV/AIDS, the emerging European bovine spongiform encephalitis (BSE) crisis, and wider concerns about environmental systems collapse, antibiotic apocalypse warnings reflected surging AMR and an emerging crisis of antibiotic innovation (Greenwood, 2008).

When *Science* dedicated a whole issue to 'The Microbial Wars' in 1992 (Koshland, 1992), it did so to stress that for the time being it was the microbes who had won. Antibiotics that had once promised a bright future for human medicine and food production now appeared as a precarious artefact of a jeopardized historical future, a powerful but fast eroding resource (Lie and Podolsky, 2016). In a marked change of outlook, the future for the post-war wonder drugs began to be seen in the preservation of the existing pharmacopeia rather than in an expansion of its usage. Fired by popular science treatments like Stuart Levy's *The Antibiotic Paradox* (Levy, 1992) and campaigning by the Alliance for the Prudent use of Antibiotics (est. 1981), therapeutic rationalists began to find a more receptive audience. Meanwhile, an increasing number of influential Western expert reports began to frame AMR as a major threat to national security (IoM, 1992). In 1996, the term antibiotic stewardship was coined as a catchphrase to capture practices devised to contain the development and spread of AMR (McGowan and Gerding, 1996).

Similar to calls from the 1960s, the first target of national and international action lay in the creation of comprehensive surveillance of AMR and antimicrobial usage. In a late echo of the work begun by Ericsson and Sherris, WHONET from 1985 (<https://whonet.org>). provided an integrated electronic data platform to input global AMR data. Under the impression of new forms of vancomycin-resistant enterococci (VRE) and pressure to license further antibiotics for non-human use, high-income countries in North America, the European Union, and Asia also began to launch integrated AMR surveillance systems at the national level (Bud, 2007; Kirchhelle, 2021).

The decline of the formerly utopian framing of antibiotics coincided with a changing political climate. From the 1960s onwards, the international rise of environmental movements had facilitated a political reframing of the planetary environment from a space to conquer into a delicate and finite resource in need of protection (Uekötter, 2011). Although concerns about 'polluting' residues in food and AMR as an ecological threat dated back to the 1950s and 1960s, the 1990s saw antibiotics increasingly described as a form of environmental pollution that emanated from farms, factories, and human wastewater (Kirchhelle, 2020). The combined effect of these changing popular and political perceptions of antibiotics was a discernible rise in policy documents focusing on usage and AMR across the human, animal, and environmental domains, which had previously been treated separately (Overton et al., 2021).

A well-known initial result of such discussions was the 1998 Copenhagen summit, during which the EU began to aim at creating an explicit policy on antibiotics and integrated surveillance systems across the agricultural and human domains (Thamdrup Rosdahl and Børge Pedersen, 1998). Another tangible result of the 1998 conference was an expansion of 1970s European bans to encompass all low-dosed antibiotic feeds by 2006 (Bud, 2007; Kahn, 2016; Kirchhelle, 2020). At the scientific level, the EU conference and parallel WHO-led expert consultations provided the impetus for new collaborative behavioural, microbiological, and epidemiological research on antibiotic consumption and AMR in different settings (Goosens et al., 2005).

In addition to creating pressure on other governments to implement similar measures, the burst of European transnational action facilitated a gradual shift of engagement by international organizations. In a new era of Global Health, United Nations organizations like the WHO, Food and Agriculture Organization (FAO), and the World Organisation for Animal Health (OIE) shifted from merely assisting nation state coordination and publishing expert reports to acting as centres of governance, fund-raising, and progressive action via surveillance programmes and policy frameworks in their own right. In an early sign of this new ambition, the WHO and partners de-cided to launch a global strategy to contain AMR. However, the announcement of the launch on 9/11 2001 and subsequent scares about bioterrorism and the 2003 SARS pan-demic meant that AMR-focused initiatives were drowned out by other policy priorities (Overton et al., 2021).

Globalizing AMR

It was only in the years around 2010 that political momentum for internationally co-ordinated AMR policies re-emerged (see Chapters 4 and 14). The multiple immediate factors for this resurgence included a concerted attempt by the UK's government to assert international leadership in Global Health via AMR, concerns about the inter-national spread of *NDM-1*, a worsening drug innovation crisis, and an increasing focus of governmental and non-governmental donors like the Wellcome Trust and Gates Foundation on biosecurity risks emerging from the Global South (Overton et al., 2021). Amongst the most prominent reports and initiatives were the 2016 AMR Review (O'Neill report) (O'Neill, 2016), the WHO's global action plan of 2015, and the parallel launch of GLASS, a platform for global surveillance of antimicrobial resistance (<https://www.who.int/initiatives/glass>). Following policy and stewardship templates provided by high-income countries and the UK Fleming Fund, this initial wave of at-tention was followed by a surge National Action Plans to combat AMR at the national and local level by low- and middle-income countries (LMICS) from around 2015 on-wards (Rogers Van Katwyk et al., 2020).

Seen from a more long-term perspective, additional causal factors for the surge of international AMR attention and action emerge. Two of the most prominent factors are associated with processes of globalization in the pharmaceutical drug trade and the popularity of Global Health as a policy field.

With regards to the first factor, the period around 2010 brought a growing awareness by high-income countries that the centres of antibiotic production and marketing no longer aligned with those of policing. Since the 1970s, a large part of global antibiotic manufacturing had shifted from 'Northern' countries to increasingly assertive devel-oping countries of the South like India and China. Meanwhile, key pharmaceutical growth markets were no longer located in 'Western' countries. With pharmaceutical producers increasingly relying on sales of generics rather than new patented molecules for profits, industry attention increasingly focused on LMICs as growth markets—which included the aggressive marketing of cheap antibiotics (Greene, 2014). In an im-agined triangle of pills, markets and policies, the one thing that Northern countries and Northern-based donors still controlled was policy (Beaudevin et al., 2020). In the case of AMR, the result was a concerted moral and political Northern push to assert influence over LMIC antibiotic marketing, industry regulation, and other forms of 'stewardship' in international fora.

Northern initiatives to assert moral leadership at the international level took the form of appeals to protect the global 'antibiotic commons', technical aid programmes for surveillance and stewardship (see above), and public pressure on middle-income countries to reduce specific forms of antibiotic usage like polymyxin growth promoters after 2015. At the national level, they coincided with heightened biosecurity rhetoric at the national level. In an era of Global Health and under the impression of the recent SARS and swine flu pandemics, experts and activists sensitized donors and politicians to AMR by stressing the health and economic hazards resulting from the rapid global spread of resistant microbes and genes. AMR was compared to other contemporary security threats resulting from terrorism, climate change, and flooding, economic impacts were calculated, and 1990s scenarios of a post-antibiotic apocalypse rehashed.

The way in which risks were staged informed proposed solutions. With its focus on integrated surveillance, stewardship, and biotechnological innovation, the 2015 WHO Action Plan and resulting national action plans were strongly informed by 1990s reform templates originating in high-income European and North American contexts. While the years since 2015 have also seen discussions and more research on the wider factors underpinning antibiotic use and systems vulnerability to AMR, a majority of mobilized funds were spent not on broader systems strengthening but on traditional technology- and behaviour-focused interventions like surveillance, educational campaigns for 'rational' drug use, improved biosecurity, and reinvigorating biotechnological innovation. This was despite criticism of existing metrics of capturing usage and AMR burdens, concerns about the applicability of 1990s reform templates outside high-income contexts, as well as growing uncertainty about the efficacy of existing reduction-oriented stewardship interventions in curbing AMR (Kirchhelle et al., 2020; Overton et al., 2021).

Conclusion

If our historical investigation has shown one thing, it is that policing antibiotics has referred to rather different objects and activities at different times. When viewed from the perspective of preserving antibiotic efficacy, one underlying cause for this is that AMR as a dynamic challenge has changed form through history. What was primarily perceived as a problem of treatment failure in hospitalized patients and animals in the 1940s had evolved into a broadly framed global ecological phenomenon by 2010. In addition, the political intensity with which initiatives targeting the different forms of AMR were pursued has varied considerably over time. Following a phase of concerns about antibiotic scarcity, control over antibiotic use—as opposed to antibiotic quality and production—was mostly left to elite users like doctors and veterinarians and, in the case of less toxic lower-dosed applications, farmers, feed experts, and individual consumers. Out of this initial lack of attention and policing arose successive debates about diverse subjects such as unified diagnostic technologies, guidelines for human and non-human use, selective drug restrictions, and biosecurity risks arising from the global proliferation of antibiotic infrastructures and AMR.

Notably, rather than building upon each other, antibiotic policy debates seem to have been driven forward by moral panics and a somewhat scandalizing attention, which usually echoed problems resulting from specific forms of antibiotic application at a given time rather than broader concerns about the environmental phenomenon of AMR. This start-stop mode of policy evolution resulted in an uneven and incomplete apprehension of the matter in question. The pandemic spread of penicillin-resistant *Staphylococcus* in the 1950s triggered a debate on diagnostic standards and epidemiological studies. Widespread AMR in animal husbandry around 1970 resulted in high-profile controversies with regards to the question of therapeutic drug restrictions. In the 1990s, a crisis of drug innovation and AMR in high-profile pathogens opened a window of opportunity to discuss new integrated forms of AMR and usage surveillance as well as reduction-oriented stewardship schemes in human and animal health. A fourth debate since about 2010 focusses on the proliferation of antibiotics in globalization and biosecurity risks from primarily Southern overuse.

Yet, similar to previous iterations, this most recent debate has been quite narrow. Recommendations for a global export of 1990s-style stewardship programmes, surveillance frameworks, and drug innovation stimuli have fallen short of a full discussion of the policy challenges posed by antibiotic regulation in an age of globalized drug supply chains where profits are driven less by molecular innovation in the Global North than by the production and circulation of generics in the Global South. Changes in the global circulation of pills have not been mirrored in the flows of international policy-making. In an age of faltering internationalism and multipolar politics, the Northern-dominated biosecurity and stewardship rhetoric dominating international policy-making does not necessarily align with the political and economic interests of major Southern powers. And finally, this geographic misalignment of the flows of pills and policies continues to be exacerbated by stark global inequalities when it comes to food and economic security as well as health systems access. With attention for AMR beginning to fall at the international level (see Chapters 14 and 15; also Overton et al., 2021), acknowledging the growing disconnect between the geographies of pills and policies seems to be an essential prerequisite for allowing antibiotic policy-making and stakeholder engagement to catch up with the existing dynamics of use and AMR.

References

Barber, M., Dutton, A. A. C., Beard, M. A., Elmes, P. C., and Williams, R. (1960). 'Reversal of Antibiotic Resistance in Hospital Staphylococcal Infection', *British Medical Journal*, 5165, 11–17.

Beaudevin, C., Gaudillière, J.-P., Gradmann, C., Lovel, A., and Pordie, L., eds. (2020). *Global Health and the New World Order: Historical and Anthropological Approaches to a Changing Regime of Governance* (Manchester: Manchester University Press).

Bud, R. (2007). *Penicillin: Triumph and Tragedy* (Oxford: Oxford University Press).

Chandler, C., Hutchinson, E., and Hutchinson, C. (2016). *Addressing Antimicrobial Resistance Through Social Theory: An Anthropologically Oriented Report.* Retrieved from https://core.ac.uk/download/pdf/74229739.pdf (access date 25.01.2023). London School of Hygiene & Tropical Medicine.

Colquhoun, J., and Weetch, R. S. (1950). Resistance to Cholramphenicol Developing during Treatment of Typhoid Fever. *The Lancet*, 256/6639, 621–23. doi:10.1016/S0140-6736(50)91585-6.

Ericsson, H. M., and Sherris, J. C. (1971). *Antibiotic Sensitivity Testing. Report of an International Collaborative Study* (Vol. Suppl. 217) (Copenhagen: Munksgaard).

Goosens, H., Ferech, R., Vander Stichele, R., and Elsviers, M. (2005). 'Outpatient Use in Europe and Association with Resistance: A Cross-National Database Study', *The Lancet*, 365, 579–87.

Gradmann, C. (2011). 'Magic Bullets and Moving Targets: Antibiotic Resistance and Experimental Chemotherapy 1900–1940', *Dynamis*, 31, 305–21.

Gradmann, C. (2013). 'Sensitive Matters. The World Health Organisation and Antibiotics Resistance Testing', 1945–1975. *Social History of Medicine*, 26, 555–74.

Gradmann, C. (2016). 'Re-Inventing Infectious Disease: Antibiotic Resistance and Drug Development at the Bayer Company 1945-1980', *Medical History*, 59, 155–80.

Greene, J. A. (2014). *Generic: The Unbranding of Modern Medicine* (Baltimore, MD: Johns Hopkins University Press).

Greenwood, D. (2008). *Antimicrobial Drugs. Chronicle of a Twentieth Century Triumph* (Oxford: Oxford University Press).

Hillier, K. (2006). 'Babies and Bacteria: Phage Typing, Bacteriologists, and the Birth of Infection Control', *Bulletin of the History of Medicine*, 80, 733–61.

Institute of Medicine (IoM). (1992). *Committee on Emerging Microbial Threats to Health: Emerging Infections Microbial Threats to Health in the United States* (Washington DC: IOM).

Kahn, L. H. (2016). *One Health and the Politics of Antimicrobial Resistance* (Baltimore, MD: Johns Hopkins University Press).

Kirchhelle, C. (2016). 'Toxic Confusion: The Dilemma of Antibiotic Regulation in West German Food Production (1951–1990)', *Endeavour*, 40/2, 114–27. doi:10.1016/j.endeavour.2016.03.005.

Kirchhelle, C. (2018). 'Swann Song. British Antibiotic Regulation in Livestock Production (1953–2006)', *Bulletin of the History of Medicine*, 92, 317–50.

Kirchhelle, C. (2020). *Pyrrhic Progress. Antibiotics in Anglo-American Food Production (1949–2015)* (New Brunswick, NJ: Rutgers University Press).

Kirchhelle, C. (2021). 'Between Bacteriology and Toxicology—Agricultural Antibiotics and US Risk Regulation', in A. N. H. Creager and J.-P. Gaudillière, eds, *Risk on the Table: Food Production, Health, and the Environment* (New York, NY: Berghahn Books, Incorporated), 214–42.

Kirchhelle, C., Atkinson, P., Broom, A., Chuengsatiansup, K., Ferreira, J. P., Fortané, N., et al. (2020). 'Setting the Standard: Multidisciplinary Hallmarks for Structural, Equitable and Tracked Antibiotic Policy', *BMJ Global Health*, 5/9, e003091. doi:10.1136/bmjgh-2020-003091.

Kirchhelle, C., Dyson, Z. A., and Dougan, G. (2019). 'A Biohistorical Perspective of Typhoid and Antimicrobial Resistance', *Clinical Infectious Diseases*, 69(Supplement_5), S388–S394. doi:10.1093/cid/ciz556.

Koshland, D. E. (1992). 'The Microbial Wars', *Science*, 257, 1021.

Landecker, H. (2019). 'A Metabolic History of Manufacturing Waste: Food Commodities and Their Outsides', *Food, Culture & Society*, 22/5, 530–47. doi:10.1080/15528014.2019.1638110.

Lesch, J. E. (2007). *The First Miracle Drugs: How the Sulfa Drugs Transformed Medicine* (Oxford: Oxford University Press).

Levy, S. B. (1992). *The Antibiotic Paradox. How Miracle Drugs are Destroying the Miracle* (London: Plenum Press).

Lie, A. H. K., and Podolsky, S. H. (2016). 'Futures and Their Uses: Antibiotics and Therapeutic Revolutions', in F. Condrau, J. Greene, and E. S. Watkins, eds, *Therapeutic*

Revolutions: Pharmaceuticals and Social Change in the Twentieth Century (Chicago: University of Chicago Press), 18–42.

MacFarlane, J. T., and Worboys, M. (2008). 'The Changing Management of Acute Bronchitis in Britain, 1940–1970: The Impact of Antibiotics', *Medical History*, 52, 47–72.

McGowan, J. E., and Gerding, D. N. (1996). 'Does Antibiotic Restriction Prevent Resistance?', *New Horizons (Baltimore, MD)*, 4/3, 370–76. Retrieved from http://europepmc.org/abstract/MED/8856 755 (access date 25.01.2023).

McKenna, M. (2010). *Superbug: The Fatal Menace of MRSA* (New York, NY: Free Press).

McKenna, M. (2018). *Big Chicken: The Incredible Story of How Antibiotics Created Modern Agriculture and Changed the Way the World Eats* (Washington, DC: National Geographic).

O'Neill, J. (2016). *Tackling Drug-Resistant Infections Globally*. Retrieved from London: AMR Review.

Overton, K., Fortané, N., Broom, A., Raymond, S., Gradmann, C., Orubu, E. S. F., et al. (2021). 'Waves of Attention: Patterns and Themes of International AMR reports (1945–2020)', *BMJ Global Health*, 12, e006909. doi:10.1136/bmjgh-2021-006909.

Podolsky, S. H. (2015). *The Antibiotic Era: Reform, Resistance, and the Pursuit of Rational Therapeutics* (Baltimore, MD: Johns Hopkins University Press).

Podolsky, S. H. (2018). 'The Evolving Response to Antibiotic Resistance (1945–2018)', *Palgrave Communications*, 4/1, 124. doi:10.1057/s41599-018-0181-x.

Rogers Van Katwyk, S., Weldon, I., Giubilini, A., Kirchhelle, C., Harrison, M., McLean, A., et al. (2020). 'Making Use of Existing International Legal Mechanisms to Manage the Global Antimicrobial Commons: Identifying Legal Hooks and Institutional Mandates', *Health Care Analysis*, doi:10.1007/s10728-020-00393-y.

Smith-Howard, K. (2010). 'Antibiotics and Agricultural Change: Purifying Milk and Protecting Health in the Postwar Era', *Agricultural History*, 84/3, 327–51. doi:10.3098/ah.2010.84.3.327.

Smith-Howard, K. (2017). 'Healing Animals in an Antibiotic Age: Veterinary Drugs and the Professionalism Crisis, 1945–1970', *Technology and Culture*, 58/3, 722–48. doi:10.1353/tech.2017.0079.

Spink, W. W. (1955). 'Clinical Problems Relating to the Management of Infections with Antibiotics', *Journal of the American Medical Association*, 152/7, 585–90.

Thamdrup Rosdahl, V., and Børge Pedersen, K. (1998). *The Copenhagen Recommendations. Report from the Invitational EU Conference on The Microbial Threat*. Retrieved from Copenhagen: Statens Serum Institut and Danish Veterinary Laboratory.

Thoms, U. (2014). 'Handlanger der Industrie oder berufener Schützer des Tieres?—Der Tierarzt und seine Rolle in der Geflügelproduktion', in G. Hirschfelder, A. Ploeger, J. Rückert-John, and G. Schönberger, eds, *Was der Mensch essen darf. Ökonomischer Zwang, ökologisches Gewissen und globale Konflikte* (Wiesbaden: Springer Fachmedien Wiesbaden), 173–92.

Thoms, U. (2017). 'Antibiotika, Agrarwirtschaft und Politik in Deutschland im 20. und 21. Jahrhundert', *Zeitschrift für Agrargeschichte und Agrarsoziologie*, 65, 35–52.

Uekötter, F. (2011). *Am Ende der Gewissheiten. Die ökologische Frage im 21. Jahrhundert* (Frankfurt: Campus).

Woods, A. (2014). 'Science, Disease and Dairy Production in Britain, c.1927 to 1980', *Agricultural History Review*, 62/2, 294–314.

3

Global Eradication and AMR

Nancy Leys Stepan

Introduction

In January 2021, the British global chemical firm INEOS announced a gift of £100 million to the University of Oxford to establish an Institute for Antimicrobial Resistance (AMR). Estimating that AMR causes some 1.5 million excess deaths a year worldwide, a figure that could rise to over 10 million a year by 2050 as we run out of effective antimicrobial drugs to curb infections, INEOS states that AMR is 'arguably the greatest economic and healthcare challenge facing the world post-Covid' (INEOS Group, 2021).[1]

In a separate initiative, in 2019 *The Lancet* Commission on Malaria, made up of a large panel of malaria epidemiologists and research scientists, published a report announcing its endorsement of the goal of the complete eradication of malaria by 2050, presenting disease eradication as the necessary solution to the 'never-ending struggle against drug and insecticide resistance' (*The Lancet* Commission on Malaria Report, 2019: 1056).

Juxtaposing these two initiatives highlights what seems to me to be a tension at the heart of the governance of global public health.

On the one hand we have plans and programmes, as represented by the INEOS Institute and also the World Health Organization's (WHO) 'Global Action Plan on Antimicrobial Resistance' (2015), to reduce the incidence of infection through effective sanitation, hygiene and preventive measures, so as to 'optimize' the use of antimicrobials (meaning reduce misuse) and thereby reduce the emergence of antimicrobial resistance.

On the other hand, we have the pursuit of malaria eradication, with eradication meaning an absolute reduction of worldwide malaria incidence to zero as a result of deliberate effort.[2] The effort relies heavily on the mass use of insecticides and antimalarial drugs, which experience shows leads to repeated cycles of insecticide and drug resistance. The eradicationists don't ignore AMR but argue that eventually, by the end

---

[1] The donation is one of the largest ever given to a British university.

[2] The definition given by the U.S. Centers for Disease Control Eradication is distinguished from disease 'control', which refers simply to the reduction of disease incidence to a manageable level, and from 'elimination', which means the removal of a disease from a specific region or country. Eradication also makes an argument about costs: that disease eradication is expensive in the short term but cheaper in the long run than control, since once zero disease incidence has been achieved, and all transmission of the infective agent stopped, the costs of maintaining control can be given up forever. An eradication campaign also sets a start and end date to the project (usually ten to twenty years).

Nancy Leys Stepan, *Global Eradication and AMR* In: *Steering against Superbugs*. Edited by: Olivier Rubin, Erik Baekkeskov, and Louise Munkholm, Oxford University Press. © Oxford University Press 2023. DOI: 10.1093/oso/9780192899477.003.0003

of an eradication campaign, disease transmission ends forever and therefore there is no more need for the constant innovation of new insecticides and antimicrobial drugs (there are few new antimicrobials right now in the pipeline). Yet out of many eradication campaigns, absolute zero worldwide disease incidence has been achieved only once—with smallpox, in a campaign based not on antimicrobials but on a vaccine, the gold standard of preventive medicine but one that has so far eluded malariologists.[3]

There is thus a fundamental tension between recognition of AMR and the need to abandon overreliance on and misuse of antimicrobials in medicine, farming, and food production, and the pursuit of disease eradication based on the large-scale use of antimicrobial drugs and insecticides. This tension exists within WHO itself—its announcement of its Global Action Plan on Antimicrobial Resistance in 2015 was preceded by its endorsement in 2012 of an all-out yaws eradication campaign (with an end date set for 2020, already passed), despite concern about AMR emerging against the antibiotic azithromycin on which the eradication plan is based.

This chapter explores this contradiction, looking to the history of the post-World War II global malaria eradication campaign (GMEP) as a cautionary tale in the wider global fight against AMR. My focus on the malaria eradication campaign adds a different aspect to the AMR story because much of the discussion about AMR refers to hospital and clinical settings, leaving out of the story some of the largest health interventions in the history of the Global South. Also relevant is the current topicality of malaria, which in 2019 was responsible for 229 million cases and 407,000 deaths, 94 per cent of them in WHO's African Region, where malaria has been on the increase.

Eradication had its critics then and now. In this chapter I look at the ideas of the French-born American bacteriologist, René Dubos. Writing at the height of the GMEP in the 1960s Dubos articulated an ecological, evolutionary view that recognized the complexity of our microbial interactions and the impossibility of eradicating diseases. He highlighted the problem of AMR and mosquito resistance to insecticides generated by malaria eradication. His is a view that resonates today—made relevant by the fact that malaria eradication is once again on the agenda. The Bill and Melinda Gates Foundation (GF), the largest private philanthropic organization in international health, announced in 2007 that its aim was the absolute eradication of malaria. Given this, it is not surprising that today, *The Lancet* Commission on Malaria, which was funded by the Gates Foundation, pushes hard for eradication, despite the opposition of the Director-General of WHO (Ghebreyesus, 2019). This points to the power of a private philanthropy to set a global public health agenda—the resources of the Gates Foundation far outstrip those of WHO (Stepan, 2011: 252–4; also see Chapter 19).

But the GF commitment to eradication also raises the larger question of why, given that time-limited eradication based on the widespread use of antimicrobials and insecticides has proved an elusive if not impossible goal, while generating resistant strains

---

[3] Vaccines can reduce AMR by preventing infections that would otherwise require antimicrobial treatment. The most recent malaria vaccine mentioned in the news, the RTS vaccine, has about a 40 per cent protection rate and requires a demanding four-shot regime.

of microorganisms and insects, has eradicationism proved so enduring? Yes, much of what Dubos said has now been widely absorbed, yet still the question remains: why has it been so hard to organize a response to AMR along Dubosian lines? what policy changes are needed to control malaria without exacerbating AMR?

From disease control to eradication

As an approach to international efforts in public health to dealing with disease eradicationism became dominant after World War II, resulting in a series of eradication 'campaigns' launched under the auspices of the newly created WHO, founded in 1948. Arguably among the most ambitious and costly global efforts in public health ever undertaken, the campaigns against yaws, hookworm disease, yellow fever, malaria, and smallpox were based on growing confidence in the biomedical approach to public health, based on war-time innovations in antibiotics, vaccines, and long-lasting insecticides.

The GMEP, launched in 1955, was the largest and arguably the most significant of all the eradication campaigns and the first to declare failure, closing in 1969.

On the face of it, this failure was not surprising; malaria was an unusual choice for absolute eradication, owing to the disease's complexity. In fact, so complex is malaria that many pre-World War II malaria experts had come to think of it not as one disease but rather as many different diseases, shaped in different ways in different geographical spaces and human populations, posing different challenges to its control in different localities.

Microbiologically, the infective agent of malaria exists as five different species of a protozoan plasmodium (*P. vivax, falciparum, ovale, malariae,* and *knowlesi*), the plasmodia being transmitted to human beings by the bite of a female mosquito belonging to some thirty to forty species of anopheles. The *Anopheles gambiae* mosquito, widespread in Africa, is the most 'efficient' of the malaria vectors, being highly anthropophilic (preferring to feed on humans rather than other animals). In addition, in Africa, the *P. falciparum* form of malaria, the deadliest to humans, is widely distributed.

But this is only to name the biological factors in malaria transmission. Malaria also has social, economic, and environmental determinants, being closely associated with poverty, poor housing (e.g., houses without screened windows), as well as with particular geographies and economies (e.g., agricultural plantations). Human behaviours and activities, from the introduction of new agricultural crops, forest clearance and destruction, population movements and migration, constantly change the socio-biological ecology in which anopheles mosquitoes breed.

Much of this was known to malaria experts who studied malaria in the colonies. Indeed a view had been built up in the pre-World War II period of the ecological complexity of malaria, its multiple determinants, and the possibility of effective control only in limited areas of commercial importance. Eradication was not on the agenda.

World War II changed this and shifted the goal from control to eradication; and with eradication came intensified vector and microbial resistance.

The crucial factor in the development of global eradicationism was the war-time discovery of the long-lasting characteristics of the synthetic insecticide DDT, and the powerful antimalarial effects of the drug chloroquine. Both were effective and cheap. Heavy DDT-spraying had been used successfully in war-time Italy to control malaria. Of particular importance was the post-war experiment in Sardinia, where five years of spraying the island with DDT from 1946 to 1950 seemed to eliminate malaria (without exterminating the specific mosquito vector) (Hall, 2010; Stepan, 2011).

DDT shifted the argument decisively in favour of attacking mosquitoes, ignoring or bypassing the social context. A DDT-based programme was to become a universal technical measure, to be applied everywhere, thus ignoring the idea of disease localism and ignoring too the need to improve social and economic conditions. Ecological knowledge was overlooked and the complexities forgotten in the rush to apply DDT.[4]

DDT recommended itself because it was apparently simple to use by spraying inside dwellings, where most biting by mosquitoes occurred, and spraying teams could be organized in a separate service without waiting for basic health services to be set up. The feeling was that however underdeveloped a country was, and whatever the climate, it was possible to banish malaria.

Launched by WHO in 1955, by 1961 the GMEP involved some sixty-six countries. The early results were dramatic: in Venezuela, in India, in Thailand, malaria incidence plunged. So impressive did these early campaigns seem that by 1963 the Rockefeller Foundation malariologist, Paul F. Russell, was ready to declare that "Man has at last mastered malaria" (Stepan, 2011: 159).

Yet within six years of Russell's claim, WHO announced the end of the GMEP; the goal of eradication was given up; the recommendation that countries revert to malaria 'control' was in many places a recipe for the abandonment of programmes and the return of malaria, sometimes in explosive epidemics.

The emergence of resistance: Insects and plasmodia

Many factors were involved in the failure of the GMEP, from supplies of DDT running out, officials not showing up when expected, agricultural schemes altering the environment, finances proving inadequate, and politicians losing the will to make eradication

---

[4] In 1956, the WHO Expert Committee on Malaria outlined the rationale behind the eradication strategy, using the epidemiologist George Macdonald's formula, introducing the concept of the Reproduction Number, R_0 (familiar to us now because of the COVID-19 pandemic). Macdonald's formula was mathematically complex, involving many epidemiological variables concerning the character or/and number of the mosquitoes. Most experts in malaria could not follow the mathematical details but could grasp his main point, that shortening the life span of the mosquito vector and therefore the number of bites a mosquito could make in a day would interrupt malaria transmission. As Packard says, '[t]his DDT could do', but though the formula included many factors, it left out many others, for example the habits of human beings that affect the biting rate of mosquitoes. So Macdonald's formula was complex but did not capture the social complexity of malaria. As Packard says, 'It made sense in the abstract, but the devil was in the details.' (See Packard 2016: 157; Macdonald, 1956.)

work. In effect the failure was a result of the gap that existed between the idea that the world could be thought of as a single geographical space, in which a single, universal method of public health intervention would work, and the practical realities of a world made up of many different spaces, with different political, economic, and biological characteristics all with different requirements for public health policy. It was not so much that the GMEP was an 'outside' programme imposed by the west on the Global South as it was a policy geared to thinking globally but not to acting locally (contrary to René Dubos's commandment to 'Think Globally, Act Locally').

But resistance was a crucial factor in the GMEP's failure. One is struck, indeed, by how early scientific information came out about resistance in both insect vectors and plasmodia. Dr. Marcelino Candau, the Director-General of WHO from 1953 to 1973, in fact made the case for malaria eradication in 1955 precisely because, among other reasons, the evidence of vector resistance to DDT was accumulating so fast as to give urgency to action. In 1956, only a year after the launch of MEP, Russell warned that '[t]ime is of the essence because DDT resistance had appeared in six or seven years' (quoted in Garrett, 1994: 48). It seemed that the only thing to do was to press on, using DDT as rapidly and widely as possible, rather than find ways to use DDT more se-lectively or rethink the whole project (though Packard notes that DDT resistance did make Russell and others stop spraying once malaria transmission had ended, rather than persisting until no parasites were found in the population). As Packard says, '[e]radication had to be executed before the central weapon against malaria was no longer viable' (Packard, 2007: 155).

Resistance to pesticides was inevitable if spraying was repeatedly used; often, the methods employed made things worse, by incomplete spraying or using watered down insecticide to make DDT supplies go further and allow for increased coverage. The use of DDT in agriculture compounded the problem, especially, as Packard notes, when areas were cleared for new crop plantations, as happened in El Salvador, where the owners of cotton plantations used DDT to get rid of pests. By 1958, the local mal-aria vector (*A. albimanus*) had become resistant to DDT and its substitutes. By the time WHO closed the GMEP in 1969, reverting instead to the goal of control, fifty-six species of anopheles mosquitoes exhibited resistance. The turn to other insecticides, mainly pyrethroids such as malathion, was problematic, as they were so much more costly than DDT that all spraying was reduced (Packard, 2007: 163, 164).

Initially the GMEP was planned around the spraying of insecticides alone, but it was soon realized that, against original expectations and to many, regrettably, this was not enough, that anti-malarial drugs had to be part of the GMEP, as no large area in Africa had seen the elimination of malaria by residual spraying alone (Bruce-Chwatt, 1956). The use of antimicrobials then presented a parallel problem to the use of insecticides—drug resistance developed inexorably in *P. falciparum*, the deadliest form of malaria; resistance then led to the same repetitive search for alternatives as had occurred with insecticides in relation to mosquito vectors. The same underlying social and genetic mechanisms were involved in both kinds of resistance—that is, fast-reproducing and evolving insects and plasmodia—with the overuse and/or inconsistent use of chemicals in the environment, leading to the spread of resistant variants through selective pressure (Knobler et al., 2003).

By the 1960s, resistant strains of *P. falciparum* to the front-line drug, chloroquine, were becoming widespread in Southeast Asia and the Amazon. The resistance of *P. falciparum* was at first received with incredulity, and then with disquiet, as though the constant variation and adaptation of plasmodia had been forgotten (Peters, 1969). Packard shows that there is a strong correlation between the geographical areas where mass drugs were administered and where chloroquine resistance first appeared (Packard, 2016). The distribution of cooking salt saturated with chloroquine (adopted in Brazil and elsewhere as a practical way to encourage the routine use of the drug as a malaria preventative) exacerbated the problem of drug resistance.

With WHO recommending the continuation of malaria control efforts after eradication was abandoned, AMR did not go away; anti-malarials were widely used, with each new drug eventually generating plasmodium resistance, leading to the search for yet further drugs. Combination therapy (CT), based on sulfadoxine/pyrimeamine, was introduced as a substitute for chloroquine, but by the mid-1990s this too had met with parasite resistance which spread from Southeast Asia to the world, leading to a large increase in *P. falciparum* deaths. The newest therapy is artemisinin, derived from the Asian plant *Artemisinin annua*, and promoted by WHO in 2004 and used in combination with other anti-malarials. But in turn this too has led to parasite resistance, especially in Asia and Latin America.

In some countries, such as India, the low incidence of malaria achieved by the GMEP was sustained for many years, sometimes decades, after the end of the eradication programme. In others, many with weak or no basic health systems, control measures disappeared, with the result that epidemic malaria returned.

From the start, Africa was in a category by itself. Malaria is so deeply embedded in the tropical African regions that it was felt at the time, when the possibility of malaria eradication was being discussed, that all that could be initially aimed for was pilot programmes to assess whether modern tools were adequate to achieving malaria elimination (let alone eradication). The answer seemed to be 'no'.[5] The intensity of malaria, and the lack of basic health infrastructure in many newly independent African countries, meant that the attack phase of the GMEP, designed to interrupt transmission, might be endless and require an efficiency in insecticide spraying beyond what science and political will could achieve. Moreover, DDT was found to repel rather than kill the *A. gambiae* vector, so that spraying inside homes was not effective. Eradication in Africa was considered 'premature'. Eradication could not therefore be global, since Africa was in effect left out of the GMEP.

Chloroquine was nonetheless widely used as a prophylactic and a therapeutic, and slowly drug resistance emerged in *P. falciparum*, resulting in what James Webb calls a

---

[5] The Garki Project in Nigeria, conducted by WHO between 1969 and 1976, showed that malaria transmission could not be interrupted by systematic indoor spraying with insecticide and mass administration of an anti-malarial drug (Molineaux and Gramiccia, 1980).

'silent resurgence' of malaria, silent because it was 'hidden in plain sight', so low was the priority given to health in Africa (Webb, 2014: 119–20, 130). Africa had anyway never seen the dramatic declines in malaria incidence achieved in some of the countries in the Global South, but in the 1980s and 1990s drug resistance led to a surge in malaria incidence in Africa to levels not seen since colonial days.

A complicating factor in Africa was and is acquired immunity, the immunity adult Africans acquire in intensely endemic areas via repeated infections of malaria in childhood. This immunity is partial and tied to specific localities; the immunity is lost if people migrate to new places. The immunity also comes at a high cost in childhood illness and deaths. Nevertheless, acquired immunity gives significant protection from malaria. When anti-malaria projects are abandoned, malaria can rebound, sometimes in epidemic form, sickening and killing populations that have lost their immunity. This poses an ethical dilemma in malaria control and/or eradication in Africa that is rarely addressed; in highly endemic areas, anti-malaria efforts must be long-term and sustainable, otherwise they put at risk the very population the malaria control effort is meant to protect (Graboyes, 2015; Stepan, 2011).

René Dubos' anti-eradicationism and AMR

Dubos was a French-born bacteriologist working at the Rockefeller Institute in New York City as a research scientist who, at the height of the eradication campaigns in the 1950s and 1960s, was emerging as the leading eradication sceptic (Moberg, 2005). His anti-eradicationism was part of a larger view, that perfect health was an illusion, a mirage, as the title of his book *Mirage of Health* indicated (Dubos, 1959). Instead, in his second popular work, *Man Adapting*, he argued that we humans have to learn to adapt to the microbes which share the natural world with us.

A pioneer of the antibiotic era, who identified the first anti-bacterial agents from microorganisms in the soil, Dubos was among the first to warn about the emergence of AMR, based on his understanding of the facts of bacterial adaptation (Moberg, 1999). This insight led him to question whether infectious diseases could ever be eliminated. Dubos was also more generally critical of the germ theory of disease, not because he doubted the reality of germs but because he thought that the over-emphasis in medicine on attacking microbial agents with antibiotics led to the neglect of the wider social and economic factors in disease. His special interest was in tuberculosis, whose decline in the West, he argued, predated the discovery of the TB bacillus (in 1882) and was the result of improved sanitation and rising standards of living (and not drugs).

Dubos was especially alert to the complex dynamic interactions that exist between human populations and microbial pathogens—the constant ecological and evolutionary dimensions in living things. The theme is the coexistence of ourselves with micro-organisms that evolve and adapt to changes in the environment, many of them made by humans. In *Man Adapting*, Dubos referred to latent infections, showing how infectious microbes like the TB bacillus can be retained in individuals without causing manifest disease until some factor, such as physiological or social stress, leads the ba-cillus to erupt and cause symptoms. In several regards, as Warwick Anderson shows, Dubos's views were close to those of pre-World War II scientists who emphasized dis-ease complexity, such as Macfarlane Burnet (who studied myxomatosis in Australia), where multiple factors, such as latent infections, carriers, and variations in human sus-ceptibility had to be factored in to understand disease.[6]

The hallmark of Dubos's viewpoint was to link the social and the biological within an evolutionary framework, with an emphasis on complexity: there are multiple points of inter-connection between all living things, their natural environments, and their social environments (human beings and their activities). From his ecological point of view, it was impossible to extract one element—a vector or a pathogen—and try to deal with it in isolation from all the other organisms to which it is connected in its ecological niche.

To Dubos, environmental/ecological realities necessarily undermined projects such as eradication of pathogens or vectors, since such projects failed to take into account the dynamic processes by which pathogens interacted and adapted through genetic modifications.

This was not a matter of saying 'diseases are always with us', or that vectors and pathogens are hard to eliminate. It was suggesting that any public health policy that did not engage with the ecological aspects of disease was inadequate and misguided. Addressing eradication head-on in *Man Adapting*, Dubos drew attention specifically to insect vector resistance resulting from the overuse of insecticides in malaria eradi-cation, as well as adaptations to the chemicals by avoidance behaviours in mosqui-toes. His point was that malaria eradication campaign generated a repetitive cycle of synthesizing, at an ever-increasing cost, more and more insecticides to which vectors become progressively resistant. In addition, there was growing evidence that insecti-cides accumulated in animal and plant tissues, with negative effects.[7]

AMR was another problem. Dubos pointed out that in several parts of the world mu-tant forms of *P. falciparum* had appeared that were resistant to all the available drugs except quinine. In Dubos's opinion, disease eradication would fail and the environment would be made toxic (Dubos, 1965: 374, 379–82).

Control or reduction of disease, in this regard, was far preferable to eradication. Dubos thought that detailed knowledge of microbial ecology would allow subtle ma-nipulations of the environment (such as planting shady trees to reduce the popula-tions of sun-loving anopheles mosquitoes) that would help control infectious diseases without the brutal sledgehammer of chemicals. 'Proper skillful handling of ecological situations makes it possible to create environments in which diphtheria, tubercu-losis, leprosy, malaria, poliomyelitis, smallpox, etc. are converted from major diseases into minor public health problems' (Dubos, 1965: 381). Dubos pointed out that while

---

[6] Historians have only recently begun to uncover these ecological traditions in biomedicine and in public health more widely (Anderson, 2004; Honigsbaum and Méthot, 2020).

[7] Rachel Carson's *Silent Spring* (1962), whose target was the overuse of DDT in agriculture, included a chapter on the problem of insect resistance caused by the overuse of synthetic insecticides in public health (Carson, 1962).

vaccination would control many diseases (e.g., polio), we must expect mutant forms to continue to emerge.

Dubos's contribution, then, was to point in the direction of a different understanding of disease than that embedded in the eradicationist framework, and in biomedicine generally—an understanding that would reduce the endless cycle of synthesizing new insecticides and drugs to which vectors and microbes become progressively resistant. The resulting policies would be 'biosocial', linking knowledge of microbial and animal genetic evolution, variation, and adaptation to the social environments created by human activity. The basic problem with WHO's GMEP strategy was that it did not change mosquito ecology through larval source reduction, nor human ecology through the provision of adequate housing with screens.

Over time, Dubos became a visionary public figure and a radical critic of public health as it was practised at the time, as well as a critic of urban life and capitalism more generally. Given the shifting meaning of 'ecology', commentators disagree as to what kind of ecologist Dubos was. What is certain is that through him a generation of biologists and doctors were alerted to the limitations of eradicationism and the importance of basic health services and the social causes of ill-health.

But Dubos's bio-social model never fully coalesced into a prescriptive paradigm, which restricted his ability to shake the biomedical model. He is probably best understood as a medical environmentalist—a patron saint of the environmental movement and, as noted earlier, the author of the command to 'Think Globally, Act Locally'.[8]

The return of eradication and AMR

With the return of malaria eradication on the agenda, it is fair to ask whether anything has been learned from the failure of the first global malaria eradication campaign. Why has malaria, arguably a uniquely complex disease, with multiple determinants, been selected by the GF for eradication, that most stringent of goals, once again?

One reason is no doubt the progress that has been made since 2000 in reducing malaria cases and deaths in many countries, using long-lasting insecticide-treated bed nets and combinations of anti-malaria drugs. On the other hand, progress has stalled since 2015, with increased drug and vector resistance resulting in increases of malaria incidence cases and deaths, especially in the Americas, Asia, the Western Pacific, and above all in Africa, where the highest burden of malaria has always fallen.

It is in the context of these developments—optimism that tools to tackle malaria are at hand or will be developed in the future, but worry about setbacks—that we need to situate *The Lancet* Commission on Malaria's call in 2019 for a second try at malaria eradication (exactly fifty years after the MEP ended in failure). Setting a goal of

---

[8] What kind of ecologist Dubos was is much debated; the term's meaning had not stabilized in Dubos' lifetime; at one point he rejected the idea that he was an ecologist.

eradication is, the Commission declares, 'ambitious, achievable, and necessary' (*The Lancet* Commission on Malaria, 2019: 1056).

Necessary, according to the Commission, because of biological resistance in vectors and parasites. Indeed, what is striking about *The Lancet* Commission is how central AMR and vector resistance is to the case being made, and yet it is the opposite of Dubos's.

Whereas Dubos argued that eradication projects based on anti-malarial drugs and insecticides generate endless cycles of resistance in micro-organisms and vectors, harming the environment with chemicals in pursuit of a chimerical goal, *The Lancet* Commission maintains that it is only by achieving complete termination that the cycle can be stopped, claiming that 'eradication is the only way to overcome the relentless evolution of malaria drug and insecticide resistance' (*The Lancet* Commission, 2019: 1058).

This is, of course, the crux of the AMR/vector resistance paradox: if there is no transmission left, there is no need to kill mosquitoes and parasites with chemicals, so the cycle of resistance ends. But to get the end point of eradication, the project inevitably constantly creates biological resistance. As with the original GMEP, resistance frames the current project of the eradication of malaria, giving to the end goal its extra urgency. But will setting a goal of eradication this time around reintegrate the bio-social with the bio-technical and reduce reliance on drugs and insecticides?

In fact, on the evidence, it is striking how 'bio-tech' and similar to the first GMEP the methods of the proposed scheme of malaria eradication are. Long-standing socio-political determinants are barely touched upon in *The Lancet* Commission's report. The Commission refers only in passing to possible socio-economic factors in the recent rise in malaria, such as heavy rainfall in sub-Saharan Africa and India, and decreased access to interventions—that is, to climatic, political, and economic factors (see Chapter 7 for the socio-economic challenges of the Global South). But dealing with such factors is seen as lying outside or largely beyond the remit of the Gates Foundation. As some critics of *The Lancet* Commission's report point out, the fact that Nigeria accounts for 25 per cent of the global burden of malaria, and the Democratic Republic of Congo 11 per cent, and that these are also the two countries with the highest number of people living in extreme poverty, is not a coincidence (Kennedy and McCoy, 2020). The reality is that '[m]alaria cannot be understood or eliminated without changes in the social factors that drive it (Packard, 2007, p. xvii, quoting Rosenberg). Housing with screens is better than biocides.

Instead *The Lancet* Commission premises the chance of success in eradication on financial, operational, and especially biological innovations. Faith in biotechnology is as strong as ever—in new drugs, new insecticides, potentially an effective vaccine (a long-standing but thus far unattained dream). Since the arrival of the viral era, starting with HIV-AIDS in the 1980s and followed by SARS, Ebola, Zika, and now COVID-19, molecular genetics has become fundamental to modern medicine; it has led to a hugely increased understanding of the genetics of the microbial world, of gene reassortment and gene drives, allowing such innovations as using CRISPR technology to modify the genes of anopheles mosquito vectors so as to inhibit the transmission of plasmodia.

Apart from the ecological risks that might ensue from releasing genetically modi-fied mosquitoes into the environment, we have to be concerned that these innovations have tended to add to the bio-technical arsenal of tools, rather than lead to the kind of bio-social-ecological approach to public health Dubos had in mind and which many in public health are today calling for; an example would be the One Health model (see Chapters 11, 12, and 13 for discussions of the One Health model; see also Lang and Rayner, 2015; Wallinga et al., 2015).

No-one doubts that AMR is difficult to deal with; we have known about resist-ance since the 1940s, yet the world today struggles to find solutions to the overuse of antimicrobials and chemical insecticides in agriculture, pharmaceuticals, and medi-cine. Some people liken the task of dealing with AMR to that of acting on climate change (see Chapters 14 and 15 for a discussion of climate change in relation to AMR); the challenge with both is the complexity of the determinants and the multiplicity of different steps that need to be taken now, in very different domains simultaneously, in order to reach a better future that still seems to many a long way off, despite all the warnings by WHO and other organizations.

Eradicationism as a model or paradigm in public health is only one part of a much larger issue that has many parts. Yet to this historian, the commitment to eradication, as an answer to the growing threat of AMR and vector resistance, is misguided; history shows eradication is almost always impossible to achieve and in regard to both anti-microbial and insect vector resistance, is more likely to be part of the problem rather than the solution.

On a positive note, the One Health approach, involving multiple disciplines—social science, economics, anthropology, ecology, etc.—suggests an alternative to eradication by emphasizing sustainability and control in place of eradication. But taking the larger view, and on a more pessimistic note, AMR is an under-appreciated problem, despite its seriousness, and I think that unless WHO is given both adequate funding and the necessary powers to manage the global response to AMR, along with other threats to global health, no new policies to overcome AMR, however well adapted to local condi-tions, are likely to succeed (see Chapter 19 for discussion of WHO funding).

References

Anderson, W. (2004). 'Natural Histories of Infectious Disease: Ecological Vision in Twentieth-Century Biomedical Science', *Osiris*, 19, 39–61.
Bruce-Chwatt, L. J. (1956). 'Chemotherapy in Relation to Possibilities of Malaria Eradication in Tropical Africa', *Bulletin of the WHO*, 15/3–5, 852–62.
Carson, R. (1962). *Silent Spring* (New York: Houghton Mifflin).
Dubos, R. (1959). *Mirage of Health: Utopias, Progress, and Biological Change* (New Brunswick, NJ: Rutgers University Press).
Dubos, R. (1965). *Man Adapting* (New Haven, CT: Yale University Press).

Garrett, L. (1994). *The Coming Plague: Newly Emerging Diseases in a World Out of Balance* (New York, NY: Picador).

Ghebreyesus, T. A. (2019). 'The Malaria Eradication Challenge', *The Lancet*, 394/10203, 990–91.

Graboyes, M. (2015). *The Experiment Must Continue: Medical Research and Ethics in East Africa, 1940–2014* (Athens, OH: Ohio University Press).

Hall, M. (2010). 'Environmental Imperialism in Sardinia: Pesticides and Politics in the Struggle Against Malaria', in M. Armerio and M. Hall, eds, *Nature and History in Modern Italy* (Athens, OH: Ohio University Press), 70–86.

Honigsbaum, M., and Méthot, P.-O. (2020). 'Introduction: Microbes, Networks, Knowledge—Emerging Infectious Diseases in the Time of COVID-19', *History and Philosophy of the Life Sciences*, 42/3, 28. doi:1007/s40656-020-00318-x.

INEOS Group. (2021). 'INEOS Donates £100 Million to Create new Oxford University Institute to fight Antimicrobial Resistance', 19 January 2021. <https://www.ineos.com>. July 2015, 2021.

Kennedy, J., and McCoy, D. (2020). 'Malaria Eradication', *The Lancet*, 395/10233, e70 http//doi.org/10.1016/S0140-6736(20)30221-X>.

Knobler, S. L., Lemon, S. J., Najafi, M., and Burroughs, T. (eds). (2003). *The Resistance Phenomenon in Microbes and Infectious Disease Vectors: Implications for Human Health and Strategies for Containment* (Washington, D.C.: National Academies Press).

The Lancet Commission on Malaria. (2019). 'Malaria Eradication within a Generation: Ambitious, Achievable, and Necessary', *The Lancet*, 394/10203, 1056–112. <http://dx.doi.org/10.1016/S0140-6736(19)31139-0>.

Lang, T., and Rayner, G. (2015). 'Beyond the Golden Era of Public Health: Charting a Path from Sanitarianism to Ecological Public Health', *Public Health*, 129, 1369–82.

Macdonald, G. (1956). 'Theory of the Eradication of Malaria', *Bulletin of the WHO*, 15/3–5, 369–87.

Moberg, C. L. (1999). 'René Dubos, a Harbinger of Microbial Resistance to Antibiotics', *Perspectives in Biology and Medicine*, 42/4, 559–80.

Moberg, C. L. (2005). *René Dubos. Friend of the Good Earth: Microbiologist, Medical Scientist, Environmentalist* (Washington, D.C.: ASM Press).

Molineaux, L., and Gramiccia, G. (1980). *The Garki Project. Research on the Epidemiology and Control of Malaria in the Sudan Savanna of West Africa* (Geneva: WHO).

Packard, R. M. (2007). *The Making of a Tropical Disease: A Short History of Malaria* (Baltimore, MD: Johns Hopkins University Press).

Packard, R. M. (2016). *A History of Global Health: Interventions into the Lives of Other Peoples* (Baltimore, MD: Johns Hopkins University Press), 157.

Peters, W. (1969). 'Chemotherapy and Drug Resistance in Malaria—A Perspective', *Transactions of the Royal Society of Tropical Medicine and Hygiene*, 63/1, 25–40.

Stepan, N. L. (2011). *Eradication! Ridding the World of Diseases Forever?* (Ithaca, NY: Cornell University Press).

Wallinga, D., Rayner, G., and Lang, T. (2015). 'Antimicrobial Resistance and Biological Governance: Explanations for Policy Failure', *Public Health*, 129, 1314–25.

Webb, L.A. Jr. (2014). *The Long Struggle Against Malaria in Tropical Africa* (Cambridge: Cambridge University Press).

WHO. (2015). *Global Action Plan on Antimicrobial Resistance* (Geneva: WHO).

4

Conceptualizing AMR as a Creeping Disaster in Terms of Pace and Space

Reidar Staupe-Delgado, Alina Engström, and Sebastián Andres Frugone Cádiz

Introduction

Antimicrobial resistance (AMR) has been labelled one of the greatest threats to life and well-being currently faced by modern society (Baekkeskov et al., 2020). At the global level, the annual death toll associated with AMR is estimated at over 700,000 and, if current resistance trends should continue, this number is projected to hit upwards of 10 million by 2050 (UK Review on Antimicrobial Resistance, 2016). Affecting the entire biosphere as a process of biological evolution, AMR is one example of a truly transboundary process calling for planetary-scale disaster risk governance (Boin et al., 2021; Peoples, 2021). It has been claimed that we are headed towards a 'post-antibiotic' age, or a new dark age, signalling a return to a time when minor infections become increasingly severe or even impossible to treat. From a global health governance perspective, AMR is recognized as a global health threat and a perpetual one at that, and will require holistic responses ranging from vigilance in use of antimicrobials as well as innovations within existing and new paradigms of treatment. However, its status as a global public health emergency remains unclear. For example, a European Union-level policy mechanism was agreed upon only a decade ago, in 2011, whilst a global-level initiative at the World Health Organization (WHO)-level was agreed upon as late as 2015. These initiatives certainly do not appear to be like declarations of an emergency. One impediment for action is perhaps the realization that the challenge of AMR can never truly be overcome. The ever-pervasive nature of AMR as a fact of biology and as a problem across microbes and contexts also means that AMR and its management is closely connected to how societies declare emergencies and conceptualize disasters. How to approach AMR as one of the defining challenges of our time is a question that ultimately will guide responses to it and will increasingly become a discussion of vital importance.

In the natural world, microbes and antimicrobial substances have always coexisted and competed against one another—be it inside human or animal bodies or in the wider environment. The slow accumulation of resistance to antimicrobials is part of the very evolutionary process in which all organisms operate. From an anthropocentric viewpoint, only a handful of microbes have lethal potential. Most bacteria, parasites, fungi,

Reidar Staupe-Delgado, Alina Engström, and Sebastián Andres Frugone Cádiz, *Conceptualizing AMR as a Creeping Disaster in Terms of Pace and Space* In: *Steering against Superbugs.* Edited by: Olivier Rubin, Erik Baekkeskov, and Louise Munkholm, Oxford University Press. © Oxford University Press 2023. DOI: 10.1093/oso/9780192899477.003.0004

and viruses are non-lethal, many even harmless, yet all of them evolve in distinct ways over time, which includes the evolutionary process by which some microbes acquire varying degrees of resistance to antimicrobials (see Chapter 3 for AMR challenges pertaining to malaria). Antimicrobials refer to the broad range of treatments that eliminate or hinder microbe threats. They have become central to maintaining current levels of prosperity associated with modern society. At the same time, the widespread use of antimicrobials also accelerates the AMR problem. It is a dilemma by definition. AMR is an archetypical crisis of modernity (Beck, 1992), a threat that is at the same time instrumental to current levels of prosperity and also threatens to partially undermine our hard-won gains in mortality and morbidity reduction.

There exists no automatic relationship between the severity of a hazard and attention devoted to it (Rubin, 2015). Serious consequences are rarely a necessary or a sufficient condition for a problem to be elevated to emergency status (Spector, 2019). Politics and culture always play a role. So too do characteristics of the hazard itself. Diffuse risks with temporally stretched onsets as well as spatially dispersed impacts do not provide fertile ground for social mobilization and efforts at casting such problems as approaching emergencies often take a long time to take hold and do not always succeed. Building on similar previous work (e.g., Engström, 2021; Viens and Littmann, 2015), this chapter thus argues for the fruitfulness of conceptualizing AMR not just as a global health challenge but as a creeping form of disaster. Whilst the disaster concept has typically been associated with forms of destruction and suffering that are more immediate and concentrated in time and space, our aim here is to reconcile classical and newer perspectives on disasters and the usefulness of considering the notion of creeping disasters. We argue that a disaster lens centred on the onset dynamics of AMR provides a better understanding of why AMR receives disproportionately low attention compared to other defining challenges of the twenty-first century, and also adds nuance to how one can think about feasible responses.

The chapter is structured as follows. In the next section we unpack the disaster term to highlight the need for considering disasters not as necessarily time-bound or place-bound phenomena. The third section then places the global threat of AMR with this discussion, reflecting on how AMR can be fruitfully understood as a creeping disaster. The fourth and concluding section summarizes the salient points raised in the chapter and discusses its wider implications for AMR scholarship and disaster research, including how AMR and similar creeping phenomena can be more effectively tackled.

Considering creeping disasters

Disaster researchers have typically centred on the study of disasters associated with immediate, material, and geographically limited forms of destruction (Dynes, 2004; Lindell, 2013; Hsu, 2019), with some notable exceptions (for an overview, see Staupe-Delgado, 2019a). A considerable body of literature has emerged over the decades attempting to address the question of what constitutes a disaster (e.g., Perry, 2018; Perry and Quarantelli, 2005; Quarantelli, 1998). A common feature of suggested definitions is that a 'disaster' occurs in a geographically limited area and is of a limited duration. Disaster management manuals often organize disasters in terms of 'phases', where disasters consist of a pre-disaster phase, an acute-disaster phase, and a post-disaster phase, with some degree of variation (cf. DHS, 2021; IFRC, 2021). A common denominator across many manuals is that disasters are approached according to an onset–impact–aftermath logic. A seminal definition of disaster that emphasizes the temporal delimitation of disastrous phenomena is provided by Charles Fritz (1961: 655), who sees a disaster as:

> an event concentrated in time and space, in which a society or one of its subdivisions undergoes physical harm and social disruption, such that all or some essential functions of the society or subdivision are impaired.

As may be read from this oft-cited definition, disasters are typically understood as distinct occurrences or 'events', as opposed to more pervasive societal issues. AMR breaks with this pattern in quite obvious ways as AMR does not conform to sequence patterns of disaster as they are normally typologized according to classical disaster definitions. Differently put, more elusive phenomena in terms of pace and space, albeit more deadly, are often construed as something other than disasters (e.g., 'social problems' (as sociologists call them), challenges, crises, or epidemics). For example, a flooding disaster killing two dozen people will typically be a more salient occurrence (and conform more to how we understand the disaster term) than the slower and more elusive accumulation of hundreds of local deaths per year due to driving, drowning, infectious disease, or other less event-like killers (Lindell, 2013).

Although noting that we may be headed towards a time characterized by a blurring between acute conditions and more slow-onset and chronic conditions, Quarantelli noted in the concluding remarks of a roundtable on the topic that the field of disaster research is better served by a spatially and temporally bound disaster concept (Quarantelli, 1998). Several roundtable participants underlined that whilst there are many disastrous phenomena that are neither geographically delimited nor temporally bound, extending the denotational scope of the disaster term to cover chronic and gradual forms of destruction would dilute or add unnecessary ambiguity to the disaster term. Although later roundtables also challenged these claims (Perry and Quarantelli, 2005), a majority of disaster researchers seemed to agree that time-delineated acuteness remains a defining feature of disasters. In other words, the benefits of having a neatly defined disaster concept in terms of denotation (the kinds of phenomena it refers to) has become an accepted argument for restricting the focus of the disaster concept to the sudden and acute, leaving little room for discussing many of the greatest crises faced by modern society.

Recent conceptual work on disasters has begun to question the appropriateness of disregarding gradual processes from definitions of the term. In an attempt to broaden the field without upsetting the terminological landscape, sociologist Eric Hsu (2019) argues for an expanded temporal understanding of disasters. Noting that previous work has tended to exclude diffuse and creeping phenomena from their focus on the grounds that it would create an unnecessarily imprecise concept, Hsu (2019: 904) argues that 'there are ways of theorizing disasters as involving a protracted component that do not completely threaten the wholesale integrity of the concept'. While the problem associated with diffuse phenomena is precisely that they often fail to attain emergency status, their cumulative toll can in many cases be manifold that of conventional time-bound and localized disasters. The significant and arguably increasing toll of slow-onset phenomena can thus be considered a good reason for labelling them disasters (Hsu, 2019). This argument is supported by the work of Matthewman (2015) or more recent work on 'creeping crises' (Boin et al., 2021), underlining the increasingly complex nature between cause and effect, distribution of losses, and onset dynamics. This has also been increasingly recognized in emerging work aiming to discuss whether AMR can be said to constitute a disaster or crisis and with what implications (e.g., Engström, 2021; Viens and Littmann, 2015). The present chapter builds on this work but we take as our point of departure a conceptualization centred on the spatial and temporal dynamics of the creeping disaster of AMR and how these dynamics may shape its governance.

AMR as a creeping disaster: Pace and space

The classical definition of a disaster, as we have seen, has a temporal and spatial aspect. It suggests a relatively clear beginning and end to disasters, where it is possible to trace when and where they started, at least in hindsight. This temporal and spatial aspect also pertains to common health disasters, such as epidemics, which are temporally and spatially bound, at least until becoming endemic (Viens and Littmann, 2015). Thus, the traditional definitions of crises or disasters fail to grasp ambiguous adversities without such pace- and space-based delineations. AMR is but one case in point. AMR progresses slowly, incubates in various sectors, and occasionally punctuates normalcy by escalating into random large-scale community outbreaks (Engström, 2021). Rather than constituting a uniform disastrous phenomena, it is more like an umbrella concept for emerging resistance in a number of contagions (much like climate change is perhaps not one disaster but an 'augmenter of disasters'). Inherently global phenomena, one common challenge for the governance of AMR and similar societal threats is the difficulty of pointing out when and where exactly the emergency began and even more difficult to conceive of a potential end-point to emerging hardships as well as global distributions of burden and responsibility.

In this section, we will consider some advantages to be derived from conceptualizing AMR not merely as a global public health challenge but as a creeping disaster, recognizing that it lacks some of the temporal and spatial boundaries typically associated with disasters. Following the argument of Viens and Littmann (2015), we argue that AMR is unquestionably a slowly emerging disaster unfolding before us, and that it should be treated as such regardless of typical urgency-based understandings of disasters and emergencies. We are also mindful of the trade-offs, however, as disaster framings may be counterproductive in the context of permanent problems, as a problem may not be able to maintain disaster or emergency status indefinitely (Patterson et al., 2021). An analysis based on pace and space also implies an understanding of the threat as inherently 'glocal' (Robertson, 1995), seeing it as a problem operating across levels of governance (e.g., 'transboundary' (Ansell et al., 2011). The idea of perpetual disaster or emergency risks more than diluting the concepts, it also risks bringing about the paralysing effects of disaster fatigue. It is in many ways precisely the failure of seeing creeping phenomena as emergencies or disasters that cause them to become large-scale disasters in the first place.

The creeping disaster of AMR can be considered a multifaceted phenomenon unfolding across sectors and according to different and intersecting spatial and temporal horizons (depending on evolutionary processes in each type of contagion), rendering it quite distinct from disasters falling under the classical definition. For example, the kinds of actors involved vary greatly as few traditional emergency management authorities, as such, are involved in AMR governance as 'first responders'. In the following analysis we will centre on the pace of the disaster, its spatial dynamics as well as its multi-level nature (see Figure 4.1). Our approach explicitly employs a disaster study lens, grounded in vulnerability analysis. Thus, our conceptualization will centre on some of the root causes of AMR as well as obstacles to effective action.

In Figure 4.1, we can observe that the temporal and spatial attributes of AMR poses distinct challenges and is driven by processes occurring across levels. At the meta-level we find the drivers of AMR disaster risk. The globalization process augments the disaster risk picture in the form of migration, cross-border integration as well as the internationalization of public health governance. These processes are also related to patterns

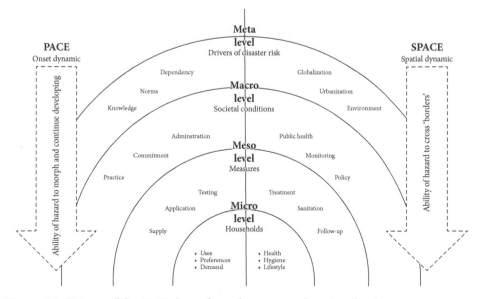

Figure 4.1 Drivers of the AMR threat from the meta- to the micro-level.

of urbanization and changes in the environment, including at the microscopic level, where interactions and interchanges are increasingly sped up due to the acceleration of society which in turn increases the potential for new strains to spread quickly and widely. These spatial aspects are part of what characterizes transboundary and global-scale crises in general (Ansell et al., 2010). Socio-cultural patterns of antimicrobial dependency and overuse, in turn related to norms and knowledge, also play a major part in driving both the pace and the scope of the problem. The onset dynamics associated with AMR can thus best be understood in terms of the interaction between its spatial dynamics and the pace of its onset(s), depending on if we consider the overall AMR process or degrees of AMR displayed by distinct contagions (AMR as overall phenomenon or varying degrees of AMR as attributes of distinct disease agents).

The threat agents at the heart of this disaster are the various microbes that mutate into resistant or extensively resistant 'superbugs' (Burki, 2018). While this mutation is a natural phenomenon, it is being accelerated by the mis- and overuse of antimicrobials, speeding up its pace. Such acceleration is facilitated by numerous conditions. To mention a few, one crucial concern is the ineffective governance of the excess, access, use, and limited discovery of antimicrobials. Another is regulation that does not sufficiently target responsible production, distribution, and usage of microbes in the systems of healthcare, food production, and pharmaceutical dispensing (World Bank, 2019), but conditions also pertain to market forces (the supply and demand for cheap meat) (Laxminarayan et al., 2015) and the individual use of antimicrobials, which is closely related to norms, knowledge of correct use, and, as we will explain below, culture. All these conditions exist in increasingly complex and interconnected systems, which makes it difficult or even impossible to trace or identify precisely when and where the disaster came into existence. This impossibility to trace the incubation phase (see Turner, 1976) illustrates clearly that AMR needs to be conceptualized as a disaster that is not temporally bound, instead qualifying as a slow-onset, or creeping disaster, evolving in time, unstoppably, perpetually—at least in the absence of a paradigm shift in infectious disease medicine.

Whilst not being temporally bound, the phenomenon also defies national borders (Boin, 2019), allowing for the slow progress of the disaster to continue despite local responses in one place. While the previous paragraph discussed the incubation period and slow accumulation of the problem over time, it is crucial also to outline the process of transmission, which not only contributes to the disaster moving across the human, animal, and natural world but also to its progress towards quick escalation. When antibiotics are then used to treat an infection, only the antibiotic resistant bacteria will survive, leaving them without competitors (Ali et al., 2018). Resistance in this way builds up and accumulates over time, within and between bodies and borders. In the context of the current study, this is the process where the threat agent at the heart of the crisis morphs and develops its threat potential over time.

One aspect that makes the phenomenon of AMR hard to respond to is precisely the temporal aspect. This is because it is an endemic condition, influencing other endemic diseases. Endemic diseases, as opposed to epidemic or pandemic diseases, evolve constantly and change at a slow rate—sometimes over months or years. They are our timeless maladies. While it can influence large numbers in a population and cause a high burden of disease, it does not cause immediate burden on health systems that stress them beyond normal operating capacity. Epidemic or pandemic diseases can cause a rapid increase of cases within a short period of time, as recent pandemic experience illustrates. Although AMR in itself is not an epidemic or pandemic condition (it may be better understood as an umbrella term covering a number of distinct but related processes), the phenomenon of AMR is recognized as a considerable disaster risk for the future as a growing number of common infections become increasingly difficult to treat. In terms of severity, we can consider the growing health disaster potential of AMR on a continuum ranging from resistant microbes that are possible to address with small changes to existing treatment practices on one side of the scale to truly resistant 'superbugs' that do not respond to any treatment on the other.

At the macro level, societal conditions connected to how public health administration functions nationally or regionally impacts not only the degree of commitment to international attempts at formulating treaties to address the emerging disaster but also forms practice and ultimately upholds norms operating at the meta level. Policy guidance at the national level, albeit often lagging behind international commitments at the WHO level (Engström, 2021), lays the foundation for better monitoring and a culture of integrating AMR concerns within wider discussions of public health within the national health system.

Because of the complexity and interconnectedness of systems, several possibilities exist for the threat to transmit across levels as well as between individuals, humans, and the environment, making it difficult to tie the issue to a distinct spatiality (see discussions of One Health in Chapters 11, 12, and 13). This means that mitigation, much like with any disaster risk, begins at the local level with support and incentives from higher levels, but with more issues related to issue ownership (Engström, 2021). Further, AMR as an endemic condition changes the existing disease landscape and associated morbidity dynamics. While resistant infections can influence large numbers in a population and cause a high burden of disease, it does not cause an immediate burden on health systems that stress them beyond normal operating capacity. In fact, without high-quality data, slowly simmering health disasters can be difficult even to detect and conceptualize in terms of emergency (Staupe-Delgado, 2019b). These kinds of elusive outbreaks of resistant microbes may well be more susceptible to the politics of attention and prevailing cultural frames in a society, as their existence as emergencies only become clear after deliberately looking for them.

Indeed, the emergence of resistant bacteria has been growing rapidly over the last seven decades. The first case of methicillin-resistant *Staphylococcus aureus* (MRSA) was first discovered in the United Kingdom in 1961 (Sengupta et al., 2013; see also Chapter 2). However, resistance has accumulated, and all pathogens have now developed resistance towards one or multiple antibiotics. Some bacteria already show concerning resistance levels—such as *Klebsiella pneumonia*, *Escherichia coli* (*E. Coli*), and *Staphylococcus aureus* (UK Review on Antimicrobial Resistance, 2016). What currently is believed to pose the largest threats are the pathogens *Staphylococcus aureus* and *Enterococcus*. MRSA kills more people in the United States annually than HIV/AIDS, emphysema, Parkinson's disease, and homicide combined (Gross, 2013), but AMR is not even among the top 100 risks and threats dreaded by the US public (Friedman, 2019).

So how does the threat agent constantly evolve and morph at a slow rate over time? Although the development of antimicrobial resistance is a natural phenomenon, it is being facilitated by and accelerated by conditions related to antimicrobial exposure and inappropriate use. This entails the excess, access, use, and governance across different sectors, industries, and institutions. As formerly mentioned, the more antibiotics we use, the more resistance we will develop. This gives the agent time to morph over time. We can refer to this as 'AMR incubation'. The irrational use of antimicrobials is facilitated not only by macro-level conditions, but also by meta-level and lower-level conditions, as shown in the previous figure.

The agent at the heart of the disaster emerges in complex systems containing a high number of parts with relations between them. Meanwhile, as these complex systems are increasingly interconnected, transmission is facilitated. The more complex the system, the more relations between its parts, the more likely it will be that the threat agent moves across the systemic parts. It is in these complex systems that such minor disturbances occur—initially slowly—and before long, potentially reaching all corners of the world. In the case of AMR, the disturbances are the mis- or overuse of antimicrobials, which in turn allows for 'AMR incubation', hence time for the threat agent to morph over time, between sectors, people, and places.

After morphing, societal and environmental conditions often facilitate and accelerate the epidemic potential of the contagion. The disaster risk will have built up over time and will be further shaped by opportunities and constraints related to the lives of the contagion's hosts. Because of the complexity and connectedness of different systems, there is not only enough time for microbes to develop resistance unnoticed but also several possibilities for the agent to spread across different individuals, systems, and sectors. Once resistance is observed these strains are often found all over the world shortly thereafter. Certain societal conditions also facilitate the spread of contagion. Such spatial conditions are those conditions that facilitate the agent's onward transmission and pose a challenge for efforts to limit the prevalence of resistance locally. These conditions are associated with prevailing urbanization trends, mobility patterns, migration, international travel, and so on. Metropolitan cities are generally connected in such a way that contagions appearing in one of them can appear in one or all of them in less than a day (Zhou and Coleman, 2016).

Although AMR is an endemic creeping disaster that simmers under the surface, constantly changing and evolving over a long period of time, there might be sudden outbreaks of resistant infectious diseases that appear more like sudden ruptures. These outbreaks hit local communities and hospitals at the meso level and below but may well originate in distant lands or other communities. In 2019, for instance, the WHO was informed about several cases of infections caused by antibiotic-resistant *Pseudomonas aeruginosa* in US hospitals. The majority of the patients were hospitalized due to complications associated with infections that they have obtained following invasive procedures in Tijuana, Mexico (WHO, 2019). Hospital outbreaks have been reported from different geographical areas. However, far from all cases of superbug infections and deaths caused by such infections are reported and many thus go unnoticed.

The multilevel efforts to combat the AMR issue began over two decades ago but gained momentum only recently with the Global Action Plan on Antimicrobial Resistance process under the auspices of the World Health Assembly in the mid-2010s (see Chapter 2). There are some outbreaks that might have influenced the increased attention by the international community at this time, one being the Pakistani Typhoid fever outbreak in 2016 that quickly transmitted internationally. The Enterobacteriaceae *Klebsiella pneumoniae* is also a superbug that has caused several outbreaks throughout the United States and worldwide during the last two decades, beginning in New York City in the early 2000s. This superbug has also been deemed as one of the highly critical superbugs by US authorities and the WHO and vividly illustrates the transboundary characteristics of the threat.

It is not only that particular outbreaks seem to have influenced the high-level political actors—individual superbugs also might have influenced their sudden action in the 2010s. *Candida auris* and the so-called *Iraqibacter* are examples of two that have been portrayed in the media as being invasive enemies to humans. The Indian superbug *NDM-1* was also portrayed as being dangerous for humans in the UK and US print media. Judging from news reports alone, it appears that AMR is increasingly gaining an emergency status in the press. In fact, research suggests that the media discourse on superbugs began to shift in the late 1990s (Capurro, 2020). Earlier media reports had mainly reproduced rhetoric from the medical literature but increasingly started to portray the superbugs in apocalyptic terms (Brown and Crawford, 2009). The late 1990s was also the time when WHO first started addressing the AMR issue, although initially only modestly.

The AMR issue is complex as it follows transboundary trajectories and occasionally explodes in local concentrated manifestations in the form of 'outbreaks'. These outbreaks are precursor events that might have the potential to draw attention to the problem, albeit only momentarily. However, as many outbreaks are not reported, occurring in distant lands, the origin and pathways of the threat are hard to follow and attention is difficult to sustain. The spatially and temporally diffuse nature of the emergency render it difficult to cast the threat in disaster terms, at least when classical definitions are applied. Nevertheless, casting the threat in emergency terms clearly also seems to increase its salience in the press, in politics, and in public discourse, and yet the fact that AMR is rather an umbrella term for a number of individual health emergencies related to all kinds of contagions and associated diseases does not help in conceptualizing AMR in disaster terms. All these factors ultimately contribute towards rendering the threat elusive and making it difficult to manoeuvre the menacing threat in the policy world. As we have seen, AMR does not even feature on most lists of threats that the general public fear or worry about. There is a clear interface of the spatial and temporal aspects of AMR. Both the beginning of the accumulation and paths of transmission are difficult to trace and define. This prompts the discussion whether this disaster should rather be conceptualized as a creeping disaster despite having temporal and spatial attributes that challenge classical conceptions of disaster. Because creeping disasters can be understood as separate from the kinds of occasions we normally conceive of in disaster terms, the term 'creeping disaster' opens up for analyses more explicitly centred on the elusive, slow, and largely invisible effects of AMR and similar issues (such as climate change), with important health governance implications. Principal among these may be the challenge of how to spark action despite the fact that AMR lacks many of the traits we typically associate with disasters, while at the same time constituting a looming disaster in terms of its expected future impact on human health and prosperity.

Concluding remarks

One obstacle to overcoming response and attention inertia in the context of creeping disasters is the lack of clearly observable precursor events, lack of direct experience of accumulating disaster impact, and the elusive and spatio-temporally diffuse nature of the onset. We noted in the introduction that AMR is a crisis of modernity. It is precisely its importance and usefulness that has also exacerbated the problem in the form of overuse. Antimicrobials have in many ways improved the life of humans, including food security, but has at the same time contributed to risky dependency. This renders AMR as a societal issue highly influenced by prevailing cultural frames in society as many of the key obstacles to addressing it are interwoven into the fabric of society itself. Many health systems around the world are ill-equipped to deal with global health crises, particularly these crises are elusive and ambiguous. This has important implications for how we think about disasters generally and AMR particularly.

A disaster theory lens clearly offers a fresh perspective on the mounting AMR crisis. When it comes to complex cultural and social aspects of the creeping disaster, the issues related to the misuse of antibiotics and posterior resistance, is greatly connected to the behavioural aspects of the society, which in turn is conditioned by their cultural, political, and economic dynamics. As we have seen, the societal structure as well as the modernization process itself shape vulnerabilities to AMR in important ways. For one, failures in global health have caused self-medication with over-the-counter antibiotics to be an easy way to sidestep diagnosis and responsible treatment. Cultural practices associated with illness and treatment thus directly shapes AMR as a problem and solutions to it. In the contemporary culture of care there is a significant focus on 'taking something' to feel better or 'giving something' as a way of caring. These notions tend to develop into misuse, which becomes integrated into the local culture.

Similarly, societal addiction to cheap meats and dairy exacerbates the disaster in the agricultural sphere. The market-centred logic of most cultures in the twenty-first century has given rise to a demand for practices that speed up the onset of AMR in contagions. The agricultural sector is structurally dependent on antimicrobials in many parts of the world. This issue goes beyond simply altering how livestock is raised. Demand structures in many ways restrict how supply-side issues can be meaningfully addressed. For example, reducing antimicrobial use in agriculture would, for one thing, require increased space and hygiene as an alternative to combating germs through pharmaceutical means. In other words, AMR is both an inevitable disaster in the sense that resistance is a fact of biology, whilst at the same time being a societally constructed disaster risk in the sense that we have allowed ourselves to simultaneously become overly dependent on abundant antimicrobial use without sound AMR stewardship across levels. Reducing AMR disaster risk would thus hinge on also making structural changes affecting the demand side of the equation, or behaviours, cultures, and practices, which essentially is true for all kinds of disasters. AMR can be approached as a disaster that operates across multiple sectors and temporalities, as well as at different levels of governance. The root causes of the problem are woven into our increasingly complex and interconnected market and cultural systems, which makes it hard to determine concrete solutions within the prevailing cultural manoeuvring space. In this way, AMR demonstrates a number of similarities with other disasters looming on the horizon, including climate change and other creeping phenomena.

References

Ali, J., Rafiq, Q. A., and Ratcliffe, E. (2018). 'Antimicrobial Resistance Mechanisms and Potential Synthetic Treatments', *Future Science*, 4/4, FSO290.

Ansell, C., Boin, A., and Keller, A. (2010). 'Managing Transboundary Crises: Identifying the Building Blocks of an Effective Response System', *Journal of Contingencies and Crisis Management*, 18/4, 195–207.

Baekkeskov, E., Rubin, O., Munkholm, L., and Zaman, W. (2020). 'Antimicrobial Resistance as a Global Health Crisis' in *Oxford Research Encyclopedia of Politics* (Oxford: Oxford University Press).

Beck, U. (1992). *Risk Society: Towards a New Modernity* (London: Sage).

Boin, A. (2019). 'The Transboundary Crisis: Why We Are Unprepared and the Road Ahead', *Journal of Contingencies and Crisis Management*, 27/1, 94–9.

Boin, A., Ekengren, M., and Rhinard, M. (2021). *Understanding the Creeping Crisis* (Cham, Switzerland: Palgrave Macmillan).

Brown, B., and Crawford, P. (2009). '"Post Antibiotic Apocalypse": Discourses of Mutation In Narratives of MRSA', *Sociology of Health & Illness*, 31/4, 508–24.

Burki, T. K. (2018). 'Superbugs: An Arms Race Against Bacteria', *The Lancet Respiratory Medicine*, 6/9, 668.

Capurro, G. (2020). '"Superbugs" in the Risk Society: Assessing the Reflexive Function of North American Newspaper Coverage of Antimicrobial Resistance', *SAGE Open*, 10/1, 1–13.

DHS (2021). Disasters Overview. <https://www.dhs.gov/disasters-overview> accessed 27 August 2021.

Dynes, R. (2004). 'Expanding the Horizons of Disaster Research', *Natural Hazards Observer* 28/4, 1–2.

Engström, A. (2021). 'Antimicrobial Resistance as a Creeping Crisis', in A. Boin, M. Ekengren, and M. Rhinard, eds, *Understanding the Creeping Crisis* (Cham, Switzerland: Palgrave Macmillan), 19–36.

Friedman, J. A. (2019). 'Priorities for Preventive Action: Explaining Americans' Divergent Reactions to 100 Public Risks', *American Journal of Political Science*, 63/1, 181–96.

Fritz, C. E. (1961). 'Disasters', in R. K. Merton and R. Nisbet, eds, *Social Problems* (New York: Harcourt Brace & World), 651–94.

Gross, M. (2013). 'Antibiotics in Crisis', *Current Biology*, 23/24, 1063–5.

Hsu, E. L. (2019). 'Must Disasters be Rapidly Occurring? The Case for an Expanded Temporal Typology of Disasters', *Time & Society*, 28/3, 904–21.

IFRC (2021). About Disasters. <ttps://www.ifrc.org/our-work/disasters-climate-and-crises/what-disaster> accessed 25 January 2023.

Laxminarayan, R., van Boeckel, T., and Teillant, A. (2015). *The Economic Costs of Withdrawing Antimicrobial Growth Promoters from the Livestock Sector* (Paris: OECD).

Lindell, M. K. (2013). 'Disaster Studies', *Current Sociology*, 61(5–6), 797–825

Matthewman, S. (2015). *Disasters, Risk and Revelation: Making Sense of Our Times* (Cham, Switzerland: Palgrave Macmillan).

Patterson, J., Wyborn, C., Westman, L., Brisbois, M. C., Milkoreit, M., and Jayaram, D. (2021). 'The Political Effects of Emergency Frames in Sustainability', *Nature Sustainability*, 4/1, 841–50.

Peoples, C. (2021). 'Global Uncertainties, Geoengineering and the Technopolitics of Planetary Crisis Management', *Globalizations*, 1–15.

Perry, R. W. (2018). 'Defining Disaster: An Evolving Concept', in H. Rodríguez, W. Donner, and T. E. Trainor, eds, *Handbook of Disaster Research* (2nd edn, Cham, Switzerland: Springer), 3–22.

Perry, R. W., and Quarantelli, E. L. (2005). *What is a Disaster? New Answers to Old Questions* (Philadelphia: Xlibris).

Quarantelli, E. L. (1998). *What is a Disaster? Perspectives on the Question* (London: Routledge).

Robertson, R. (1995). 'Glocalization: Time-Space and Homogeneity-Heterogeneity', in M. Featherstone, S. Lash, and R. Robertson, eds, *Global Modernities* (London: Sage), 25–44.

Rubin, O. (2015). 'Natural Disasters and Politics', in R. Dahlberrg, O. Rubin, and M. T. Vendelø, eds, *Disaster Research: Multidisciplinary and International Perspectives* (London: Routledge), 82–96.

Sengupta, S., Chattopadhyay, M. K., and Grossart, H. P. (2013). 'The Multifaceted Roles of Antibiotics and Antibiotic Resistance in Nature', *Frontiers in Microbiology*, 4, 47.

Spector, B. (2019). *Constructing Crisis: Leaders, Crises, and Claims of Urgency* (Cambridge: Cambridge University Press).

Staupe-Delgado, R. (2019a). 'Progress, Traditions and Future Directions in Research on Disasters Involving Slow-Onset Hazards', *Disaster Prevention and Management*, 28/5, 623–35.

Staupe-Delgado, R. (2019b). *Overcoming Barriers to Proactive Response in Slow-Onset Disasters. Contributing Paper to GAR 2019* (Geneva: UNDRR).

Turner, B. A. (1976). 'The Organizational and Interorganizational Development of Disasters', *Administrative Science Quarterly*, 21/3, 378–97.

UK Review on Antimicrobial Resistance (2016). *Tackling Drug-Resistant Infections Globally: Final Report and Recommendations* (London: UK Review on Antimicrobial Resistance).

Viens, A. M., and Littmann, J. (2015). 'Is Antimicrobial Resistance a Slowly Emerging Disaster?', *Public Health Ethics*, 8/3, 255–65.

WHO (2019). Carbapenem-resistant Pseudomonas aeruginosa infection—Mexico. <https://www.who.int/emergencies/disease-outbreak-news/item/5-march-2019-carbapenem-resistant-p-aeruginosa-mex-en> accessed 27 August 2021.

World Bank (2019). *Drug-resistant Infections: A Threat to Our Economic Future* (Washington, D.C.: World Bank).

Zhou, Y. R., and Coleman, W. D. (2016). 'Accelerated Contagion and Response: Understanding the Relationships among Globalization, Time, and Disease', *Globalizations*, 13/3, 285–99.

PART II
COORDINATION AND LEADERSHIP IN AMR GOVERNANCE

5

Combatting AMR in the EU

Governmental Dimensions

Carsten Strøby Jensen

Introduction

This chapter focuses on the European Union (EU) and its initiatives to combat antimicrobial resistance (AMR). The EU has been an active international player with regard to AMR for the past twenty years. It is especially in the last ten years that the EU has increased its efforts to manage the problems caused by AMR. A number of action plans have been developed with the goal of reducing misuse of antimicrobial in both the human medical and livestock sectors, these being the main users of antimicrobial products in the EU. These action plans focus on developing an overview of antimicrobial consumption and to introduce initiatives to reduce overall antimicrobial consumption in the entire EU area.

In this chapter, I begin (in the second section) by presenting the EU antimicrobial 'landscape' by describing which countries and sectors are the main users of antimicrobials. We can observe major variations in consumption levels and consumption patterns among the different EU Member States. This overview describes some of the differences in antimicrobial consumption within the human and veterinarian sectors in the EU countries. A full picture of antimicrobial consumption is essential because consumption is closely correlated with levels of AMR. Countries with high consumption tend to have high levels of AMR.

The third section of the chapter discusses how the EU governmental structures manage the challenges posed by AMR. The EU has probably the most developed transnational cooperation between independent countries in the world. It has developed a sophisticated decision-making structure that contains elements of both national and transnational character, thus forming common governmental structures. EU policies to control consumption of antimicrobials and combat AMR are embedded primarily in the health policy area.

However, within the EU, health policy is defined as a policy area with national competence and only scant transnational competence. This limitation is discussed in the overview of the important initiatives taken by EU.

The fourth section of this chapter discusses the EU from a more global perspective. Focus is on how the EU contributes to global governance initiatives to manage AMR.

Carsten Strøby Jensen, *Combatting AMR in the EU* In: *Steering against Superbugs*. Edited by: Olivier Rubin, Erik Baekkeskov, and Louise Munkholm, Oxford University Press. © Oxford University Press 2023. DOI: 10.1093/oso/9780192899477.003.0005

The fifth and concluding section of the chapter discusses the policy implications of the governmental initiatives emanating from the EU.

A recurring theme in this chapter is the extent to which we can observe trends towards convergence or divergence in levels of consumption of antimicrobials in different EU countries and at the global level. Much of the European and global governmental effort to combat AMR is oriented towards reducing the overall consumption of antimicrobials. If these governmental efforts are successful, we will see a convergence in the consumption patterns (e.g., overall reduction in the use of antimicrobials) among the EU countries and in other regions. Using institutional theory, the drivers (or the dynamics) behind such trends towards convergence towards reduced consumption of antimicrobials could be differentiated into 'coercive drivers', 'mimetic drivers', and 'normative drivers' (DiMaggio and Powell, 1983; Scott, 1995). The three types of drivers or types of isomorphism indicate the extent to which governmental instruments pushing convergence rely on 'coercions/force' (e.g., legislation), on 'mimetic/inclination' (e.g., adaptation in order to create legitimation), or on 'norms/appropriateness' (e.g., promoting what is considered to be 'good behaviour').

Use of antimicrobials in the EU Member States

Studies have shown that how and to what extent antimicrobials are used in treatment is not only a result of purely medical decision-making. How and to what extent are antimicrobials prescribed by doctors and veterinarians depend to a large degree on the societal context of which they are a part. The national economy, legislation, and social norms all influence decisions about how, when, and where antimicrobials are prescribed (Jensen et al., 2019).

In the EU, antimicrobials are utilized in both the human medical sector and in livestock production. Table 5.1 gives an overview of differences in levels of antimicrobial consumption in EU Member States (and some European Economic Area (EEA) countries). Table 5.1 presents human and livestock consumption both in absolute amount of consumption of active substance in each country and relatively, in relation to biomass.

Table 5.1 shows huge differences in consumption levels among the Member States. While the overall level of consumption is closely correlated to population size and to size (and type of species) of livestock production, analysis of antimicrobial consumption in terms of biomass (humans/animals) shows major differences among countries.

Examining the human medical sector, we find that the average EU/EEA use of antimicrobials per milligram/kilogram (mg/kg) of human biomass was 130 in 2017. However, this average hides a range of variations. In Germany, antimicrobial use was only 63.8 per mg/kg human biomass and in the Netherlands 52.8. In other countries, antimicrobial use reached 212.6 mg/kg in Greece and 191.1 in Spain.

Similar country differences in antimicrobial consumption are in the livestock sector. The average EU/EEA consumption of antimicrobials was 108.3 mg/kg in 2017. Iceland (4.6) and Norway (3.3) had very low levels of antimicrobial use in their livestock

Table 5.1 Consumption of antimicrobials by humans and food-producing animals in tonnes, with estimated biomass of the corresponding population in 1,000 tonnes and consumption expressed as milligrams consumed per kilogram biomass in twenty-eight EU/EEA countries in 2017.

Country	Consumption in tonnes of active substance			Estimated biomass in 1,000 tonnes			Consumption in mg/kg biomass	
	Humans	Animals	Total	Humans	Animals	Total	Humans	Animals
Austria*	41	45	85	548	954	1502	74.4	46.8
Belgium	104	221	325	709	1683	2393	146,3	131,3
Bulgaria	52	50	101	444	375	819	116,7	132,3
Croatia	33	21	54	260	296	555	122.8	71.5
Cyprus	8	45	54	53	107	161	153.1	423.1
Denmark	49	94	143	359	2398	2757	135.3	39.4
Estonia	6	6	12	82	111	193	73.2	56.7
Finland	41	10	51	344	507	851	118.8	19.3
France	762	483	1244	4175	7039	11214	181.6	68.6
Germany*	339	767	1106	5158	8609	13766	63.8	89.0
Greece	143	117	260	673	1243	1916	212.6	93.9
Hungary	51	147	199	612	771	1383	84.0	191.0
Iceland*	2	1	3	21	125	146	111.4	4.6
Ireland	44	98	143	299	2114	2413	148.8	46.6
Italy	560	1058	1618	3787	3864	7651	147.9	273.8
Latvia	11	6	17	122	176	298	88.6	33.3
Lithuania	19	12	31	178	333	511	107.3	34.8
Luxembourg	6	2	8	37	55	92	158.4	35.0
Malta	4	2	6	29	15	43	140.6	121.0
Netherlands	58	188	246	1068	3341	4408	52.8	56.3

(continued)

Table 5.1 Continued

Country	Consumption in tonnes of active substance			Estimated biomass in 1,000 tonnes			Consumption in mg/kg biomass	
	Humans	Animals	Total	Humans	Animals	Total	Humans	Animals
Norway	45	6	50	329	1861	2190	136.0	3.3
Poland	294	750	1044	2373	4539	6912	123.9	165.2
Portugal	78	135	213	644	1002	1646	133.3	134.8
Romania	207	263	470	1228	2916	4144	168.8	90.1
Slovakia	38	14	52	340	225	564	111.6	61.9
Slovenia	13	7	19	129	184	313	97.8	36.5
Spain	556	1770	2326	2908	7684	10592	191.1	230.3
Sweden	70	9	79	625	804	1429	122.1	11.8
UK	488	234	722	4115	7202	11317	118.6	32.5
EU/EEA mean (**population weighted)	4122	6558	10680	31649	60532	92181	130.0**	108.3**

Source: ECDC, 2021: 16.
* Consumption in hospitals is not included. Consumption in hospitals typically accounts for about 10 per cent of the overall human antimicrobial consumption in a country.

production, no doubt related to the fact that livestock production in those countries is non-intensive. In Iceland, sheep roaming freely in highland plateau areas is the primary form of livestock production, which entails only limited veterinary intervention. Antimicrobial use in Denmark (39.4) and the Netherlands (56.3) lies well below EU average, while Italy (273.8) and Spain (230.3) consume more than twice the EU average.

From Table 5.1, we can see that two-thirds of the overall consumption in the EU/EEA zone is linked to livestock production. In 2017, 10,680 tonnes of active substance were consumed in the EU of which 6,558 tonnes was used in connection with livestock production. The remaining 4,122 tonnes was used in the human medical sector. In this respect, livestock production is by far the main antimicrobial-consuming sector in the EU.

Comparing the different levels of consumption in the human and livestock sectors, there is a tendency towards both a north–south and an east–west axis. Countries in the northern part the EU/EEA tend to have lower levels of antimicrobial use than do countries in the south. Similarly, countries in the west tend to have lower levels of use than countries in the east. There are a number of exemptions, of course. Nevertheless, the AMR data show much the same geographic variation. A report by the European Center for Disease Prevention and Control (ECDC) concludes that 'the AMR situation in Europe displays wide variations depending on bacterial species, antimicrobial group and geographical region. For several bacterial species–antimicrobial group combinations, a north-to-south and west-to-east gradient is evident' (ECDC, 2019: 1). Overall antimicrobial consumption levels correlate highly with levels of AMR.

Seen from a governmental perspective, it is obvious that the differences in levels of consumption of antimicrobials in the EU Member States reflect very different national situations. However, the differences derive not only from factors such as type of livestock production (e.g., pigs versus chickens) but also differences in prescription practices, legislation, economy, etc., within both the human medical and livestock sectors. Dealing with these differences is one of the challenges when trying to propose common EU initiatives, as common regulation will invariably interfere with existing national practices. From a convergence/divergence perspective, the figures from the different Member States indicate that they have had quite different and divergent approaches to the use of antimicrobials in both the human and livestock sectors. The norms and legislation relating to antimicrobial use have historically been quite different across the Member States.

During the last three to four years, however, we have seen a dramatic decrease in antimicrobial consumption within livestock production across the EU. According to the ECDC (ECDC, 2021), the average use of antimicrobials in animals in EU/EEA has fallen from 151.5 mg/kg biomass in 2014 to 108.3 mg/kg in 2017. This overall decrease in antimicrobial consumption reflects huge reductions in antimicrobial use in Germany (149,3 in 2014; 89 in 2017) and France (107 in 2014; 68.6 in 2017) (ECDC et al., 2017: 31; ECDC, 2021: 16). The ECDC report notes that '[t]his change is the result of a significant decrease in AMC among food-producing animals, suggesting that the measures taken at country-level to reduce the use of antimicrobials in food-producing animals are effective' (ECDC, 2021: xix).

This development indicates that there are converging trends in EU with regard to antimicrobial use. Within livestock production, use of antimicrobials has declined dramatically in just a few years. Not all countries have contributed equally to this development, but it indicates that initiatives taken at EU level have indeed had some kind of impact at national levels. In the next section, we describe some of these initiatives.

EU initiatives to combat AMR in Europe

In this section, I will firstly present a brief overview of the EU's governmental possibilities to take initiatives regarding AMR with a point of departure in the Treaty of the Functioning of the European Union (TFEU). I then describe some of the most important EU initiatives within the last ten years to reduce antimicrobial consumption and AMR.

Governmental initiatives regarding the combat of AMR at EU level spills into a number of different EU policy fields. First and foremost, AMR as a policy field relates to 'health policy' because its primary purpose is to secure the European population against sickness. Secondly, it also relates to 'agricultural policy' because antimicrobials are widely used in livestock production (cf. the previous section on consumption of antimicrobials in EU). Thirdly, policies regarding antimicrobials spill into 'the internal market policy area', as trade with and authorization of medical products (like antibiotics) to a large extent are dealt with in accordance with internal market regulation.

The fact that combatting antimicrobials spills into these quite different policy areas implies that the EU's potential governmental instruments in the field are quite complex because these policy areas hold rather different positions in the EU cooperation framework.

Health policy is in principle a policy area offering only limited possibilities for EU institutions (such as the EU Commission) to develop policy initiatives. The TFEU (Article 168 No. 7 TFEU) explicitly states that health policy is primarily an area of national competence. EU institutions are therefore restricted in the opportunities they have to implement initiatives in relation to antimicrobials, especially if these are seen as interfering with or intervening in national health policies (Böhm and Landwehr, 2014; Greer, 2006; Lamping, 2013; see also Chapter 6).

Agricultural policy, in contrast to health policy, is more embedded in the EU and in the TFEU. The agricultural policy area affords opportunities for the EU to create regulation. Agriculture has always been high on the EU agenda. Some of the first EU-level initiatives regarding AMR were related to agriculture. In 2006, the EU enacted a regulation banning the use of antimicrobials as growth promoters in livestock production (Kahn, 2016). Traditionally, antimicrobials have been used as growth promoters (and are still used for this purpose in the United States and in many other countries).

Medicines and medical products are to a large extent subject to regulation at EU level. The EU has tried to create a common market for medicine and medical products in order to create competition between pharmaceutical companies and establish a common market the size of which would make it attractive for the pharmaceutical industry to develop new products (Lamping and Steffen, 2009). All medical products undergo a process of authorization either at national level or at EU level (Hauray, 2016).

Despite the complexity in the legal basis for EU initiatives regarding AMR, since around 2010, the EU has systematically developed a political strategy focusing on combatting AMR. First and foremost, the EU Commission has presented two action plans 'against the rising threats from antimicrobial resistance'. The first plan was presented in 2011 and the second in 2017 (European Commission, 2011, 2017). In both these action plans, the Commission—after consulting with the European Parliament and the Council of Ministers (European Commission, 2011; European Parliament, 2018)—outlined the main political initiatives that had been and will be taken in relation to AMR.

The Commission initiatives in the action plans are divided into three specific areas: (i) prevention of AMR in the human and the veterinary sector by focusing more on reducing antimicrobial consumption in EU; (ii) marketing and sales of antimicrobials within the EU; and (iii) innovation and research in new types of antimicrobials (European Commission, 2017).

The initiatives regarding reduction in the use of antimicrobials in EU contain a number of more specific policy initiatives that can be summarized under the heading 'establishing prudent use of antimicrobials'. To establish prudent use of antimicrobials implies that both the human and livestock sectors become more hesitant to use antimicrobials and use them only in situations where there is a clear need. Among the concrete initiatives that the Commission has proposed to is that of developing more surveillance and monitoring of the actual consumption of antimicrobials in the EU. Today, few EU countries have precise estimates of their consumption of antimicrobials. The Commission has called for more and better data. Another important proposal is the development of national action plans. Each Member State has been asked to develop national action plans for reducing their consumption of antimicrobials (in both the human and veterinary sectors).

Another initiative coming from the Commission is that of increasing the level of biosecurity in livestock production. Increased biosecurity means that farmers should be made more aware of the risk of bacterial transmission from the environment into livestock stables/barns. Farmers should avoid transmitting bacteria when they enter their stables by taking simple measures such as changing clothes.

Other proposals focus on introducing stewardship principles in vulnerable venues such as hospitals. Antimicrobial stewardship has been introduced in a number of hospitals in many countries over the last decade. A specific organizational structure has been established, the purpose of which is to create more transparent standards for how antimicrobials should be used under different circumstances (Charani et al., 2013; Rynkiewich, 2020). The overall objective is that a stewardship system can help reduce overall antimicrobial consumption.

Most of the initiatives presented by the Commission in the antimicrobial area are non-binding proposals, recommendations only. The lack of mandatory regulations reflects the fact that according to the TFEU, health is an area reserved national, rather than EU-level, competence. This makes it difficult for the Commission to suggest regulations or directives as legal instruments for health initiatives, although the effects might be more directly felt at Member State level. The establishment of national action plans can be seen as an example of what is called the 'open method of co-ordination', where the EU uses soft law and normative pressure to motivate Member States to take specific forms of action (Hodson and Maher, 2001; see Chapter 19 for a discussion of the World Health Organization's (WHO) use of soft law in global health governance). Member States are expected to present plans for how they will reduce their national consumption of antimicrobials, and they are asked to establish timetables for this implementation. Member States should report on their results on an annual basis.

From a governmental perspective, marketing of antimicrobial products in the EU is a key competence area of direct EU policy as it concerns the (free) movement of goods. Hence, the legal instruments used for implementing EU policies in the market area are much stronger than in the health area. Unlike the health area, internal market-related regulations and directives are primarily used in this policy area as they can be more directly implemented in Member State legislation.

Every medical product sold in EU must undergo an authorization process, either at Member State or EU level. Medical products authorized at EU level can be sold in every Member State without any national process of authorization. Authorization of medical products applies to both humans and animals, although the actual processes and systems differ. In relation to veterinary medical products, the EU has played an active role in an effort to reduce antimicrobial consumption. In 2018, the EU issued two regulations on veterinary medical products (European Union, 2018) which in certain areas limit the use of antimicrobials in livestock production. Use of 'critically important antimicrobials' in livestock production was hereby restricted. 'Critically important antimicrobials' are those used in humans when all other antimicrobials do not work (WHO, 2019).

Innovation and research in new types of antimicrobials are high on the agenda, both in the EU and at a more global level. Only a few new types of antimicrobials have been identified and created over the past twenty to thirty years, and this has contributed to the increasing problem with AMR. One explanation for the lack of development of new types of antimicrobials is that the pharmaceutical industry has become less engaged in antimicrobial research (Drlica and Perlin, 2011). To a certain extent, this lack of engagement can be explained by the lack of economic incentives for investing in research (Mossialos, 2010). Antimicrobials are generally sold quite cheaply and pharmaceutical firms find more profitable investments in other medical areas (such as diabetes). In order to increase the research and development incentives and manage AMR, the EU has taken initiatives to create creating more innovation and research in antimicrobials.

The EU effort involves creating common interests across the EU to develop new types of antimicrobials. More money is being spent on managing the AMR problem through research in the Seventh Framework Program on research. One important research area relates to developing vaccines that can decrease the need for antimicrobial treatment by preventing the outbreak of diseases. Another important area relates to the development of tests that can identify the need for antimicrobial treatment. Sometimes antimicrobials are used as a preventive measure because physicians or veterinarians are unable to identify the specific character of an infection. Tests that can identify the specific need for treatment can therefore help reduce antimicrobial use, especially use of what are known as 'broad spectrum antimicrobials'.

There is no question that over the past decade, the EU has increased its efforts to combat AMR; this has become an important EU policy area. The EU has become a driver for initiatives focusing on reducing overall consumption of antimicrobials and for stimulating research that can help develop new types of antimicrobials and new types of tests. These measures, plus the quite impressive reduction in consumption of antimicrobials in livestock production in EU (shown in Table 5.1) indicate a trend towards convergence in patterns and levels of antimicrobial consumption in Member States. This convergence entails an overall reduction in antimicrobial consumption and hence a reduction of AMR. Considering this convergence trend and in view of the logic behind this development with reference to the three aforementioned types of isomorphism (or drivers) identified by DiMaggio and Powell (1983), we can see that coercive measures have played only a minor role. Health policy, as we have mentioned, is primarily a policy area with Member State competence, which thus limits the Commission's ability to introduce more binding and far-reaching measures (Jensen, 2020). Hence, it is not any new, binding legislative initiatives coming from the EU that have compelled Member States to reduce their antimicrobial use in the livestock sector. The potential to reduce antimicrobial consumption in the EU depends to a large extent on Member States' willingness to accept EU initiatives and to their own national interests in developing national AMR policies. The mimetic and normative types of drivers seem to have been much more important than the coercive.

EU initiatives in a global perspective—the EU as a global player

'To deal with the cross-border health threat of AMR, it is crucial to identify and share best practices and politics, so that a lack of action in one region or sector does not undermine progress made in others' (European Commission, 2017: 7–8).

This quotation is from the latest action plan against AMR, presented by the EU Commission in 2017. It gives an indication of the importance that the EU Commission and the other EU institutions attach to global cooperation. The fight against AMR needs to be embedded in a global institutional context because of the cross-national character of resistant bacteria. A reduction in the amount of AMR in the EU will be effortlessly minimized if AMR increases and develops in other parts of the world. We live in a globalized world where humans, animals, and goods cross borders and regions continuously, thereby contributing to the spread of AMR.

A key element of the EU action plans on AMR, therefore, is for the EU to act as a global player in the AMR field. The EU is endeavouring to shape the entire global AMR agenda. It has thus established strategic cooperation agreements with major international organizations and AMR-relevant countries (European Commission, 2021).

The main international and global actors—besides the EU—in relation to AMR are the United Nations and the WHO, the World Organisation for Animal Health (OIE), the UN Food and Agriculture Organization (FAO), and in some cases the Organisation for Economic Co-operation and Development (OECD), the Transatlantic Taskforce on Antimicrobial Resistance (TATFAR, which includes the EU, the United States, Canada, and Norway), and the G7 and G20 states. Besides these forums, large countries such as the United States and China also have a more or less direct impact on global governance initiatives on AMR.

In 2015, WHO adopted a global action plan on AMR (WHO, 2015). The proposals coming from global actors such as WHO are in many ways similar to those presented in the EU Commission action plans. The need for further research into antimicrobial development and the need to develop national action plans to reduce antimicrobial consumption are common elements in both the WHO and EU plans. This alignment between EU initiatives and the WHO action plan indicates a close interaction between the EU institutions and global actors such as the WHO.

One specific area where the EU has tried to impact the global consumption of antimicrobials is through trade agreements between the EU and other regions (or countries) or within the World Trade Organization (WTO) framework. Trade agreements sometimes contain standards or types of regulations that would prohibit the use of specific chemicals in certain products or the use of child labour in the production process. AMR issues are being increasingly dealt with in trade agreements (George, 2019), and the EU is a strong proponent of this kind of conditionality. Such regulations in trade agreements could entail that meat produced using specific antimicrobials (e.g., the 'critical antimicrobials') be banned from importation into the EU (see Chapter 18 for a further discussion of supply chain regulation). To what extent such types of regulation should be implemented in trade agreements has been controversial, as some countries perceive these initiatives as nothing short of trade barriers.

Due to the different patterns of antimicrobial use in various regions of the world, regional differences can also be observed. In all the EU countries, antimicrobials can be obtained (with only few exceptions) only by prescription from either a medical doctor or veterinarian. In other parts of the world, antimicrobials are sometime obtained without any prescription. This is the case in India, China, and many other countries. The challenges involved in reducing the use of antimicrobials are also quite different in different regions in the world due to the differences in the factors that trigger the need to administer antimicrobials. In some countries—especially low-income countries—antimicrobials are widely used among humans in connection with infectious diseases such as diarrhoea or lung diseases (e.g., tuberculosis). The high incidence of these types of infectious diseases in low-income countries is a direct result of poverty in these countries and of global inequality (Barreto, 2017; WHO, 2020). Poor housing conditions, lack of access to clean water, and poor sanitation create favourable conditions for the spread of bacteria and infections. Use of antimicrobials becomes the immediate solution to these infections for the population; antimicrobials also help reduce child mortality and other harmful effects of the infections. However, a reduction in antimicrobial consumption would be possible and responsible only if poverty were also reduced, meaning that people need access to clean water, sanitation, etc. It indicates that the fight against AMR it not solely a question of the prudent use of antimicrobials. Antimicrobial consumption is also embedded in more general global societal structures (WHO, 2020).

Conclusion—challenges and possibilities for EU and global governance initiatives on AMR

In many ways, the EU can be viewed as a driver in the struggle to control AMR. The EU's role is important both within Europe and for the global situation as a whole. For example, in connection with the ban on use of antimicrobials as growth promoters in livestock production, the EU has for many years been at the forefront of efforts to reduce antimicrobial consumption. The last ten years have seen increased efforts to develop policies which could reduce antimicrobial consumption in both the livestock production and in the human medical sectors. The two EU action plans have focused on reducing antimicrobial consumption and on developing new types of antimicrobials. Some success has already been observed. The dramatic reduction in the use of antimicrobials in livestock production from 2014 to 2017 from 151 mg/kg to 108.3 mg/kg is a clear indication that governmental initiatives taken at both EU and Member State level are working (ECDC, 2021). Antimicrobial consumption in livestock production is converging among EU countries at a lower level. At a global level, the EU has proposed that trade agreements should include binding standards on antimicrobial use applied to agricultural products sold on the global market or in the EU. This should prevent farmers in countries with low levels of regulation from using antimicrobials as growth promoters.

Nevertheless, a major challenge to the development of a common EU AMR policy is that health policy is primarily an area of national competence. National control over health policy means that most initiatives coming from EU remain only at the level of recommendations to Member States. Learning from best practices of other Member States is the key element in many of these initiatives. The challenge posed by this kind of health initiative is that an individual Member State might be reluctant to make changes if there is opposition by national stakeholders. In such situations, the EU's ability to intervene or impose policy is greatly restricted. The EU is at the mercy of national-level factors.

The EU has sought to contribute not only to Europe-wide but also to the global campaign against AMR. Hence, the EU has established close cooperation with other international organizations such as the WHO in order to support and contribute to the development of AMR policies.

It is unclear whether we will see lower levels of antimicrobial consumption at a global level in the coming years. Increasing wealth in formerly poor parts of the world has led to increased demand for livestock products, a demand that often leads to increased use of antimicrobials in the agricultural sector (Van Boeckel et al., 2015). Global governmental initiatives can counteract this trend. These global initiatives are not likely to be based on coercion. We have no 'global government' than can enforce binding forms of legislation or similar compulsory measures. Initiatives must be expected to be of what DiMaggio and Powell call 'mimetic' or 'normative' character. Nation states in different regions of the world will try to reduce their antimicrobial consumption not because of coercion but because global norms indicate this to be the most appropriate way to behave and because they have a national interest in reducing local presence of AMR. This normative 'push' could be seen as a weak form of global governance. Nevertheless, this strategy can be successful, as we have seen in connection with the EU initiatives in the agricultural sector.

References

Barreto, M. L. (2017). 'Health Inequalities: A Global Perspective', *Ciência & Saúde Coletiva*, 22/7, 2097–108.

Böhm, K., and Landwehr, C. (2014). 'The Europeanization of Health Care Coverage Decisions: EU-Regulation, Policy Learning and Cooperation in Decision-Making', *Journal of European Integration*, 36/1, 17–35.

Charani, E., Castro-Sanchez, E., Sevdalis, N., Kyratsis, L., Drumright, N. Shah, and Holmes, A. (2013). 'Understanding the Determinants of Antimicrobial Prescribing Within Hospitals: The Role of "Prescribing Etiquette"', *Clinical Infectious Diseases*, 57/2, 188–96.

DiMaggio, P. J., and Powell, W. W. (1983). The Iron Cage Revisited: Institutional Isomorphism and Collective Rationality in Organizational Fields', *American Sociological Review*, 48/2, 147–60.

Drlica, K., and Perlin, D. (2011). *Antibiotic Resistance: Understanding and Responding to an Emerging Crisis* (Upper Saddle River, NJ: FT Press).

ECDC. (2019). *Surveillance of Antimicrobial Resistance in Europe 2018* (Stockholm: ECDC).

ECDC, European Food Safety Authority (EFSA), and European Medicines Agency (EMA). (2021). 'Third Joint Inter-Agency Report on Integrated Analysis of Consumption of Antimicrobial Agents and Occurrence of Antimicrobial Resistance in Bacteria from Humans and Food-producing Animals in the EU/EEA: JIACRA III 2016-2018', *EFSA Journal*, 19/6, 1–166.

ECDC/EFSA/EMA. (2017). *ECDC/EFSA/EMA Second Joint Report on the Integrated Analysis of the Consumption of Antimicrobial Agents and Occurrence of Antimicrobial Resistance in Bacteria from Humans and Food-Producing Animals* (Parma: European Food Safety Authority).

European Commission. (2011). *Communication from the Commission to the European Parliament and the Council—Action Plan Against the Rising Threats from Antimicrobial Resistance*. European Commission, Com (2011), 748.

European Commission. (2017). *A European One Health Action Plan against Antimicrobial Resistance (AMR)* (Brussels: European Commission).

European Commission. (2021). *Progress Report 2017 EU AMR Action Plan* (Brussels: European Commission).

European Parliament. (2018). *Report on a European One Health Action Plan against Antimicrobial Resistance (AMR) (2017/2254(INI))* (Brussels: European Commission).

European Union. (2018). Regulation (EU) 2019/6 of the European Parliament and of the Council of 11 December 2018 on veterinary medicinal products and repealing Directive 2001/82/EC.

George, A. (2019). 'Antimicrobial Resistance (AMR) in the Food Chain: Trade, One Health and Codex', *Tropical Medicine and Infectious Disease*, 4/1, 54. doi:10.3390/tropicalmed4010054. PMID: 30917589; PMCID: PMC6473514.

Greer, S. L. (2006). 'Uninvited Europeanization: Neofunctionalism and the EU in Health Policy', *Journal of European Public Policy*, 13/1, 134–52.

Hauray, B. (2016). 'The European Regulation of Medicines', in S. L. Greer and P. Kurzer, eds, *European Union Public Health Policy: Regional and Global Trends* (London: Routledge), 81–94.

Hodson, D. and Maher, I. (2001). 'The Open Method as a New Mode of Governance: The Case of Soft Economic Policy Co-ordination', *Journal of Common Market Studies*, 39(4): 719–46.

Jensen, C. S. (2020). 'While We Are Waiting for the Superbug: Constitutional Asymmetry and EU Governmental Policies to Combat Antimicrobial Resistance', *Journal of Common Market Studies*, 58/6, 1361–76.

Jensen, C. S., Nielsen, S. B., and Fynbo, L. (2019). 'Risking Antimicrobial Resistance: A One Health Study of Antibiotic Use and Its Societal Aspects', in C. S. Jensen, S. B. Nielsen, and L. Fynbo, eds, *Risking Antimicrobial Resistance: A Collection of One-Health Studies of Antibiotics and Its Social and Health Consequences* (Cham, Switzerland: Palgrave Macmillan), 127–42.

Kahn, L. H. (2016). *One Health and the Politics of Antimicrobial Resistance* (Baltimore, MD: Johns Hopkins University Press).

Lamping, W. (2013). 'European Union Health Care Policy', in S. L. Greer and P. Kurzer, eds, *European Union Public Health Policy: Regional and Global Trends* (London: Routledge), 19–35.

Lamping, W., and Steffen, M. (2009). 'European Union and Health Policy: The "Chaordic" Dynamics of Integration', *Social Science Quarterly*, 90/5, 1361–79.

Mossialos, E. (2010). *Policies and Incentives for Promoting Innovation in Antibiotic Research*. European Observatory on Health Systems and Policies.

Rynkiewich, K. (2020). 'Finding "What's Wrong with Us": Antibiotic Prescribing Practice Among Physicians in the United States', *Frontiers in Sociology*, 5/5.

Scott, W. R. (1995). *Institutions and Organizations* (London: Sage).

Van Boeckel, T. P., Brower, C., Gilbert, M., Grenfell, B. T., Levin, S. A., Robinson, T. P., Teillant, A., and Laxminarayan, R. (2015). 'Global Trends in Antimicrobial Use in Food Animals', *Proceedings of the National Academy of Sciences*, 112/18, 5649–54.

WHO. (2015). *Global Action Plan on Antimicrobial Resistance* (Geneva: WHO).

WHO. (2019). *Critically Important Antimicrobials for Human Medicine—6th Revision 2018*. (Geneva: WHO).

WHO. (2020). *World Health Statistic: Monitoring Health for the SDGs, Sustainable Development Goals* (Geneva: WHO).

World Organisation for Animal Health (OIE). (2016). *The OIE Strategy on Antimicrobial Resistance and the Prudent Use of Antimicrobials* (Paris: OIE).

6

Contested Governance of Collective Action against AMR in the EU

Daniel Carelli, Jon Pierre, and Björn Rönnerstrand

Introduction

This chapter reports an ongoing study on the coordination of the efforts to contain and reduce antimicrobial resistance within and among the European Union (EU) Member States. There are (at least) three models of governance in the antimicrobial resistance (AMR) field in the EU: networks of national senior public servants (human health sector); a strong EU mandate (veterinarian sector); and the higher profile of EU control in the human health sector as outlined in the 'EU4Health' programme, at the time of writing under public consultation. In addition, there are numerous other actors and institutions such as the World Health Organization (WHO); networks aimed to disseminating knowledge on AMR across the EU; research networks; professional associations; administrative networks; and so on. In 2022, AMR governance in Europe is at a formative moment and it is extremely difficult to assess the long-term outcomes of the institutional transformation currently underway.

The global governance of AMR is a struggle. AMR is often seen as a quintessential global collective action problem (Hoffman et al., 2015; Jørgensen et al., 2016; Laxminarayan et al., 2013; Sandler et al., 2015). A key aspect of AMR is its cross-border nature; through trade and travel multi-resistant bacteria move swiftly from one country or continent to another. This means, first, that despite the collective and long-term threat of antibiotic resistance, individual states may avoid investment in policy that limits the resistance problem within its borders. Unless all countries commit to, and deliver, a concerted effort to reduce the use and accessibility of antibiotics, measures taken by any individual country will be futile (see Chapters 14 and 19).

Secondly, international exchanges will expose countries to AMR and exacerbate the antibiotic resistance problem, regardless of their domestic performance. Therefore, countries have significant stakes in the performance of other countries. Collaboration facilitates learning and support to countries lagging in their AMR work. Thus, a successful AMR strategy needs to build on some form of cross-national collaboration.

For most economists, the theory is that utility-maximizing actors have no incentives to devote resources to common or public goods. Social scientists, for their part, tend to view the problem as more related to risks of defection and free-riding. Our

Daniel Carelli, Jon Pierre, and Björn Rönnerstrand, *Contested Governance of Collective Action against AMR in the EU* In: *Steering against Superbugs*. Edited by: Olivier Rubin, Erik Baekkeskov, and Louise Munkholm, Oxford University Press. © Oxford University Press 2023.
DOI: 10.1093/oso/9780192899477.003.0006

understanding of the collective action problem is less deductive or driven by expected outcomes. Instead, our main interest is to understand the extent to which collaboration among the EU Member States is prevented by diversity in terms of the AMR challenge, or by different administrative systems and traditions, or by national and regional cultural values and behaviours which obstruct political and administrative action to curb the use of antibiotics.

All these approaches to collective action acknowledge that in order to be effective, AMR must be addressed as a global problem. If, as we argue, collaboration is a requirement for a successful struggle to reduce AMR in the EU, the configuration and leadership of that collaboration is a contested issue at the mass level, the national administrative level, and at the international and institutional level. The chapter first reviews these patterns before we turn to the EU's 'EU4Health' programme to see how it is likely to alter the governance arrangements in the EU. In 2022 we are at a formative moment of EU AMR governance and our concluding discussion will by necessity be tentative and speculative.

Who should lead the work against AMR in Europe?

When citizens in the EU twenty-seven Member States, Norway, and the United Kingdom were asked about the most effective level to tackle AMR, they tended to favour the national level, the global level, and the individual/family, but not the EU. Public health experts agree. When public servants in the EU27, Norway, and the United Kingdom were asked the exact same question, they too favoured the global level and the national level over the EU. Interestingly, even public servants working with AMR in the animal sector where the EU already exercises considerable authority (see Chapter 5) think that a global solution is the most effective level to tackle resistance (see Figure 6.1).

However, while AMR experts favour a global solution in terms of how best to tackle resistance to antibiotics, they seem to make a virtue out of necessity. Figure 6.2 compares experts' views on the extent to which the EU, the World Health Organization (WHO), networks or civil servants or experts, or a group of national politicians are best suited to take a leading role in European coordination of the AMR field. The survey responses, which were made on scale was from 1 (Not well suited) to 7 (Very well suited), show that 85 per cent of the experts think that the EU is well suited to play a leading role in AMR coordination in Europe (response alternatives 5 to 7). The group of experts negative towards EU leaderships over AMR is very small; only about 5 per cent selected the response alternative 1 to 3 on the seven-point scale.

Most of the experts are also in favour of network solutions to AMR leadership. About two-thirds—67 and 68 per cent, respectively—believe that a network of civil servants or a network of experts are well suited to take the lead. Almost one in four (23 per cent) think a network of experts are very well suited to lead AMR coordination in Europe (response alternative 7). By contrast, only 55 per cent believe that the WHO is a suitable

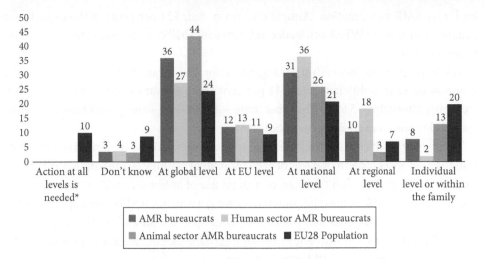

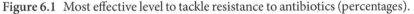

Figure 6.1 Most effective level to tackle resistance to antibiotics (percentages).

Comment: Question wording: "At what level do you believe it is most effective to tackle the resistance to antibiotics?". Response alternative as in figure. Responses from EU28 population comes from the Special Eurobarometer 478, in field between the 8th and 26th September 2018. The number of responses: 27 747. Responses from AMR public servants in EU27, the UK and Norway come from the European AMR expert survey in field between 8ths of October 2020 and February 22nd 2021. The number of responses: 117 (human sector 55, animal sector 62.) *Respondents of the two surveys were presented with the same response alternatives, except for that respondent of the Special Eurobarometer survey could spontaneously say that action at all levels is needed.

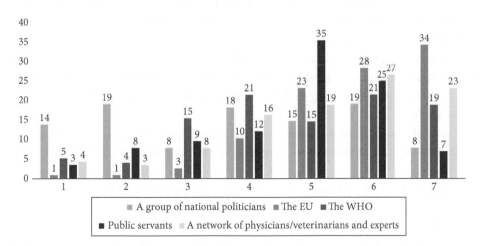

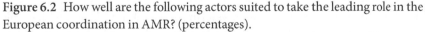

Figure 6.2 How well are the following actors suited to take the leading role in the European coordination in AMR? (percentages).

Comment: Question wording: "How well are the following actors suited to take the leading role in the European coordination in AMR?". Response scale: 1 (Not well suited) to 7 (Very well suited). Responses from the European AMR expert survey in field between 8ths of October 2020 and February 22nd 2021. The number of responses: 117

leader in AMR coordination. Almost one out of four (24 per cent) of the experts are negative towards the WHO as a leader in European AMR coordination (response alternatives 1 to 3).

The least popular leadership arrangement for European AMR coordination is a group of national politicians. Only 41 per cent are in favour of such AMR leadership (response alternatives 5 to 7). The same share—41 per cent—are against national politicians as leaders (response alternatives 1 to 3).

The survey results mirror the collective action dynamic of AMR. Since the contribution to the global problem of AMR of each individual country is limited, they often lack sufficient incentives to limit human or animal use of antibiotics within their borders. This feature of AMR shapes the preferences for governance and leadership; instead of a leadership involving national politicians, who may defend and prioritize the interests of their domestic constituency over an international collaboration, experts want a 'third party' to step in as AMR leader in Europe.

The results also point to an interesting mismatch between the perceived ideal solution to the AMR problem on the one hand, and the political and institutional realities of transboundary health governance on the other. One possible explanation is that AMR experts acknowledge that international cooperation will not grow out of toothless institutions. Like most other issues in politics and administration, collective action will not 'just happen' (see Goldfinch and t'Hart, 2003) unless there is leadership and drivers.

The survey responses from citizens and AMR experts neatly illustrates the dilemma of global collective action problems. Both European citizens and AMR experts across the continent seem to agree that the most effective level to tackle AMR would be at the global level, and yet, when experts are asked about which actors they believe are suitable to lead European coordination in AMR, they tend to favour the EU over the WHO. Thus, although AMR is a truly global problem, experts prefer a regional leader over a global leader.

One likely cause of the discrepancy between the 'ideal' level to tackle AMR and the most suited system of governance is related to institutional strength and capacity for enforcement of binding agreements. A basic assumption in rational choice approaches to collective action is that cooperation for the common good will not happen without institutions with the capacity change the incentive structure in favour of collective action (Olsen, 1965).

In contradiction to the WHO, the EU has the authority to issue binding agreements in the AMR domain, at least in the case of veterinary use of antibiotics, which falls under the Common Agricultural Politics, but in theory this could be expanded to human use of antibiotics. Meanwhile, WHO governance arrangements on AMR are all based on 'soft law' steering (see Chapter 19). For example, the Global Action Plan and the corresponding national action plans (NAPs) are based on voluntary compliance (Baekkeskov et al., 2020).

A second factor that may explain the tendency of experts to favour the EU over the WHO as a leader in AMR has to do with the nature of the AMR problem. Some large-scale challenges have direct global consequences. For example, regardless of where it is emitted, greenhouse gas emissions immediately contribute to climate change as a global problem. However, for some global problems, the spill-over consequence can be constrained (Buchholz and Sandler, 2021). Limiting antibiotic use in Europe makes a larger regional difference for AMR in Europe, as compared to other continents. Thus, in contrast to, for example, climate change mitigation, action to limit AMR in Europe can provide an excludable regional benefit to individual states in Europe, at least temporarily. Via the logic of subsidiarity, it is likely that this temporal 'quasi-regional' aspect of AMR contributes to support for EU as a leader of coordination over AMR.

A regional European solution instead of a global institutional panacea is also consistent with the polycentric approach to the governance of global collective action problems, as suggested by Elinor Ostrom (Ostrom, 2010). A system of collaboration between multiple regional authorities—a polycentric system of AMR governance—can benefit from the strengths of 'bottom-up' approaches, such as local knowledge, adjustments to heterogeneity of actors, and allowing for experimentation and policy learning across different nodes in the polycentric system (cf. Rubin, 2019).

Thus, the overall picture coming out of the surveys is that citizens and experts see a need for institutional authority and regulatory capacity to address the AMR problem successfully. Equally important, there is a perception of a need for less formal governance arrangements to engage experts and the broader public in the AMR work. In the EU context, notions about networks operating in 'the shadow of hierarchy' have been employed to integrate formal authority with informal governance models (Héritier and Lehmkuhl, 2008; Héritier and Rhodes, 2011).

The rise of the European Health Union

Health policy in the EU Treaty is defined as 'national competence'. Thus, the EU's role in the human health sector was quite limited when the coronavirus hit Europe. Only a small fraction of the huge health policy domain, like the obligation to harmonize national laws on pharmaceuticals and medical devices, was enforced through EU treaties. In crisis preparedness, procurement, and hospital surveillance, to name only some of the bigger domains, the role of the EU has been to support Member States' domestic policies and to encourage European coordination (Brooks and Geyer, 2020).

The COVID-19 pandemic uncovered significant variation in the health crisis preparedness among the EU Member States. In a move reminiscent of Churchill's famous quote of 'never letting a good crisis go to waste', the EU Commission saw the COVID pandemic and the problems in forming a coherent response among the Member States as a window of opportunity to assume a higher profile in the human health sector (Schmidt, 2020). As Brooks and Greyer (2020; see also Schmidt, 2020) argue, the COVID-19 pandemic and the very limited preparedness among the EU Member States that it uncovered helped break the 'national competence' path dependency in the public health arena.

The initial responses to the pandemic played out very differently across the Member States. However, the pandemic response gradually succeeded in increasing coordination among Member States, first by the consensus on the imperative to 'flatten the curve' (Alemanno, 2020), and later by the joint advancement of procuring vaccines. The Commission has increasingly become more dominant in pandemic response management, a development which has evoked a consensus among scholars that the EU is now moving towards a 'Health Union' (Beaussier and Cabane, 2020; Brooks and Geyer, 2020; Schmidt, 2020). As Schmidt (2020) puts it, 'in light of the Commission's proposed new health agency, EU4Health [HERA], we may very well see paradigmatic change and deepening integration made possible by the deal between the Council and the European Parliament (EP) on the budget in November 2020'.

Such a scenario would be path dependent with several historical examples of health-related crises over the last two decades leading to a further expansion of the Commission's authority on human healthcare (Brooks and Geyer, 2020; Greer, 2006). As a senior public servant in the European Commission's DG Santé put it in an interview (18 November 2021) with the present authors, 'we have made "progress by catastrophe" so that with each major problem there was progress'. Thus, the creation of the European Centre for Disease Prevention and Control (ECDC), just as routines for joint procurement of vaccines were the direct outcome of the SARS outbreak in 2003 and the Swine flu epidemic in 2009.

There are also examples of how the EU has acquired increasing authority in other policy fields. In macroeconomic policy, where the EU always has had extensive authority over the Member States, the deep economic crises after the 2007–2008 global financial crisis led—or justified—the Commission to assume a bigger role in economic governance to implement extensive policy learning on existentialist threats and to foster an environment of policy entrepreneurs well trained to create policy in an abrupt fashion (Bauer and Becker, 2014; Ladi and Tsarouhas, 2020). Thus, the EU has for some time pursued a general plan to expand its authority across the board over the Member States. In the public health sector the COVID pandemic was the cue to apply that strategy.

Thus, in 2021, the Commission proposed the 'EU4Health' programme (Samarasekera, 2021). In a similar vein, the 'Europe's Plan to Beat Cancer', also launched in 2021, accords the EU a high profile in the public health sector. An extensive debate ensued concerning the role and function of such investments in Member States' healthcare infrastructure. The commission, one argument goes, should increase its authority in the area of surveillance by obligating Member States to compile and share data on health infrastructure to develop the joint procurement programmes (McEvoy and Ferri, 2020), to beef up and increase the capacity of the ECDC, and to assess the cooperative arrangements with the WHO (Clemens and Brand, 2020).

Indeed, a reinforced ECDC and better coordinated national policies would, according to Beaussier and Cabane (2020: 820), 'preserve Member States' decision-making powers while making coordination more binding and the substance of it more detailed'. Interestingly, the ECDC is currently 'a weak agency in a position to make great claims … almost one hundred times smaller than the US CDC, but if it becomes the hub of Europe's communicable disease capacity, it might in the long term speak with comparable authority' (Greer, 2012: 1025).

A similar approach to increasing the coordination among the Member States is summarized by Christopher Bickerton and associates (Bickerton et al., 2015) by the concept of 'the new intergovernmentalism'. They argue that 'EU policy-makers remain willing to pursue collective solutions to shared policy problems but they have become more reluctant to delegate new powers to supranational institutions along traditional lines' (Bickerton et al., 2015: 3). Also, coordination within the existing legal EU framework can be strengthened by using soft policy instruments such as EU guidance (Pacces and Weimar, 2020).

The 'EU4Health' programme, it must be noted, will be rolled out within the boundaries of EU control in the human healthcare sector as defined in the Treaty. A senior DG Santé public servant (interview, 18 November 2021) describes the programme's design thus:

> The 'health union' package stretches the possibilities in the Treaty to the limit, if you wish. Also, proposing the HERA [Health Emergency Preparedness and Response Agency] agency is qualitatively a step forward, but all this is done within existing Treaty provisions so it does not require any new Treaty provisions. In that sense, the Commission does not claim any new prerogatives but you could say that the prerogatives in the Treaty are fully used. That has not been the case earlier. Previously there was a lack of resources to do that.

A fundamental aspect of the 'EU4Health' programme is that it rests on voluntary participation of the Member States. For instance, the programme invites countries to join groups to facilitate 'best practice' learning and the dissemination of successful practices. Such participation would make the member states eligible for considerable financial support from the programme. The same combination of voluntary participation and significant financial compensation can also be found in other areas of the programme. Again, joining the programme's agenda is voluntary although several EU Member States may find the financial incentives too big to resist. In some ways, the programme design squares the circle of 'national competence' in the public health sector; as the senior DG Santé official put it, 'the system works without the EU having a legal basis to impose anything on the member states because it is all voluntary'.

Thus, when the president of the European Commission, Ursula von der Leyen, told the G7 Summit in Rome in October 2021 that 'HERA will take cooperation to a new level', she envisaged a significantly more active role and higher profile of the Union in European public health albeit embedded in the framework of the existing EU Treaty. HERA, the new EU agency charged with detecting major health threats and coordinating Member States' responses to pandemics and other health crises is one manifestation of this bigger role for the EU in this sector. Arguably, strengthening the role of EU institutions is facilitated not just as 'progress through catastrophes' but also by the UK's departure from the EU, as Britain was one of the strongest critics of encroachments on national sovereignty.

However, increased EU authority on health policy could work against the principle of subsidiarity, which is at the heart of EU politics (De Ruijter, 2019; Renda and Castro, 2020). Shifting power to the supranational level can also provide fertile ground for mass populist protests against centralization at the cost of national sovereignty (see e.g., Mudde, 2007). Here, however, we note that a survey experiment among 4,000 Dutch citizens conducted before the pandemic on the issue of more EU authority on stock-piling of medicines, pharmaceutical procurement, and policies to combat infectious diseases found strong support (De Ruijter et al., 2020). Thus, public health politics might not be as politically controversial as, for instance, more distributive policy areas.

Under the current EU leadership, however, cooperation will only be reached by strengthening the role and authority of the EU's institutions. The subtext to Ursula Von der Leyen's statement is that coordination is contingent on a growing role and increasing leverage of EU over the Member States without altering the treaties between the EU and its member states. Indeed, scholars have criticized the EU and many academic observers for interpreting the EU's legal space in the public health area as too narrow. Commenting on the management of the COVID-19 pandemic, Purnhagen et al. (2020: 306) maintain that 'the Union has powers that permit more actions than it has taken to date. Union competencies, properly understood, support many of the actions the Commission has proposed and executed, *and* more' (italics in original).

The question remains exactly how the new health union will be organized, and for the sake of this chapter, how it will affect the work against AMR. Commenting specifically on the linkages between the work against AMR and the 'EU4Health' programme, the DG Santé senior public servant pointed out that 'this is clearly a step forward in the EU policy domain concerning AMR. In 2018, the EU established a One Health program in order to link the environmental, animal, and human health.'

A key element of the 'EU4Health' programme is the creation of the agency HERA. HERA is evidently an emulation of the Biomedical Advanced Research and Development Authority (BARDA) in the United States, responsible for intervening during pandemics, for building reserves of medicines and medical devices, for funding research and development, and for coordinating various health-involved infrastructures (Anderson et al., 2021; see Chapter 11 for a broader discussion of US initiatives on AMR). HERA will become the hub of all current EU Member State health agencies, as illustrated in the image below. In a recent *Lancet* review, Anderson et al. (2021: 2) point out that

[b]eyond pandemics, the impeding threats of climate change, and antimicrobial resistance will also guide thinking over the next decades. Increasingly, these issues are acknowledged as interlinked, with environmental disruption driving zoonotic events that have the potential to cause pandemics, and climate change impacting the proliferation and dissemination of antimicrobial resistance. To fully understand future and impeding threats to health, HERA will be required to take a One Health approach, and

foster closer collaboration across human, animal, and environmental health disciplines and international organisations.

This is clearly a step forward in the EU policy domain concerning AMR. The EU's One Health programme (OHEJP), adopted in 2018 to improve targeting the environmental, animal, and human health aspects of the issue, has been described as 'an exemplary One Health initiative' (Brown et al., 2020), and the 'EU4Health' with HERA as the key agency is clearly continuing along this successful path.

We mentioned previously the WHO as a potentially important centre of governance in the AMR field but also an organization with limited financial resources and no coercive mandate. The WHO has spent decades building partnerships and networks in the EU and beyond and there is a long history of coordination between the WHO and the EU. 'EU4Health', however, is to some extent seen by WHO staff as a paradigmatic change in the EU's role in the public health sector, partly because of the vast financial resources it brings, partly because of the new regulatory style that the EU play, and partly because of the expanded geographical reach of the EU's programme. Voicing personal opinions rather than official WHO standpoints, a senior WHO official in a European WHO office is moderately concerned that the EU's limited experience in the public health area might be a problem when the 'EU4Health' programme is rolled out:

> So far it is good news that there is now a substantial increase in funding for AMR-related research and activities. That said, I think that the EU4Health program means that the EU expands both geographically and also in terms of technical areas, and a lot of that is something which the ECDC is expected to take on ... They [the EU] have a long history of dealing with agriculture and trade and it is easier to put legislation around that. It is not the same situation in health and it would be catastrophic if they were to suggest something like that without consulting us. (Interview 15 October 2021)

An important issue moving forward with the programme will be how best to align the substantive knowledge and networks built by the WHO over decades with the EU's agenda to support public health programmes in the Member States. The senior WHO official again:

> I hope to see us as a strong partner and that is also what they [the EU] are saying ... I hope they acknowledge that we have both the connections and the experience and with the right resources we can actually do a lot of things, and of course we can share the credit as we do now with co-funded projects with very little involvement from the Commission. If they are OK with that I think it is OK with us. (Interview 15 October 2021)

Here is a fascinating governance and coordination problem. The EU and the WHO should have significant synergies in the public health area in Europe and beyond. Although—or perhaps because—these are two very different types of organizations in almost all important aspects, current public health issues require a variety of measures that neither organization can provide alone. However, as there is some contestation, both at the mass and elite level, in Europe as to which organization is best positioned and resourced to lead, those synergies may be hard to exploit in the short term. Also, the history of cooperation between the two organizations appears to be characterized by both positive and negative experiences. Recently, the WHO official told us, there has been an 'equilibrium' with an efficient division of labour and responsibilities and little duplication. The big question for the future is to what extent that 'equilibrium' can sustain the implementation of the 'EU4Health' programme.

Concluding discussion

This chapter provides a brief overview of the governance and coordination of AMR work in Europe. The EU's growing role in the public health area, built not least on massive funding, is quite likely to be a game changer in European AMR governance. Launched in the wake of the COVID-19 pandemic, the 'EU4Health' programme justifies this move by reference to the apparent lack of coordination and cross-border collaboration, particularly in the early phases of the pandemic. 'EU4Health' replaces firm reliance on Member States to deliver public health services domestically and to be active partners in voluntary collaborative efforts in the public health field with a more distinct model of governance combining top-down directives with bottom-up processes to disperse knowledge and facilitate learning.

It is difficult to assess *ex ante* exactly how the programme will alter governance of public health in general and AMR in particular. While the programme does not accord the EU any more formal authority than it had before the pandemic, it does offer the Union substantive leverage in terms of powerful financial incentives to Member States to join various specific projects.

There are different opinions about the extent to which the 'EU4Health' programme is appropriately designed to address the diversity among the Member States in terms of their public health performance. It is no secret that such diversity exists, and our research suggests that Member State experts' views on national competence versus EU control corresponds to some extent with domestic AMR conditions. A somewhat broad-brushed account of expert opinion on the governance of the work to address AMR is that in countries where the work to reduce AMR is going relatively well—the Scandinavian countries and the Netherlands for instance—there is a distinct preference for governance arrangements drawing on expert autonomy. Experts in these countries sometimes voice criticism towards the political leadership, less for not providing the resources but more for a lack of strong and sustained commitment to the AMR problem.

AMR experts in countries that are struggling with AMR, mainly countries in Eastern and Southern Europe, by contrast, take a more positive view on a stronger EU mandate. They see the leverage of international institutions like the EU and the WHO as critical to drive the domestic political leadership to engage the AMR problem to produce and update NAPs, to provide the resources requested by the public health experts, and to show leadership and commitment. A top AMR official in a southern European country in an interview saw a key role for the political leadership: 'What we need from the Ministry is that they give greater relevance to the topic' (interview 13 October 2021).

Internationally, the EU, partly through the ECDC, will engage in data collection and capacity building, areas where the WHO has spent the last couple of decades developing networks and data reporting systems. Moreover, as the 'EU4Health' programme appears to cover not just the EU Member States but also EEA countries and some countries in the Caucasus, the ECDC's geographical jurisdiction will expand. Some initial friction between the EU and the WHO should probably be expected.

Domestically in the Member States, the EU's institutional expansion in the public health sector may support the lagging countries in modernizing their public health infrastructure and assist their AMR work. At the same time, the leading countries may find the stronger role of the EU frustrating as they have for a long time been able to set and implement their own objectives.

References

Alemanno, A. (2020). 'The European Response to Covid-19: From Regulatory Emulation to Regulatory Coordination?', *European Journal of Risk Regulation*, 11/2, 307–16.

Anderson, M., Forman, R., and Mossialos, E. (2021). 'Navigating the Role of the EU Health Emergency Preparedness and Response Authority (HERA) in Europe and Beyond', *The Lancet Regional Health*, 9/100203, 1 4.

Bauer, M., and Becker, S. (2014). 'The Unexpected Winner of the Crisis: The European Commission's Strengthened Role in Economic Governance', *Journal of European Integration*, 36/3, 213–29. doi:10.1080/07036337.2014.885750.

Beaussier, A., and Cabane, L. (2020). 'Strengthening the EU's Response Capacity to Health Emergencies: Insights from EU Crisis Management Mechanisms', *European Journal of Risk Regulation*, 1–13.

Baekkeskov, E., Rubin, O., Munkholm, L., and Zaman, W. (2020). 'Antimicrobial Resistance as a Global Health Crisis', in in *Oxford Research Encyclopedia of Politics* (Oxford: Oxford University Press).

Bickerton, C. J., Hodson, D., and Puetter, U., eds. (2015). *The New Intergovernmentalism: States and Supranational Actors in the Post-Maastricht Era* (Oxford: Oxford University Press).

Brown, H. L., Passey, J. L., Getino, M., Pursley, I., Basu, P., Horton, D. L., and La Ragione, R. M. (2020). 'The One Health European Joint Programme (OHEJP), 2018–2022: An Exemplary One Health Initiative', *Journal of Medical Microbiology*, 69/8, 1037–39.

Brooks, E., and Geyer, R. (2020). 'The Development of EU Health Policy and the Covid-19 Pandemic: Trends and Implications', *Journal of European Integration*, 42/8, 1057–76.

Buchholz, W., and Sandler, T. (2021). 'Global Public Goods: A Survey', *Journal of Economic Literature*, 59/2, 488–545.

Clemens, T., and Brand, H. (2020). 'Will Covid-19 Lead to a Major Change of the EU Public Health Mandate? A Renewed Approach to EU's Role is Needed', *European Journal of Public Health*, 30/4, 624–5.

De Ruijter, A. (2019). *EU Health Law & Policy: The Expansion of EU Power in Public Health and Healthcare* (Oxford: Oxford University Press).

De Ruijter, A., Beetsma, R., Burgoon, B., Nicoli, F., and Vandenbroucke, F. (2020). 'EU Solidarity and Policy in Fighting Infectious Diseases: State of Play, Obstacles, Citizen Preferences and Ways Forward'. *Research Paper No. 2020/06*, Amsterdam Centre for European Studies.

Goldfinch, S., and t' Hart, P. (2003). 'Leadership and Institutional Reform: Engineering Macroeconomic Policy Change in Australia', *Governance*, 16/2, 235–70.

Greer, S. L. (2006). 'Uninvited Europeanisation: Neofunctionalism and the EU in Health Policy', *Journal of European Public Policy* 13/1, 134–52.

Greer, S. L. (2012). 'The European Centre for Disease Prevention and Control: Hub or Hollow Core?', *Journal of Health Politics, Policy and Law*, 37(6), 1001–1030.

Héritier, A., and Lehmkuhl, D. (2008). 'The Shadow of Hierarchy and New Modes of Governance', *Journal of Public Policy*, 28/1, 1–17.

Héritier, A., and Rhodes, M., eds. (2011). *New Modes of Governance in Europe: Governing in the Shadow of Hierarchy* (Basingstoke: Palgrave).

Hoffman, S. J., Caleo, G. M., Daulaire, N., Elbe, S., Matsoso, P., Mossialos, E., et al. (2015). 'Strategies for achieving global collective action on antimicrobial resistance', *Bulletin of the World Health Organization*, 93, 867–76.

Helmke, G., and Levitsky, S. (2004). 'Informal Institutions and Comparative Politics: A Research Agenda', *Perspectives on Politics*, 2/4, 725–40.

Jagers, S. C., Harring, N., Löfgren, Å., Sjöstedt, M., Alpizar, F., Brülde, B., et al. (2019). 'On the Preconditions for Large-scale Collective Action', *Ambio*, 49/7, 1282–96.

Jørgensen, P. S., Wernli, D., Carroll, S. P., Dunn, R. R., Harbarth, S., Levin, S. A., et al. (2016). 'Use Antimicrobials Wisely', *Nature*, 537/7619, 159.

Ladi, S., and Tsarouhas, D. (2020). 'EU Economic Governance and Covid-19: Policy Learning and Windows of Opportunity', *Journal of European Integration*, 42(8), 1041–56.

Laxminarayan, R., Duse, A., Wattal, C., Zaidi, A. K. M., Wertheim, H. F. L., Sumpradit, N., et al. (2013). 'Antibiotic Resistance—The Need for Global Solutions', *The Lancet Infectious Diseases*, 13/12, 1057–98.

March, J. G. and Olsen, J. P. (1989). *Rediscovering Institutions: The Organizational Dimension of Politics* (New York, NY: Free Press).

McEvoy, E., and Ferri, D. (2020). 'The Role of the Joint Procurement Agreement during the Covid-19 Pandemic: Assessing Its Usefulness and Discussing Its Potential to Support a European Health Union', *European Journal of Risk Regulation*, 11/4, 851–63.

Mudde, C. (2007). *Populist Radical Right Parties in Europe* (Cambridge: Cambridge University Press).

North, D. (1990). *Institutions, Institutional Change and Economic Performance* (Cambridge: Cambridge University Press).

Olson, M. (1971). *The Logic of Collective Action: Public Goods and the Theory of Groups* (Cambridge, MA: Harvard University Press).

Ostrom, E. (1990). *Governing the Commons: The Evolution of Institutions for Collective Action* (Cambridge: Cambridge University Press).

Ostrom, E. (2010). 'Polycentric Systems for Coping with Collective Action and Global Environmental Change', *Global Environmental Change*, 20/4, 550–57.

Pacces, A., and Weimar, M. (2020). 'From Diversity to Coordination: A European Approach to Covid-19', *European Journal of Risk Regulation*, 11/2, 283–96.

Renda, A., and Castro, R. (2020). 'Towards Stronger EU Governance of Health Threats after the Covid-19 Pandemic', *European Journal of Risk Regulation*, 11/2, 273–82.

Rubin, O. (2019). 'The Glocalization of Antimicrobial Stewardship', *Globalization and Health*, 15/1, 54.

Sandler, T. (2015). 'Collective Action: Fifty Years Later', *Public Choice*, 164/3, 195–216.

Samarasekera, U. (2021). 'New EU Health Programme Comes into Force', *The Lancet*, 397/10281, 1252–3.

Schmidt, V. A. (2020). 'Theorizing Institutional Change and Governance in European Responses to the Covid-19 Pandemic', *Journal of European Integration*, 42/8, 1177–93.

7

What Would It Take to Move the Global AMR Agenda Forward in the Global South?

Mirfin Mpundu, Philip Mathew, Raphael Chanda, and Francesca Chiara

Introduction

This chapter considers the steps needed to move global antimicrobial resistance (AMR) up the agenda in low- and middle-income countries (LMICs) (see also Chapter 12). Specifically, it focuses on three central governance challenges as limiting factors for the effective progression and implementation of AMR national action plans (NAPs). It calls for the design of solid leadership structures, comprehensive advocacy, and awareness campaigns to drive policy-making, and strengthening of resources and capabilities as bases for the creation of functional health systems. Finally, it proposes solutions to overcoming existing gaps in a bid to promote the development and implementation of effective policies for AMR containment in LMICs.

AMR has been recognized as a global problem of public health concern (Ramanan Laxminarayan et al., 2013). AMR is an existential threat that leads to treatment failure, increased costs related to treatments, longer hospital stays, predisposal of patients to healthcare-associated infections (HAIs) especially in those who are immunosuppressed, and affects both morbidity and mortality (Dadgostar, 2019). Left unabated, AMR threatens to reverse the major gains made in modern medicine over the past 100 years. Procedures such as surgeries, treatment of infectious diseases, and neonatal and maternal health will be difficult to perform and manage. While it is well known that the interconnectedness of human, animal, plant, and the environment contributes to the spread of resistance, very few initial steps have been taken to address AMR in its entire complexity (Destoumieux-Garzon et al., 2018; see Chapters 11, 12, and 13). In addressing AMR, the focus should not be dominated by research and development of newer antimicrobial agents but should also target public health interventions which are essential in addressing the emerging threat of superbugs (Boucher et al., 2009). The veterinary and human sectors largely share the same antimicrobial classes and consequently when resistance is developed in one context, it can quickly spread to other species and environments (Woolhouse et al., 2015). Transmission can happen through the food chain, environment (especially sewage), and direct contact. Recently, the Global Leaders Group on AMR called for an urgent reduction of the use of antimicrobials in animals, including significant investment in infection prevention

Mirfin Mpundu, Philip Mathew, Raphael Chanda, and Francesca Chiara, *What Would It Take to Move the Global AMR Agenda Forward in the Global South?* In: *Steering against Superbugs.* Edited by: Olivier Rubin, Erik Baekkeskov, and Louise Munkholm, Oxford University Press.

and control in the food system (WHO, 2021). The biggest challenge for controlling the spread of AMR is to limit infections happening in the first place, thus reducing the need to use antimicrobials in all sectors (Klein, Levin, et al., 2018; Klein, Van Boeckel, et al., 2018). Overuse and misuse, including inadequate access to the correct treatments, are still considered to be major drivers of AMR. Poor hygiene and sanitation and inadequate infection prevention measures pose the highest risk to increased burden of resistant infections. The greatest effect has been felt by LMICs, whose water, sanitation, and hygiene (WASH) infrastructures and health systems are weak, and which suffer from chronic stock-outs of critical and essential antimicrobials, critical human resources, and weak laboratory systems.

The World Health Organization (WHO) during the sixty-eighth World Health Assembly (WHA) of 2015 adopted the global action plan on AMR with five key strategic areas: raising awareness and knowledge of AMR; strengthening the knowledge base through surveillance; using infection prevention practices to reduce infections; optimizing the use of antimicrobials in both the human and animal sectors; and making an economic case for sustainable investment (WHO, 2015). Member states agreed to develop and implement NAPs within two years of this resolution to address and contain AMR in their countries. Additionally, in recognition of the complexity of addressing AMR as a One Health issue, across sectors, the WHO, Food and Agriculture Organization (FAO), and World Organization for Animal Health (OIE) together formed the Tripartite that is responsible for AMR governance across all sectors. According to WHO Regional Office for Africa, thirty-six countries have developed NAPs and are at different stages of implementation (WHO, n.d.).

Five years down the line it has become apparent that in addressing AMR, the challenge for LMICs does not rest in development of NAPs but rather in securing sufficient political interest, public attention, and financial support for implementation, as concluded by the Interagency Coordination Group (IACG) on AMR (Frumence et al., 2021; IACG, 2019; see also Chapter 14 for discussion of lack of NAP implementation). Reasons include lack of knowledge and data on the burden of AMR and inability to translate its impact on both human and animal health effectively (Pokharel et al., 2019). Describing consequences related to AMR has always proven to be a challenge due to a number of factors which include involvement of diverse pathogens, unique mechanism of transmission, and its association with a variety of clinical syndromes. Since antibiotic resistance is not a disease entity by itself, these factors provide a cloak of invisibility obscuring its impact on health (Cars and Nordberg, 2005). Additionally, AMR has a language problem: it is a term commonly used in clinical practice among health professionals with an assumption that its meaning is well understood by patients and policymakers (Mendelson et al., 2017). Several surveys conducted worldwide in different settings have concluded that knowledge and understanding of antibiotics is lacking and an innovative approach is required to address these problems in order to create awareness in the community (Bakhit et al., 2019; Brookes-Howell et al., 2012; Mokoena et al., 2021). Until very recently, AMR did not feature in the UN's 2030 Sustainable Development Goals (SDGs) but it now has one indicator (percentage of bloodstream infections due to selected antimicrobial-resistant organisms) although many of the SDGs are dependent on AMR being curbed for their delivery (WHO, 2018). If we fail to frame and communicate the dramatic impact that AMR could have beyond the health sector, as happened successfully for other global health challenges, the issue will not win the support of politicians and the public.

Governance challenges for LMICs

This section discusses three central governance challenges for LMICs. First, we look at political will and leadership, then: advocacy and awareness, and third: resources and capabilities.

1. Political will and leadership

Addressing a cross-cutting public health issue such as AMR requires strong functional governance structures. Governance of AMR at the global, regional, and country level has become a huge and complex problem, and is a relatively weak link at the country level. Though most countries in Africa have moved forward and developed their NAPs, there are issues with implementation. As NAPs are legally non-binding, most countries are not persuaded to follow through with implementation. Many countries have made very little efforts to develop operational and budget plans for implementation of NAP activities, and many have limited themselves to a strategic action plan only (FAO, 2018).

On paper, most countries may have good structures for NAP implementation that include a ministerial committee across sectors, an AMR Secretariat with a National AMR Focal Point, technical/thematic working groups across sectors, and sector-specific AMR focal points, but these are dysfunctional and rarely meet. There is no accountability, clear scope of work, nor terms of references for some of these committees and positions. Lack of the needed coordination across sectors and absence of robust engagement with various stakeholders is contributing to inaction or misaligned implementation of NAPs. Where some activities for AMR are taking place, these are largely donor driven and often not guided by country priorities. In addition, most AMR Focal Points or coordinators have other primary responsibilities that make it very difficult to focus and concentrate on AMR functions. Depending on the professional background of the national AMR Focal Point, the implementation efforts around NAPs will be skewed in favour of that domain. There are also regulatory constraints that drive the issue of AMR at country level. Medicines regulation in both human animal and agriculture sectors ensures appropriate use of antimicrobials but unfortunately, most LMICs lack appropriate legislation and policies. Even in countries with policies in place, monitoring and enforcement mechanisms are often lacking (Pokharel et al., 2019; Roth et al., 2018).

As AMR is a complex multi-sectorial problem it requires the involvement of multiple stakeholders in animal, human, agricultural, and environmental sectors. It requires intersectoral planning and implementation, a true One Health approach (Destoumieux-Garzon et al., 2018; Queenan et al., 2016; see also Chapters 11, 12, and 13). This One Health approach to AMR, however, is challenging because it requires concerted actions across different ministries and sectors, especially for LMICs. The political will at global level has minimal impact at country level and does not always translate into action, mainly due to the absence of effective governance structures and wholehearted commitment that leads to a lack of provision of resources and problems with ownership and accountability. In most cases, the governments or regulators fail to appreciate or they do not have enough data to appreciate the true extent of the burden and impact of AMR at country level (Iskandar et al., 2021). The scientific community has also not been able to frame the AMR issue in a way that can interest the policy community at the country level. All these factors hinder the translation of AMR policy from paper to action in LMICs. AMR requires long-term actions which are more challenging to achieve compared to short-term and one-sector focused solutions. As highlighted in earlier work, AMR is identified as a super wicked problem with a global impact that requires willingness of national states to collaborate internationally. The change needed represents an overwhelming challenge at the political and policy level (Baekkeskov et al., 2020; Levin et al., 2012).

In general, most LMICs have failed to move away from vertical programmes towards more integrated systems that could move AMR interventions into the mainstream. Most developing countries are implementing projects directed at WASH, HIV, TB, maternal and child health, and non-communicable diseases. However most of these programmes are still siloed with very few efforts to integrate AMR interventions in them. Beyond line ministries, there are very few that co-develop activities such as intervention activities on AMR. The way budgeting is done typically by various ministries contributes to the failure of ministries to work together. Governments need to take leadership in creating the platform and forum for interministerial planning.

Monitoring and evaluation systems are important in NAP implementation as these systems help track performance indicators. Surveillance data improve accountability and transparency, facilitate regular monitoring and evaluation, and highlight progress achieved in attaining goals laid out in the global action plan. This ensures continued stakeholder support and ultimately contributes to the global momentum on the AMR issue. However, few LMICs have developed such functional and integrated systems, highlighting potential gaps that need to be addressed (Kariuki et al., 2018).

Among the recommendations of the IACG on AMR was accelerating progress in AMR actions, a focus on innovation to secure the future, collaboration and engagement of various stakeholders, increased investments for sustainable response, and a focus on strengthening accountability and global governance (IACG, 2019). While some progress has been made in this area, a lot needs to be done through appropriate monitoring and evaluation.

2. Advocacy and awareness

Some scholars describe AMR as an advocacy crisis, building on the argument that in comparison to other well-established global health programmes directed, for instance, at tuberculosis, HIV, and malaria, AMR has not received enough support from civil society, national advocacy associations, and the general public (Fraser et al., 2021). The high burden of communicable and non-communicable diseases (NCDs) with better advocacy and visibility profiles displaces AMR positioning on national agendas, with AMR coordinators in most countries having little influence, which leads to poor integration of activities (Baekkeskov et al., 2020). Most of the advocacy and policy work on AMR has been driven by high-income countries (HICs), which have represented the issue at a high political level, although experiencing a lower burden of resistant infections compared to LMICs (see Chapters 2 and 14). In particular, health agencies, international funders, and a few HIC governments with a high stake in global health have set the AMR agenda. This raises questions on how well needs and challenges facing LMICs have been truly represented.

A good example comes from stewardship and responsible use of antimicrobials campaigns, which have proven effective in HICs but yielded poor outcomes in low-resource settings.

First, excess versus access to antibiotics is a critical dilemma in LMICs (Cox et al., 2017). Although increased used of antimicrobials has been recently documented, suggesting better access to these life-saving medicines, it is also true that many people still suffer and die due to lack of their availability (Browne et al., 2021). The recently published AMR Benchmark (Access to Medicine Foundation, 2021) shows that only 54 producers of antibacterial, antifungals, and vaccines out of the 166 tracked have a strategy to ensure provision of these products in LMICs. This leads prescribers to use inappropriate treatments, despite the existence of guidelines or awareness campaigns pointing to the correct drug of choice. Campaigns designed to promote responsible use of antimicrobials should be adjusted to the needs of the contexts where they have been implemented (Laxminarayan et al., 2016). Secondly, lack of reliable surveillance data in LMICs is also an important limiting factor to the design of advocacy, stewardship, and awareness campaigns. HICs collect and have access to reliable surveillance data that can inform on changes in drug resistance patterns and consumption of antimicrobials. However, these programmes do not often take into account the heterogeneity of health systems in LMICs, the interrelationship between patients and doctors and the role of other healthcare professionals such as pharmacists and community workers as prescribers, and lack of access to basic services such as microbiology labs, sanitation facilities, clean water, and cold supply chains, to name a few. While targeting behaviour seems to be the primary focus of many programmes, this might have little effect in contexts plagued by lack of widespread access to healthcare services and other health inequalities (Charani et al., 2021; see also Chapter 8). The COVID-19 pandemic and the slow distribution and scarce availability of vaccines in the Global South has been a painful reminder of the reality that many resource-limited settings face.

Thirdly, AMR has been described as a slow-moving pandemic. While politically this definition serves well the purpose of creating urgency on political agendas, it might dangerously shift the focus from strengthening health systems to epidemic preparedness. While epidemic preparedness obviously plays a very important role in strengthening the capacity of health systems, what many LMICs need is to lay the basis of functional and sustainable health systems rather than building capacity on a system, which lacks the foundation.

Finally, the epidemiological transition that many LMICs have experienced in the last few decades, has also resulted in a reduced interest in infectious conditions and subsequently AMR. Many agendas have shifted to raise awareness on the health impact of NCDs. As the gross domestic product (GDP) of countries has increased, habits have changed including around food and nutrition.

The consumption of animal protein and processed food has increased. The demand for animal protein is being fuelled by a general understanding that its quality is better than plant-based alternatives and the increase in per-capita income seen over time in low-resource settings. Agricultural intensification has increased production dramatically and this has also brought down the effective price of animal products. Most of the intensification is not supported by robust infection control measures and is therefore propped up by the use of antibiotics in livestock (Godfray and Garnett, 2014). The small/medium farmers in LMICs often do not have access to resources or incentives to improve the adoption of infection prevention (biosecurity) measures, which might be common practice in HICs. The price discovery process for farm products in low-resource settings also has several structural flaws, which results in poor farmer incomes. The inability of the scientific community to decipher the AMR issues for the public results in poor awareness across the board. In most countries, consumers are not willing to pay a premium for products made without routine use of antibiotics.

3. Resources and capabilities

AMR-focused funding opportunities for LMICs are few and not accessible for most countries. As a result, most countries report the lack of financial resources as one of the major hindrances to NAP development and implementation. Equally, countries are at different stages of NAP development/implementation and challenges in comparing progress indicators may arise. Among the critical roles of the national AMR Secretariats is resource mobilization that would facilitate NAP implementation. However, most AMR Secretariats at the national level are understaffed and lack the skills needed for resource mobilization.

As mentioned above, the lack of involvement from different stakeholders is another area of concern. In developing NAPs, inclusion of key stakeholders and use of local data conducted through a comprehensive situational analysis are important. Aligning AMR activities with country priority areas, in addition to advocacy efforts, may play an important role, especially in resource limited settings. These can only be achieved through governance and delegated activities.

In general, LMICs have limited capacity to conduct AMR surveillance in all sectors, and where data are collected they are mostly fragmented and lacks reflection of the true burden of AMR (WHO, 2020). Besides, quality assurance is a concern in many of the existing laboratory facilities, thereby limiting the insights which can be generated from the laboratory results (see Chapter 12 for an illustrative example of this specific challenge in Malawi). Contributing factors include poor infrastructure, lack of human resources, and reliance on external funding (Iskandar et al., 2021). AMR surveillance systems are an important component in management of infectious diseases and they form the basis of understanding the dynamics of AMR transmission. The data collected contribute to improved public health services, inform policy formulation, and act as an early warning mechanism for monitoring emerging resistance trends (Hay et al., 2018). A true One Health approach requires the integration of human surveillance systems with environmental, animal, and food systems to track the spread of resistant pathogens and antibiotic residues to identify areas of risk and priority for action (WHO, 2013). The limited capacity to conduct surveillance in LMICs impacts the ability to conduct situational analysis and generate country level data, and the absence of the data presents a further challenge for most countries to document and build a case for funding of AMR activities. In order to overcome this challenge in LMICs, innovative approaches to improving resources and financing of laboratory services are required. In 2020, Zambia developed a framework for an integrated surveillance approach which follows the lead example of high-income countries such as Canada, Denmark, United Kingdom, and Sweden, to name a few, with already established systems. Though it is too early to judge its success, it is an important step. Lack of technical capacity to implement novel stewardship interventions in human, animal, and environmental sectors is also a problem which drives the global AMR issue.

An often overlooked cause of AMR is the impact of antimicrobial residues and resistant genes in wastewaters on the spread of resistant pathogens. Contamination can happen from hospitals, households, farms, and pharmaceutical manufacturing facilities. Drug-resistant organisms have been systematically detected in communities living around manufacturing plants in India and China, which manufacture most of the world antibiotics (Rutgersson et al., 2014). In 2020, India was set to become one of the first countries to set limits for levels of antibiotic effluents in wastewater, however the India Drug Manufacturers Association successfully argued against the implementation of the policy (Schaaf, 2020). There is a need to strengthen surveillance capacity to include monitoring of the impact of wastewaters on human health and investing in innovative solutions to develop wastewater treatment plants for LMICs (see also Chapters 17 and 18 for a discussion of regulations of pharmaceutical industries).

Recommendations

Foundations of strong governance structures requires the appreciation of AMR as a public health threat that needs urgent attention. Currently few political leaders and other key decision-makers are aware of AMR as a public health problem and the proportionate response it requires. More efforts should be targeted towards political leaders and the policy community to take up AMR as a critical public health issue. National AMR secretariats must be empowered and funded to carry out the many activities including AMR NAP implementation. The COVID-19 pandemic has demonstrated that with good advocacy and leadership AMR can be placed on the global and national agenda (Cars et al., 2021). Though COVID-19 has taken away some of the political capital available to the AMR issue, the increased interest in health among the public and policy community could yield rich dividends if the AMR issue is placed strategically on the political landscape.

For coordinating the efforts around the UN SDGs, most LMICs have an expert on the issue who generally sits in the head of state's office. Engaging with these experts will gain AMR the necessary visibility for resource mobilization. Rather than supporting the creation of yet another AMR coordination body or office, we advocate for appropriate funding being made available with recruitment of dedicated AMR staff at country level. The AMR national focal points should be intended as full-time jobs and their positions supported by staff to spearhead NAP implementation, engage with stakeholders, convene technical and thematic working groups, liaise with funders, and leverage on current programs such as WASH, infection prevention and control (IPC), and vaccination programmes.

Provision of finances

Implementing AMR NAP activities is cost-intensive and requires planning and apportioning the necessary funds after thorough costing of the action plan activities. AMR should be viewed as a development issue and security threat that requires funds and it should be integrated in SDG agendas. It has been twenty years since African governments signed the Abuja declaration pledging to allocate 15 per cent of annual budgets to the health sector. However, this target has been elusive with most countries failing to honour the commitment in full; as of 2011, only South Africa and Rwanda had reached the 15 per cent target, and data from WHO Global health expenditure database showed that at the end of 2018 all South African Development Community (SADC) Member States were struggling to honour the pledge (Bwalya, 2021; WHO, 2011). Increased public health financing is also required for countries to attain universal health coverage; as highlighted during the COVID-19 pandemic, disparities in access to health still exist in LMICs. In addressing AMR it is important to frame the issue more broadly, articulating it not only as a health issue but also as a development issue as part of the SDG agenda.

Accountability

Like any national programmes or interventions, there is need for the government to build in accountability measures in AMR progress. The relevant ministries have to take ownership for the action plan and allocate resources. Clear core indicators should be reported every year to ensure progress, tease out some lessons, use monitoring and evaluation strategies that track yearly activities, and present reports every year for not only political leaders but communities who are affected by AMR.

Raising awareness and knowledge

Governments working with partners and other key stakeholders need to develop novel strategies on efforts to raise awareness and knowledge within communities. With the ease that antibiotics are accessed without a prescription in most LMICs, civil society need to be engaged to effectively tackle this issue. Such public health campaigns and interventions cost money but are rewarding. Mobilizing local communities around the AMR issue is likely to contribute to behavioural changes and unwarranted antibiotic requests when they are not medically indicated. Civil society organizations could work with and support governments with this agenda. Deliberate efforts should be made towards addressing interventions that target behavioural change. Understanding social, economic, gender, cultural, and religious dimensions and related inequalities is key to AMR containment. These range from social structures and poverty affecting literacy and hindering access to healthcare as well as a lack of universal health coverage, which burdens the most vulnerable. Cultural and religious beliefs affect the relationship between patients and healthcare professionals and trust in standard medical practices. Holistic and symbolic form of healings are still common and widely used in many contexts. Additionally, the effect of urbanization has shifted populations in search of better jobs from rural areas into cities in many fast-growing economies of the Global South. As a result, in emerging economies there are huge income disparities with a high level of poverty forcing many to live in crowded and inadequate housing with poor access to hygiene and sanitation facilities, exposing them to a higher risk of contracting infectious diseases. Women might be more susceptible as they suffer inadequate access to WASH during pregnancy and childbirth (Charani et al., 2021). The successful containment of AMR needs to address the pressing social determinants of health that still characterize LMICs.

Paradigm shift in thinking

Whilst there seem to be efforts in strengthening global leadership, through the Global Leaders Group, the Tripartite Plus, the formation of the Multi-Partner Trust Fund (MPTF), the same cannot be said for LMICs. The MPTF, for example, only has three countries that have invested funds in it, which is worrying as LMICs have indicated that AMR NAP implementation is cost-intensive and noted that they do not have funds required. We need a large resource pool which country governments can tap into for NAP implementation rather than multiple piecemeal options for financing small components of the action plans.

Sharing best practice examples from LMICs

Since most of the pioneering efforts around AMR interventions have been driven by HICs, many of these interventions may not be feasible in LMICs. As a result, governments in the developing world lack access to insights about the interventions that work in low-resource settings. Several best practices and innovative interventions which have been piloted in low-resource settings, such as the Antibiotic Smart Use project in Thailand (Sumpradit et al., 2012), suggest the need for creating a platform to share best practices and experiences between LMICs. This platform should facilitate the free flow of information on AMR interventions. Rather than being limited by methodological considerations, the platform could be used to share information on any pilots meant to contain the AMR issue in low-resource settings.

Conclusion

LMICs need to learn from some successful, disease-specific interventions such as with TB, HIV, and malaria which have been quite effective by taking a health systems approach such as investing in advocacy, raising awareness, improving surveillance systems, increasing access to quality-assured essential antimicrobials, investments in information systems, and capacity building. There is a lot to learn from the action plans to tackle climate change too, as these plans were able to mobilize adequate political capital and resources for action at the country level.

References

Access to Medicine Foundation. (2021). 'Antimicrobial Resistance Benchmark 2023' (Amsterdam: Access to Medicine Foundation).

Baekkeskov, E., Rubin, O., Munkholm, L., and Zaman, W. (2020). 'Antimicrobial Resistance as a Global Health Crisis', *Oxford Research Encyclopedia of Politics* (Oxford: Oxford University Press). Retrieved 27 January 2023, from https://oxfordre.com/politics/view/10.1093/acrefore/9780190228 637.001.0001/acrefore-9780190228637-e-1626

Bakhit, M., Del Mar, C., Gibson, E., and Hoffmann, T. (2019). 'Exploring Patients' Understanding of Antibiotic Resistance and How This May Influence Attitudes Towards Antibiotic Use for Acute Respiratory Infections: A Qualitative Study in Australian General Practice', *BMJ Open*, 9/3, e026735–e026735. doi:10.1136/bmjopen-2018-026735.

Boucher, H. W., Talbot, G. H., Bradley, J. S., Edwards, J. E., Gilbert, D., Rice, L. B., et al. (2009). 'Bad Bugs, No Drugs: No ESKAPE! An Update from the Infectious Diseases Society of America', *Clinical Infectious Diseases*, 48/1, 1–12. doi:10.1086/595011.

Brookes-Howell, L., Elwyn, G., Hood, K., Wood, F., Cooper, L., Goossens, H., et al. C. (2012). '"The Body Gets Used to Them": Patients' Interpretations of Antibiotic Resistance and the Implications for Containment Strategies', *Journal of General Internal Medicine*, 27/7, 766–72. doi:10.1007/s11606-011-1916-1.

Browne, A. J., Chipeta, M. G., Haines-Woodhouse, G., Kumaran, E. P. A., Hamadani, B. H. K., Zaraa, S., et al. (2021). 'Global Antibiotic Consumption and Usage in Humans, 2000-18: A Spatial Modelling Study', *The Lancet Planetary Health*, 5/12, e893–e904. doi:10.1016/S2542-5196(21)00280-1.

Bwalya, J. (2021). *SADC and the Abuja Declaration: Honouring the Pledge*. Policy Briefing 230. South African Institute of International Affairs.

Cars, O., Chandy, S. J., Mpundu, M., Peralta, A. Q., Zorzet, A., and So, A. D. (2021). 'Resetting the Agenda for Antibiotic Resistance through a Health Systems Perspective', *The Lancet Global Health*, 9/7, e1022–e1027. doi:10.1016/s2214-109x(21)00163-7.

Cars, O., and Nordberg, P. (2005). 'Antibiotic Resistance: The Faceless Threat', *The International Journal of Risk and Safety in Medicine*, 17, 103 10.

Charani, E., Mendelson, M., Ashiru-Oredope, D., Hutchinson, E., Kaur, M., McKee, M., et al. (2021). 'Navigating Sociocultural Disparities in Relation to Infection and Antibiotic Resistance—The Need for an Intersectional Approach', *JAC-Antimicrobial Resistance*, 3/4. doi:10.1093/jacamr/dlab123. https://www.ncbi.nlm.nih.gov/pmc/articles/PMC8485076/

Cox, J. A., Vlieghe, E., Mendelson, M., Wertheim, H., Ndegwa, L., Villegas, M. V., ... Levy Hara, G. (2017). 'Antibiotic Stewardship in Low- and Middle-income Countries: The Same but Different?', *Clinical Microbiology and Infection*, 23/11, 812–18. doi:10.1016/j.cmi.2017.07.010.

Dadgostar, P. (2019). 'Antimicrobial Resistance: Implications and Costs', *Infectious Drug Resistance*, 12, 3903–10. doi:10.2147/IDR.S234610.

Destoumieux-Garzon, D., Mavingui, P., Boetsch, G., Boissier, J., Darriet, F., Duboz, P., et al. (2018). 'The One Health Concept: 10 Years Old and a Long Road Ahead', *Frontiers in Veterinary Science*, 5, 14. doi:10.3389/fvets.2018.00014.

FAO. (2018). *Global Database for Antimicrobial Resistance Country Self Assessment* (Rome: FAO).

Fraser, J. L., Alimi, Y. H., Varma, J. K., Muraya, T., Kujinga, T., Carter, V. K., et al. (2021). 'Antimicrobial Resistance Control Efforts in Africa: A Survey of the Role of Civil Society Organisations', *Global Health Action*, 14/1. doi:10.1080/16549716.2020.1868055.

Frumence, G., Mboera, L. E. G., Sindato, C., Katale, B. Z., Kimera, S., Metta, E., et al. (2021). 'The Governance and Implementation of the National Action Plan on Antimicrobial Resistance in Tanzania: A Qualitative Study', *Antibiotics (Basel)*, 10/3. doi:10.3390/antibiotics10030273.

Godfray, H. C., and Garnett, T. (2014). 'Food Security and Sustainable Intensification', *Philosophical Transactions of the Royal Society of London, Series B: Biological Sciences*, 369/1639, 20120273. doi:10.1098/rstb.2012.0273.

Hay, S. I., Rao, P. C., Dolecek, C., Day, N. P. J., Stergachis, A., Lopez, A. D., and Murray, C. J. L. (2018). 'Measuring and Mapping the Global Burden of Antimicrobial Resistance', *BMC Medicine*, 16/1, 78. doi:10.1186/s12916-018-1073-z.

IACG. (2019). 'No Time to Wait Securing the Future from Drug Resistant Infections'.

Iskandar, K., Molinier, L., Hallit, S., Sartelli, M., Hardcastle, T. C., Haque, M., et al. (2021). 'Surveillance of Antimicrobial Resistance in Low- and Middle-income Countries: A Scattered Picture', *Antimicrobial Resistance and Infection Control*, 10/1, 63. doi:10.1186/s13756-021-00931-w.

Kariuki, S., Keddy, K. H., Antonio, M., and Okeke, I. N. (2018). 'Antimicrobial Resistance Surveillance in Africa: Successes, Gaps and a Roadmap for the Future', *African Journal of Laboratory Medicine*, 7/2, 924. doi:10.4102/ajlm.v7i2.924.

Klein, E. Y., Levin, S. A., and Laxminarayan, R. (2018). 'Reply to Abat et al.: Improved Policies Necessary to Ensure an Effective Future for Antibiotics', *Proceedings of the National Academy of Sciences of the United States of America*, 115/35, E8111–E8112. doi:10.1073/pnas.1811245115.

Klein, E. Y., Van Boeckel, T. P., Martinez, E. M., Pant, S., Gandra, S., Levin, S. A., ... Laxminarayan, R. (2018). 'Global Increase and Geographic Convergence in Antibiotic Consumption between 2000 and 2015', *Proceedings of the National Academy of Sciences of the United States of America*, 115/15, E3463–E3470. doi:10.1073/pnas.1717295115.

Laxminarayan, R., Duse, A., Wattal, C., Zaidi, A. K. M., Wertheim, H. F. L., Sumpradit, N., et al. (2013). 'Antibiotic Resistance—The Need for Global Solutions', *The Lancet Infectious Diseases*, 13/12, 1057–98. doi:10.1016/s1473-3099(13)70318-9.

Laxminarayan, R., Matsoso, P., Pant, S., Brower, C., Røttingen, J. A., Klugman, K., and Davies, S. (2016). 'Access to Effective Antimicrobials: A Worldwide Challenge', *Lancet*, 387/10014, 168–75. doi:10.1016/s0140-6736(15)00474-2.

Levin, K., Cashore, B., Bernstein, S., and Auld, G. (2012). 'Overcoming the Tragedy of Super Wicked Problems: Constraining Our Future Selves to Ameliorate Global Climate Change', *Policy Sciences*, 45/2, 123–52. doi:10.1007/s11077-012-9151-0.

Mendelson, M., Balasegaram, M., Jinks, T., Pulcini, C., and Sharland, M. (2017). 'Antibiotic Resistance Has a Language Problem', *Nature*, 545/7652, 23–25. doi:10.1038/545023a.

Mokoena, T. T. W., Schellack, N., and Brink, A. J. (2021). 'Driving Antibiotic Stewardship Awareness through the Minibus-taxi Community across the Tshwane District, South Africa—A Baseline Evaluation', *JAC-Antimicrobial Resistance*, 3/3. doi:10.1093/jacamr/dlab106.

Pokharel, S., Raut, S., and Adhikari, B. (2019). 'Tackling Antimicrobial Resistance in Low-income and Middle-income Countries', *BMJ Global Health*, 4/6, e002104. doi:10.1136/bmjgh-2019-002104.

Queenan, K., Hasler, B., and Rushton, J. (2016). 'A One Health Approach to Antimicrobial Resistance Surveillance: Is There a Business Case for It?', *International Journal of Antimicrobial Agents*, 48/4, 422–7. doi:10.1016/j.ijantimicag.2016.06.014.

Roth, L., Bempong, D., Babigumira, J. B., Banoo, S., Cooke, E., Jeffreys, D., et al. (2018). 'Expanding Global Access to Essential Medicines: Investment Priorities for Sustainably Strengthening Medical Product Regulatory Systems', *Globalization and Health*, 14/1, 102. doi:10.1186/s12992-018-0421-2.

Rutgersson, C., Fick, J., Marathe, N., Kristiansson, E., Janzon, A., Angelin, M., et al. (2014). 'Fluoroquinolones and *qnr* Genes in Sediment, Water, Soil, and Human Fecal Flora in an Environment Polluted by Manufacturing Discharges', *Environmental Science & Technology*, 48/14, 7825–32. doi:10.1021/es501452a.

Schaaf, N., Panorel, I., Caputo, A., Prakash, S., Shaw, B., Verma, N., and Veem, K. (2020). 'Reducing Emissions from Antibiotic Production'. Stockholm International Water Institute.

Sumpradit, N., Chongtrakul, P., Anuwong, K., Pumtong, S., Kongsomboon, K., Butdeemee, P., et al. (2012). 'Antibiotics Smart Use: A Workable Model for Promoting the Rational Use of Medicines in Thailand', *Bulletin of the World Health Organization*, 90/12, 905–13. doi:10.2471/BLT.12.105445.

WHO. (n.d.). *Library of AMR national action plans*. <https://www.who.int/teams/surveillance-prevention-control-AMR/national-action-plan-monitoring-evaluation/library-of-national-action-plans> (last accessed: 1 April 2023).

WHO. (2011). *The Abuja Declaration: Ten Years On* (Geneva: WHO).

WHO. (2013). *Integrated Surveillance of Antimicrobial Resistance: Guidance from a WHO Advisory Group* (Geneva: WHO).

WHO. (2015). *Global Action Plan on Antimicrobial Resistance* (Geneva: WHO).

WHO. (2018). *Global Indicator Framework after 2021* (Geneva: WHO).

WHO. (2020). *Global Antimicrobial Resistance and Use Surveillance System Report 2020* (Geneva: WHO).

WHO. (2021). *World Leaders and Experts Call for Significant Reduction in the Use of Antimicrobial Drugs on Global Food Systems* (Geneva: WHO).

Woolhouse, M., Ward, M., van Bunnik, B., and Farrar, J. (2015). 'Antimicrobial Resistance in Humans, Livestock and the Wider Environment', *Philosophical Transactions of the Royal Society of London, Series B: Biological Sciences*, 370/1670, doi:10.1098/rstb.2014.0083.

WHO. (n.d.). *Library of AMR national action plans.* <https://www.who.int/teams/surveillance-pre vention-control-AMR/national-action-plan-monitoring-evaluation/library-of-national-action-plans> (last accessed 1 April 2023).

PART III
AMR GOVERNANCE FROM BELOW

8

The Individual in Global and National AMR Governance

Mark D. M. Davis

Introduction

This chapter examines how policy and communications frame general public awareness and action on antimicrobial resistance (AMR), with particular reference to what is expected of individuals using antimicrobials in community settings. The governance of individuals, what they know and how they use antimicrobials, is a recurrent theme of global and national AMR policy discourse. The World Health Organization's (WHO) Global Action Plan on Antimicrobial Resistance had as its first objective to '[i]mprove awareness and understanding of antimicrobial resistance through effective communication, education and training' (WHO, 2015: 8), which it explained in this way:

> Steps need to be taken immediately in order to raise awareness of antimicrobial resistance and promote behavioural change, through public communication programmes that target different audiences in human health, animal health and agricultural practice as well as consumers. Inclusion of the use of antimicrobial agents and resistance in school curricula will promote better understanding and awareness from an early age. (WHO, 2015: 8)

The Action Plan goes on to describe the role of Member States in developing communications for their citizens. The second Australian national strategy framework called for 'whole of society awareness and behavioural change' (Australian Government, 2019: 9). Social marketing interventions including World Antibiotic Awareness Week (Huttner et al., 2019) operate in multiple countries to promote public action, and *AntibioticGuardian.com* (Bhattacharya et al., 2016; Kesten et al., 2018; Newitt et al., 2018, 2019) invites individuals to pledge that they will avoid antibiotics for coughs and colds, among other practices designed to reduce and rationalize the use of antibiotics. In Australia, the 2020 World Antibiotics Awareness Week focused on the theme 'Antimicrobials: Handle with care' (Australian Commission on Safety and Quality in Health Care, 2020a) and included information for consumers in a pamphlet called 'Do I really need antibiotics?' (Australian Commission on Safety and Quality in Health

Mark D. M. Davis, *The Individual in Global and National AMR Governance* In: *Steering against Superbugs*. Edited by:
Olivier Rubin, Erik Baekkeskov, and Louise Munkholm, Oxford University Press. © Oxford University Press 2023.
DOI: 10.1093/oso/9780192899477.003.0008

Care, 2020b). This pamphlet invited the reader to deliberate on their healthcare practices, and through this self-reflection reduce use of antimicrobials.

Despite this attention to individuals, global and national efforts to reduce and prevent AMR face significant challenges. Individual awareness and knowledge of AMR remains patchy (Gualano et al., 2015; McCullough et al., 2016) and is strongest amongst highly educated people with an interest in science (see Chapter 15; Davis et al., 2020; Will, 2020). Communications for the most part hail a universal individual in ways that may mean that many or even most fail to recognize the relevance of the AMR message for themselves. Policy does refer to individuals who present in primary care settings seeking antibiotics when the clinician may not believe they are warranted and accordingly argues for interventions to reduce these expectations (Australian Government, 2021), sometimes attributed to 'patient demand' (Avorn and Solomon, 2000: 128). These blind spots and emphases can be attributed to the assumptions that drive policy and communications in national and global AMR governance, among them a focus on the individual as free to act and notions that information alone will shape the required response to the threat of AMR (see Chapter 9 for a discussion of this issue in the case of Bangladesh).

This assumption of individuals as free to act on information about antimicrobial usage can be understood using the lens of Foucauldian governmentality, or the 'conduct of conduct' (Foucault, 1990). Governmentality focuses attention on how modes of advanced liberalism encourage the self-making agency of individuals to ensure biopolitical effects—that is, the sustained productivity of the population through the optimization of its health—and therefore contribute to the accumulation of material and symbolic goods. It is a form of power that produces intersubjective life as opposed to forms of power that constrain through law and coerce through punishment. In relation to AMR governance, the Foucauldian lens helps to foreground the difference between education and regulation in AMR policy settings; that is, efforts to produce individuals who themselves control their own use of antimicrobials in contrast with constraint of antimicrobial usage through surveillance, legal, and administrative structures. The previously mentioned pledge site *AntibioticGuardian.com* and the pamphlet 'Do I really need antibiotics?' can be construed as a method for encouraging self-management because they provide ways for individuals to perform endorsement of the reduction of antimicrobial use and prevention of AMR. This and similar examples exercise pastoral power, a specific form of governmentality (Rose, 2007). The individual is not directed to act in certain ways but positioned in discourse so that they are invited to consider the choices they make about their health and that of loved ones. In this mode of governmentality, individual choice to act in ways that advantage the reduction of AMR spring not from external constraint but from within (see Chapters 5 and 19 for further discussion). The genesis of autonomous action that pastoral power inspires is the ideal expression of liberalized governance of self by the self. As we will see in what follows, however, the framing of individual action in AMR governance is a somewhat inchoate mix of constraining regulation and pastoral encouragement.

This chapter, therefore, explores how individual action is framed in AMR governance with reference to critical discourse analysis of Australian AMR policy documents and qualitative interviews with members of the general public in Melbourne, Australia. First, I consider how a focus on the individual is only partly supported by the microbiology of AMR and surveillance data with implications for goals and targets in AMR policy and communications. I then problematize the concept of individual 'demand' for antimicrobials—a common element of AMR governance—in light of 'supply'; that is, the systems of healthcare delivery through which individuals are able to assert their interests. Following that, I reflect on the emergence of schisms between public health systems and the publics they serve tied to currents in AMR governance that seek to constrain the use of antimicrobials. Lastly, I make some comments about how these counterproductive approaches to AMR governance could be addressed and mitigated for more advantageous AMR outcomes in the future.

Complex AMR systems and the individual

It is reasonable to ask why attempts to reduce AMR focus on individuals and their use of antimicrobials. This is an important question in light of One Health approaches that feature in global and national AMR governance and recognize that resistant microbes are found in humans, animals and the environment (Hincliffe, 2015) and that any use of antimicrobials may contribute to the development of AMR (Australian Government, 2021). For example, streptomycin-resistant tuberculosis was observed in the first clinical trial of the antibiotic in the late 1940s (Keshavjee and Farmer, 2012) and therefore well before its widespread use. Genome sequencing has shown that methicillin-resistant *Staphylococcus aureus* emerged in the 1940s before the widespread use of methicillin in the 1960s (Harkins et al., 2017). It follows that the non-compliant use of antimicrobials on the part of individuals may not be a necessary, let alone sufficient, explanation for AMR. Improving the clinical effectiveness of the prescription and use of antimicrobials in community settings is a valuable policy goal, but it is less clear what role individuals have in the production and reduction of AMR.

The focus on the individual in AMR governance can be attributed to knowledge about patterns of antimicrobial use and AMR in community settings. The Organisation for Economic Co-Operation and Development (OECD) has reported that Australia is ninth highest of thirty-two countries for volume of prescribed antibiotics in 2017 (OECD, 2019). The Antimicrobial Use and Resistance in Australia (AURA 2019) report (Australian Commission on Safety and Quality in Health Care, 2019) analysed prescriptions in community settings made under the Pharmaceutical Benefits Scheme and the Repatriation Pharmaceutical Benefits Scheme (PBS/RPBS). These schemes subsidize the costs of prescription drugs for consumers and, due in part to expenditure tracking mechanisms, collect robust prescription data. These data show that 41.5 per cent of Australians had at least one antibiotic in 2017 (Australian Commission on Safety and Quality in Health Care, 2019). AURA 2019 shows that while the prescription of antimicrobials in community healthcare settings has declined somewhat since 2015, there is evidence of inappropriate antibiotic prescriptions. For example, high rates of antibiotic prescribing outside accepted clinical guidance was found for patients with influenza (52.2 per cent) and bronchitis (92.4 per cent).

It is important to note, too, that not all antimicrobial use in Australia is captured by surveillance systems. AURA 2019 noted that the PBS/RPBS system captures 90 per cent approximately of antimicrobials dispensed in Australia (Australian Commission on Safety and Quality in Health Care, 2019). The remaining 10 per cent can be explained in several ways. PBS/RPBS data presented in AURA 2019 for First Nations people are likely to underestimate antibiotic prescribing because some antibiotics are provided for these groups in community healthcare services. Australians are also able to acquire private prescriptions from a doctor and purchase their pharmaceuticals off the PBS/RPBS system, if they are prepared to pay for the drugs themselves. In addition, Australians travelling overseas can access antimicrobials in settings where prescriptions are not required (Davis, Lohm, Lyall, et al., 2021; Davis et al., 2020). Some citizens might also have backgrounds in international cultures where antimicrobials can be purchased off-prescription in pharmacies and markets (Whittaker et al., 2019). Families might then have members who have divergent approaches to the use of antimicrobials, revealing how transnational, cultural, and generational factors shape consumption outside of surveillance systems. These 'off PBS/RPBS' uses of antimicrobials need to be considered as additional elements of antimicrobial use and AMR production in Australia and by implication in other settings.

However, it is difficult to link any of the antimicrobial prescribing and use practices noted above directly with the AMR burden itself. AURA (Australian Commission on Safety and Quality in Health Care, 2019) noted that fluoroquinolone-resistant *E. coli* is increasing in the community even though access to fluoroquinolone in primary care settings is highly restricted. It is thought that the use of other antimicrobials to which fluoroquinolone-resistant *E. coli* is also resistant has helped to increase the prevalence of this microbe. This observation draws attention to individuals and how they use antimicrobials but equally suggests that individual behaviours are elements of the complex systems of healthcare that constitute antimicrobial use and the production of AMR (Malik and Bhattacharyya, 2019; Spruijit and Petersen, 2020; White and Hughes, 2019). These include, for example, the health status of the community in general and how much antimicrobial prescribing exists, the other antimicrobials in circulation, the genetic characteristics of *E. coli*, gene swapping between bacteria, and so on. Along with the knowledge that appropriate use of antimicrobials can contribute to AMR, the combination of these factors suggests the need to adopt a complex systems approach to reduce AMR within which the individual can be construed to make some contribution.

Individual demand (and supply) in AMR governance

Despite this system complexity, there is a tendency in the AMR field to focus on inappropriate individual demand in isolation. For example, the review of the first

Australian national strategy (Australian Government, 2021) explained AMR in the community in these ways:

> It is generally understood that consumer demand, time pressures and diagnostic un-certainty all contribute to increases in antibiotic prescribing. Tailored communication and education initiatives were identified as essential to engage consumers and profes-sionals in driving behaviour change. (Australian Government, 2021: 12)
>
> In primary health care, unnecessary prescribing for self-limiting conditions and the expectation of the community to receive antimicrobials drives over-medicalisation and inappropriate use in a cyclical fashion. (Australian Government, 2021: 20)

'Consumer demand' and the 'expectant' community are common tropes across global and national AMR governance (Avorn and Solomon, 2000). However, social research with prescribers lends only some support to these factors and tends to emphasize the organization of primary healthcare systems, including time constraints (Teixeira Rodrigues et al., 2013); and perceptions of patient anxiety, expectations and pressure, and fear of losing patients (Biezen et al., 2017). Medical practitioners have been found to prescribe against guidelines to optimize treatment and fulfil their caring role in society (Wood et al., 2007) and to reduce other health risks, particularly for children (Cabral et al., 2015), or to avoid health complications amongst patients with pre-existing condi-tions and lower socioeconomic backgrounds (Kumar et al., 2003). In addition, patient demand might make sense in settings where direct-to-consumer marketing of pharma-ceuticals is permitted, as in the United States and New Zealand (DeFrank et al., 2020), but its significance is less clear for prescribing in Australia and other countries where direct-to-consumer marketing is prohibited and access to antimicrobials is regulated.

Moreover, it is difficult to quantify the contribution of patient demand to antimicro-bial use for several reasons. As far as I am aware, there is no surveillance of antimicro-bial prescriptions that captures and disaggregates prescription events that are said to be the result of patient demand. Further, it may not be possible to collect such data through survey methods. Asking medical practitioners to collect these data may over-estimate patient demand because it might be nominated as an explanation for prescrip-tion when the respondent fears being seen to overprescribe. Likewise, patients may not be willing to report that they obtained antibiotics in these ways if they are aware that it is not appropriate. Naturally occurring prescribing events could be recorded and ana-lysed by an independent third party under conditions of consent, but in this situation, what might be construed by the prescriber as patient demand might not be seen that way by the patient. Moreover, decision-making in the clinical encounter may not be verbalized by either party. These problems indicate that claims regarding the contribu-tion of patient demand to antimicrobial consumption and therefore AMR need to be addressed with some caution.

In addition, patient demand is not necessarily an attribute of the individual. Rather, patient demand might reflect the economic organization of primary healthcare systems (Avorn and Solomon, 2000). General practices in Australia operate as small businesses so practitioners may feel pressure to ensure that their patients are satisfied with their care (Biezen et al., 2017). Unlike the UK's National Health Service, for example, patients in Australia are free to visit another general practitioner if they are unhappy with their care. However, patient demand for an unwarranted antimicrobial prescription can only succeed if the individual is able to find a medical practitioner willing to relent and/or collude with demand and therefore supply the prescription. In this light, inappropriate prescribing is not only a function of patient expectations, it reflects the organization of the business of healthcare in community settings. This economic imperative underlying prescribing has been reported by veterinarians in the United Kingdom (King et al., 2018) and Australia (Hardefeldt et al., 2018). Veterinary surgeries in these countries are fee-for-service businesses that also sell antibiotics. It is important to understand patient demand as constituted in the socio-economic relations of human and animal healthcare.

In addition, the figure of the demanding patient sits uncomfortably with currents in AMR governance that give emphasis to self-regulation. A patient who seeks antibiotics is performing self-determination. But this particular act, if not clinically justified, sits at odds with the need to reduce the use of antimicrobials. Because it is understood to expand and not reduce antimicrobial use, individual demand for antimicrobials comes into view as problematic, or worse, as worthy of condemnation and vilification (Davis, Lohm, Flowers, et al., 2021). This troublesome concept of patient demand is exemplary of an underlying tension in AMR governance: how to constrain antimicrobial use while avoiding clashes with the self-determination through which individuals are typically governed in healthcare systems.

There is need to assist doctors and vets to be able to sustain clinically justified antimicrobial prescription, even in the face of unreasonable demands from their customers. But it is less clear if there is much to be gained for the reduction of AMR, behaviourally and epidemiologically, from a focus on the knowledge and intentions of the individual, even those who seek out antimicrobials against medical advice. Moreover, the common focus on the demanding individual distracts attention away from the social and economic conditions that make unjustified prescription possible. The notion that individual demand disrupts efforts to reduce AMR reveals that AMR governance is yet to reconcile itself with the tensions that arise when liberalized self-discipline comes into contact with regulatory constraint.

Resistant individuals

Along with a mistaken focus on the individual outside of the complex system drivers of AMR and the notion of individual demand, AMR messages do not resonate particularly well with the concerns and interests of individuals. Despite AMR awareness campaigns over at least the previous twenty years (Will, 2020), general public audiences continue to report that they do not understand the microbiological concepts behind infectious diseases, how antibiotics work, and how AMR is produced. Systematic reviews of general population awareness and knowledge show that a slight majority of survey respondents were unaware that antibiotics cannot treat viral infections (Gualano et al., 2015), and majorities of survey participants mistakenly endorse the concept that resistance is a response of the individual body and not bacteria (McCullough et al., 2016). These mistaken assumptions indicate that communications have not had the desired impact (see Chapter 14 for a further discussion of shortcomings in AMR advocacy). They also suggest that AMR is framed by a long-standing concept of embodied resistance (Davis, forthcoming). From this standpoint, individuals speak of AMR as a response of their bodies to the antibiotic, suggesting that the self-management of immunity is the focus for individuals and therefore not necessarily antimicrobials. The persistence of incomplete knowledge amongst the general public and the resistant-body framing of AMR underline the limits of models of communication that focus on information provision.

In addition, information alone may not have the desired effects. In a close analysis of AMR communications in the United Kingdom, Catherine Will (2020) has noted that AMR campaign evaluations have found that respondents with more accurate AMR knowledge were also found to be more likely to seek antibiotics and access them off prescription. These findings have led some experts to argue that AMR information may itself be counterproductive, though it is likely that other factors apart from knowledge produce the association between high levels of AMR knowledge and seeking out antibiotics, including experiences of chronic illness and recurrent infections.

Will (2020) showed how these findings have led some policy framings away from information and education approaches that emphasise accurate information about antibiotics, knowledge of how AMR is produced, and reflection on the need for antibiotics, towards behavioural economics (Australian Government, 2018; Connelly and Birch, 2020), that is, setting conditions that trigger, shape, and reinforce required behaviours so that they become more or less automatic. In Australia, behavioural economics has been used to shape the behaviours of prescribers (Australian Government, 2018). Letters from the Chief Medical Officer were sent to prescribers containing data that compared their prescription of antimicrobials with other practitioners. It was expected that knowledge that one's prescribing exceeded that of peers would lead to a decrease in prescribing. As the report of this intervention said, behavioural economics assumes that individuals are 'systematically biased' (Australian Government, 2018: 10) and need assistance to make appropriate decisions. According to the authors of the report:

> Rather than expect citizens to be optimal decision makers, drawing on behavioural insights ensures policy makers design policies that go with the grain of human behaviour. For example, citizens may struggle to act in a way that aligns with their own best interests, such as saving more money in case of an emergency. Policy makers can apply behavioural insights that preserve freedom, but help people align actions with intentions. (Australian Government, 2018: 10)

The turn in AMR governance towards this kind of framing of individual behaviour recalibrates the mix of self-management and external regulation. Note for example in the above quotation the reference to freedom mingled with notional citizens who are not able to act in their own 'best interests'. In this approach, individuals are less obviously collaborators in the effort to reduce AMR, but they come into view *as* the AMR problem. Will (2020) has argued that AMR governance based on these assumptions potentially closes off opportunities for deliberative and democratic public engagement with health threats. They represent a mode of governmentality that eschews support for the self-determining subject of AMR governance and turns towards communicative architectures that assert AMR governance despite the subject. Interestingly, too, the letter intervention for prescribers supports my previous comments that the individual patient may not have much sway over prescribing in Australia and similar contexts in other parts of the world.

This turn away from individual self-discipline may further the separation of public health systems from individuals such that policy and communications have the effect of negating the provision of information, the encouragement of understanding, and assisting its citizens to act for the benefit of their health. In this mode of operation, public health systems focus on the protection of antimicrobials to reduce AMR through shaping the conduct of individuals. Individuals become the problem, in place of the rightful, though more complex, focus on the biological-social-economic systems that produce AMR. The notion of the demanding patient is a case in point. This sleight-of-hand realignment of the individual subject to object of AMR governance augurs for further problems of public trust and the management of infectious diseases.

Some reflections on possible AMR governance futures

Individuals appear in AMR governance in contradictory ways. They are sometimes encouraged to be self-determining but also problematized in AMR policy and communications as more or less 'resistant' to information and advice and, in some instances, as transgressively subverting efforts to curb AMR by demanding access to antimicrobials. Individuals are therefore asked to reduce their use of antimicrobials and comply with the advice provided by experts. AMR governance also appears to focus on either the encouragement or constraint of individuals in place of the critical examination of the governmental, scientific, economic, and healthcare structures that bring antimicrobials into human and animal bodies with consequent effects on the circulation of AMR. The ways in which individuals are addressed in policy and communications reveal how AMR governance springs from the clinical and scientific knowledge generated by professionals in the field. AMR governance is predicated on the strengthening awareness among experts that antimicrobials are disappearing and that the health threat is gradually increasing. Indeed, the term 'antimicrobial resistance' indicates its origins in biomedical science and not in life worlds of affected individuals. There is little in the field of AMR that hails individuals invested in promoting their health and expanding the means by which they can reduce AMR harms. Missing in AMR governance is a searching engagement with members of the general public to find out what it is they want in relation to the effort to avert the superbugs crisis.

As part of efforts to address this limiting habit of thought in AMR governance, some qualitative researchers have explored how individuals think and feel about antibiotics and AMR (Davis, Lohm, Flowers, et al., 2021; Davis, Lohm, Lyall, et al., 2021; Davis et al., 2020; Whittaker et al., 2019). This research found that members of the general public reported that the use of antimicrobials emerged in everyday life in multiple ways, each with distinctive antecedent contexts and rationalities. Most importantly, antimicrobials were used in circumstances that had features not all of which were under the control of the individual. These included people who used antibiotics when they had travelled overseas and were unable to obtain access to a physician and therefore a prescription. Some travellers also reported that they had obtained a prescription from doctors in Australia prior to travel to be used in case of illness. Individuals also spoke of the circumstances when antibiotics were used to care for a pet or during the management of the health of a child. In these circumstances the use of drugs had a pronounced moral loading in the sense that the individual was responsible for a child or beloved pet, for example:

With human health you can engage with it a little bit more. You can give your opinion 'cause you're experiencing it. You can learn about it. But animal health it's sort of like the vet knows and you've just gotta trust them. And there's not really much engagement when you can't ask the animal how they're feeling. And we're all scared of hurting our beautiful pets so we just do as we're told. (Jenna, 31–40, lived with her partner, suffered from chronic fatigue)

Medical staff always say, 'Oh, you've gotta do this, this and this'. And as a parent, most of the time you've kind of just gotta go, 'OK, all right. Whatever you say. Just give her whatever she needs'. Am I being a difficult parent and being overly sort of hippie and sensitive, saying, 'Oh no, my child doesn't need antibiotics'? (Trevor, 41–50, married, two young children, healthy)

For those with chronic illness such as respiratory disease, antibiotics were said to be sought out at the first symptom of infection in order to reduce the likelihood of progress to a more severe infection. For others, antibiotics were used after a period of attempted self-management using over-the-counter pain relief and remedies. These various antibiotic use situations provide an alternative to the focus on remiss individuals, demanding ones included. They draw attention to various pathways of antibiotic consumption, each with their own real-world characteristics. They imply multiple agendas for practical assistance that individuals might need if they find themselves in these situations. This and similar research lead AMR governance to focus on individual needs in ways that are less constraining and more enabling and ones that do not focus on antimicrobials separated from real world contexts.

In line with qualitative inquiry and my previous comments, to ameliorate the negative effects of assumptions about and framings of individuals in AMR governance it would be helpful to conceptualize individuals as one component of the biological, social, and economic systems that produce AMR in human health, animal care, and agriculture. On that basis, it would be helpful to establish increased specificity in AMR governance regarding which kinds of prescribing events should be a focus for reduction and rationalization and how the individual can play their part to support healthy outcomes. This systems approach combined with target specificity could shift the focus from the awareness, knowledge, and behaviour of individuals to what action they can reasonably take in the social/economic systems that enable the delivery of antibiotics in community settings. There is also benefit to be found in closer alignment of AMR governance with the life worlds of individuals and engagement with what individuals want in terms of the management of infectious diseases, self-care that may not need to include antimicrobials. Real-world alignment of AMR governance and engagement would be consistent with the emphasis most often placed in healthcare on self-management. In place of the growing tendency in AMR governance to construct the individual as the problematized object, participatory and democratic dialogue with general publics about AMR is warranted (Will, 2020).

There are also wider implications that spring from this Foucauldian analysis of self-discipline and constraint in AMR governance. For example, antimicrobial prescribing in community settings across human and animal health variously combines state-provided care and commercial enterprise where self-regulation and external regulation meet and combine. As with individuals, AMR governance needs to address itself to the conditions of the public-private mix in prescribing transactions that may compromise efforts to reduce the use of antimicrobials and therefore further AMR. In the United Kingdom, as noted, individuals might have less sway over which medical practitioners they can choose to see and therefore less purchase on any demands they might have for antimicrobials. However, conditions of austerity in the NHS might produce other economic pressures; for instance, requirements on practitioners to increase throughput efficiency and therefore prescribe antimicrobials to avoid risks for the patient and themselves. In settings where antimicrobials are easily available off prescription in marketplaces in low- and middle-income countries, the economic conditions for antimicrobial use are different again. In these contexts, it is arguable that individuals seek to manage health risks in circumstances where their own choices become more salient as to whether or not antimicrobials are used (see Chapter 9).

Antimicrobials are taken into individual bodies, great quantities of antimicrobials are prescribed in community settings in Australia and elsewhere, and resistant microbes are linked with these phenomena. The individual, however, is one element of the biological, social, and economic systems that circulate antimicrobials across species and in the environment. I have argued that while a focus on the individual in AMR governance is warranted, the individual has so far been seen in vague terms as: free to act, but not always; everyone but therefore no-one in particular; outside complex AMR systems; and sharing with scientists and public health experts a primary focus on the health impacts of AMR. Closer inspection of evidence and the critical lens of governmentality reveal some of the drawbacks of these assumptions. AMR governance needs to orient towards improved and nuanced reckoning with what individuals need to help them play their parts in the reduction and rationalization of antimicrobial use. Closer alignment of AMR governance with what individuals need to sustain their health is crucial, not only because AMR is such a serious threat but because addressing it will require sustained action for many decades to come.

Acknowledgements

This chapter is based on research supported by Australian Research Council grants (DP170100937, DP200100002). My wonderful colleague, Dr Davina Lohm, helped me to conduct interviews that provided the foundation for the some of the analyses explored in this chapter. I offer my gratitude to the key informants and interviewees who contributed to our research.

References

Australian Commission on Safety and Quality in Health Care. (2019). *AURA 2019: Third Australian Report on Antimicrobial Use and Resistance in Human Health*.

Australian Commission on Safety and Quality in Health Care. (2020a). 'Antimicrobials: Handle with Care', <https://www.safetyandquality.gov.au/publications-and-resources/resource-library/antimicrobial-awareness-week-logo> accessed 24 August 2021.

Australian Commission on Safety and Quality in Health Care. (2020b). 'Do I Really Need Antibiotics', <https://www.safetyandquality.gov.au/publications-and-resources/resource-library/consumer-brochure-do-i-really-need-antibiotics> accessed 24 August 2021.

Australian Government. (2018). *Nudge vs Superbugs: A Behavioural Economics Trial to Reduce the Overprescribing of Antibiotics* (Canberra: Department of Health and Department of the Prime Minister and Cabinet).

Australian Government. (2019). *Australia's National Antimicrobial Resistance Strategy: 2020 & Beyond* (Canberra: Department of Health and Department of Agriculture, Water and the Environment, Canberra) <https://www.amr.gov.au/resources/australias-national-antimicrobial-resistance-strategy-2020-and-beyond> accessed 18 July 2021.

Australian Government. (2021). *Final Progress Report: Australia's First National Antimicrobial Resistance Strategy 2015–2019*.

Avorn, J., and Solomon, D. (2000). 'Cultural and Economic Factors That (Mis)Shape Antibiotic Use: The Nonpharmacologic Basis of Therapeutics', *Annals of Internal Medicine*, 133, 128–35.

Bhattacharya, A., Hopkins, S., Sallis, A., Budd, E., and Ashiru-Oredope, D. (2016). 'A Process Evaluation of the UK-wide Antibiotic Guardian Campaign: Developing Engagement on Antimicrobial Resistance', *Journal of Public Health*, 39/2, e40–e47.

Biezen, R., Brijnath, B., Grando, D., and Mazza, D. (2017). 'Management of Respiratory Tract Infections in Young Children—A Qualitative Study of Primary Care Providers' Perspectives', *Primary Care Respiratory* Medicine, 27/15. doi:10.1038/s41533-017-0018-x.

Cabral, C., Lucas, P., Ingram, J., Hay, A., and Horwood, J. (2015). '"It's Safer to ..." Parent Consulting and Clinician Antibiotic Prescribing Decisions for Children with Respiratory Tract Infections: An Analysis across Four Qualitative Studies', *Social Science & Medicine*, 136–137(156–64).

Connelly, L., and Birch, S. (2020). 'Sustainability of Publicly Funded Health Care Systems: What Does Behavioural Economics Offer?', *PharmacoEconomics*, 38, 1289–95.

Davis, M. (forthcoming). *Selling Immunity: Self, Culture and Economy in Healthcare and Medicine* (London: Routledge).

Davis, M., Lohm, D., Flowers, P., and Whittaker, A. (2021). 'The Immune Self, Hygiene and Performative Virtue in General Public Narratives on Antibiotics and Antimicrobial Resistance', *Health (United Kingdom)*. doi:10.1177/13634593211046832.

Davis, M., Lohm, D., Lyall, B., Schermuly, A., Rajkhowa, A., Flowers, P., Whittaker, A., and Lemoh, C. (2021). *Promoting Australian General Public Awareness and Action on Antimicrobial Resistance* (Melbourne: Monash University School of Social Sciences). <http://doi.org/10.26180/13101491> accessed 15 June 2021.

Davis, M., Lohm, D., Whittaker, A., and Flowers, P. (2020). '"Willy Nilly" Doctors, Bad Patients, and Resistant Bodies in General Public Explanations of Antimicrobial Resistance', *Sociology of Health & Illness*, 42/6, 1394–408.

DeFrank, J., Berkman, N., Kahwati, L., Cullen, K., Aikin, K., and Sullivan, H. (2020). 'Direct-to-Consumer Advertising of Prescription Drugs and the Patient–Prescriber Encounter: A Systematic Review', *Health Communication*, 35/6, 739–46.

Foucault, M. (1990). *The Care of The Self: The History of Sexuality, Volume 3* (London: Penguin).

Gualano, M., Gili, R., Scaioli, G., Bert, F., and Siliquini, R. (2015). 'General Population's Knowledge and Attitudes about Antibiotics: A Systematic Review and Meta-Analysis', *Pharmacoepidemiology and Drug Safety*, 24, 2–10.

Hardefeldt, L., Gilkerson, J., Billman-Jacobe, H., Stevenson, M., Thursky, K., Bailey, K., and Browning, G. (2018). 'Barriers to and Enablers of Implementing Antimicrobial Stewardship Programs in Veterinary Practices', *Journal of Veterinary Internal Medicine*, 32, 1092–9.

Harkins, C., Pichon, B., Doumith, M., Parkhill, J., Westh, H., Tomasz, A., de Lencastre, H., Bentley, S., Kearns, A., and Holden, M. (2017). 'Methicillin-resistant Staphylococcus Aureus Emerged Long Before the Introduction of Methicillin into Clinical Practice', *Genome Biology*, 18, 130.

Hincliffe, S. (2015). 'More than One World, More than One Health: Re-configuring Interspecies Health', *Social Science & Medicine*, 129, 28–35.

Huttner, B., Saam, M., Moja, L., Mah, K., Sprenger, M., Harbath, S., and Magrini, N. (2019). 'How to Improve Antibiotic Awareness Campaigns: Findings of a WHO Global Survey', *BMJ Global Health*, 4(e001239). doi:10.1136/bmjgh-2018-001239.

Keshavjee, S., and Farmer, P. (2012). 'Tuberculosis, Drug Resistance, and the History of Modern Medicine', *New England Journal of Medicine*, 367, 931–6.

Kesten, J., Bhattacharya, A., Ashiru-Oredope, D., Gobin, M., and Audrey, S. (2018). 'The Antibiotic Guardian Campaign: A Qualitative Evaluation of an Online Pledgebased System Focused on Making Better Use of Antibiotics', *BMC Public Health*, 18/5. doi:10.1186/s12889-017-4552-9.

King, C., Smith, M., Currie, K., Dickosn, A., Smith, F., Davis, M., and Flowers, P. (2018). 'Exploring the Behavioural Drivers of Veterinary Surgeon Antibiotic Prescribing: A Qualitative Study of Companion Animal Veterinary Surgeons in the UK', *BMC Veterinary Research*, 14, 332.

Kumar, S., Little, P., and Britten, N. (2003). 'Why Do General Practitioners Prescribe Antibiotics for Sore Throat? Grounded Theory Interview Study', *British Medical Journal*, 326.

Malik, B., and Bhattacharyya, S. (2019). 'Antibiotic Drug-resistance as a Complex System Driven by Socioeconomic Growth and Antibiotic Misuse', *Scientific Reports*, 9, 9788.

McCullough, A., Parekh, S., Rathbone, J., Del Mar, C., and Hoffmann, T. (2016). 'A Systematic Review of the Public's Knowledge and Beliefs About Antibiotic Resistance', *Journal of Antimicrobial Chemotherapy*, 71(1), 27–33.

Newitt, S., Anthierens, S., Coenen, S., Wong, D., Salvi, C., Puleston, R., and Ashiru-Oredope, D. (2018). 'Expansion of the "Antibiotic Guardian" One Health Behavioural Campaign Across Europe to Tackle Antibiotic Resistance: Pilot Phase and Analysis of AMR Knowledge', *The European Journal of Public Health*, 28/3, 437–9.

Newitt, S., Oloyede, O., Puleston, R., Hopkins, S., and Ashiru-Oredope, D. (2019). 'Demographic, Knowledge and Impact Analysis of 57,627 Antibiotic Guardians Who Have Pledged to Contribute to Tackling Antimicrobial Resistance', *Antibiotics*, 8/21. doi:10.3390/antibiotics8010021.

OECD. (2019). *Health at a Glance 2019: OECD Indicators* (Paris: OECD Publishing) <https://doi.org/10.1787/4dd50c09-en>.

Rose, N. (2007). *The Politics of Life Itself: Biomedicine, Power and Subjectivity in the Twenty-First Century* (Princeton, NJ: Princeton University Press).

Spruijit, P., and Petersen, A. (2020). 'Multilevel Governance of Antimicrobial Resistance Risks: A Literature Review', *Journal of Risk Research*, <https://doi.org/10.1080/13669877.2020.1779784>.

Teixeira Rodrigues, A., Roque, F., Falcão, A., Figueiras, A., and Herdeiro, M. (2013). 'Understanding Physician Antibiotic Prescribing Behaviour: A Systematic Review of Qualitative Studies', *International Journal of Antimicrobial Agents*, 41/3, 203–12. <https://doi.org/10.1016/j.ijantimicag.2012.09.003>.

White, A., and Hughes, J. (2019). 'Critical Importance of a One Health Approach to Antimicrobial Resistance', *EcoHealth*, 16, 404–9.

Whittaker, A., Lohm, D., Leoh, C., Cheng, A., and Davis, M. (2019). 'Investigating Understandings of Antibiotics and Antimicrobial Resistance in Diverse Ethnic Communities in Australia: Findings from a Qualitative Study', *Antibiotics*, 8/135, <https://doi:10.3390/antibiotics8030135>.

Will, C. (2020). 'The Problem and Productivity of Ignorance: Public Health Campaigns on Antibiotic Stewardship', *The Sociological Review*, 68/1, 55–76.

Wood, F., Simpson, S., and Butler, C. (2007). 'Socially Responsible Antibiotic Choices in Primary Care: A Qualitative Study of GPs' Decisions to Prescribe Broad-Spectrum and Fluroquinolone Antibiotics', *Family Practice*, 24/5, 427–34. <https://doi.org/10.1093/fampra/cmm040>.

WHO. (2015). *Global Action Plan on Antimicrobial Resistance* (Geneva: WHO). <https://www.who.int/publications/i/item/9789241509763> accessed 18 July 2021.

9

Governing AMR

A Case for Considering Governance 'from below'

Tabitha Hrynick, Syed Shahid Abbas, and Hayley MacGregor

Introduction

Over the last decade, there has been increasing recognition of and mobilization to address the unfolding crises posed by antimicrobial resistance (AMR) around the world. Much of this mobilization has taken place at global level, with UN agencies and high-income country (HIC) governments framing both the AMR problem and defining solutions through global discourses and governance mechanisms.[1] There has been a tendency for AMR to be framed as a crisis of the global commons brought about by irrational drug usage. Although global discourses recognize AMR's complexity and the imperative of ensuring equitable access to antibiotics for all, policy solutions tend to emphasize individual-level interventions focused on antibiotic conservation in human health, especially clinical settings. This oversimplifies the multi-site, multi-scale, multi-sector, and multi-actor dimensions of AMR, and obscures the political economic systems which produce and perpetuate it (see Chapter 8 for further discussion). This is especially the case for low- and middle-income countries (LMICs) in which health and other systems do not resemble those of the HICs which have led the global discourse on AMR (see Chapter 2). Rather, addressing AMR will require much more tailored and context-appropriate approaches in LMICs.

This chapter explores tensions between the discourses around the global governance for AMR, and the realities of LMIC settings, as well as the competing priorities of the health, pharmaceutical, and livestock systems. More specifically, we consider examples from Bangladesh, which like other LMICs is at high risk for AMR (Chereau et al., 2017). Bangladesh also has characteristics common to many LMICs, including a large informal sector for drugs and health services. Our analysis draws upon an alternative conceptualization of governance (Leach et al., 2007) to the conventional legal

---

[1] Reports, action plans, and strategies at this level have primarily come from the United States, United Kingdom, and international agencies over the last decade. They include: the UK Five Year Antimicrobial Resistance Strategy 2013 to 2018 (Davies and Gibbens, 2013); the US National Action Plan for Combating Antibiotic-Resistant Bacteria (US Government, 2015); the Global Action Plan on AMR (WHO, 2015); the OIE Strategy on Antimicrobial Resistance and the Prudent Use of Antimicrobials (OIE, 2016); the FAO Action Plan on Antimicrobial Resistance 2016–2020 (FAO, 2016); *Tackling Drug-Resistant Infections Globally: Final Report and Recommendations* (O'Neill, 2016); and *Drug Resistant Infections: A Threat to our Economic Future* (Adeyi et al., 2017).

Tabitha Hrynick, Syed Shahid Abbas, and Hayley MacGregor, *Governing AMR* In: *Steering against Superbugs*. Edited by: Olivier Rubin, Erik Baekkeskov, and Louise Munkholm, Oxford University Press. © Oxford University Press 2023. DOI: 10.1093/oso/9780192899477.003.0009

and regulatory lens. It foregrounds perspectives 'from below', suggesting effective governance should be networked, deliberative, power aware, and adaptive. We argue an effective global governance for AMR is unachievable without also supporting and integrating 'governance from below'; the empowerment and leadership of people across stakeholder groups to develop and adapt their own context-appropriate solutions.

We highlight some examples of alternative AMR governance 'from below' that illustrate how these four principles can be put into practice. The examples include community-based regulation of drug shops, community-based dialogue around norms, and One Health 'competency groups' in the aquaculture sector. These initiatives illustrate the possibilities of expanding understandings of governance to include alternative models that account for local contexts and avoid transplanting blueprints into diverse settings.

Reframing governance

The conceptualization of governance advanced by Leach et al. (2007) broadly interprets 'governance' as the political and institutional processes and power relations that shape how people understand, organize, make decisions, and act within complex socio-ecological systems. Thus, 'governance' amounts to far more than the legal frameworks, formal agreements, and technical action plans of international power brokers, governments, and other formal actors emphasized in conventional approaches to governance. Through this alternative understanding, Leach and colleagues also advance a set of principles for achieving more holistic governance of critical issues, including 'wicked problems' like AMR. These hold that governance should be: (i) *networked* across a wide range of stakeholders across sectors and scales; (ii) *deliberative*, providing space to reflect and reformulate action based on inclusivity and diverse perspectives and interests of stakeholders; (iii) *power aware*, recognizing that not all stakeholders have the same agency, and ensuring mechanisms support equity; and (iv) *adaptive*, flexible, and responsive to inevitable shifts in dynamics and drivers of the problem.

Another key aspect of Leach and colleagues' approach to governance is the recognition of the diversity of framings and interpretations of a problem and its solutions, held among differently positioned, and more or less powerful, stakeholders. In the case of AMR, the dominant framing is of AMR as a healthcare issue (Wernli et al., 2017). This framing, highly visible within high-profile governance discourse, emphasizes formal clinical human health settings and patient–provider interactions. Interventions such as information and education, treatment guidelines, and other stewardship activities targeting providers and patients are seen as central to reducing unnecessary or improper use. While infection control is increasingly also advocated (e.g., hospital hygiene measures), this framing focuses on individualizing measures that shift the responsibility for making the 'right' decisions on to patients and providers (Chandler, 2019). However, this is shot through with assumptions about what is 'right' and fails to recognize the powerful ways context and wider structural factors beyond healthcare shape and constrain people's behaviour. For instance, in settings where doctors may know that their patients will return to environments where they are at high risk of infection (e.g., overcrowded informal urban settlements), or that they are unlikely to find it easy to return for follow up, the decision to provide antimicrobials outside treatment recommendations may indeed seem like the right and ethical decision to ensure patient health in the short term (Kotwani et al., 2012). Norms and expectations from patients—real or perceived—to provide antimicrobials may also influence provider prescribing behaviour, along with myriad other factors (Wilkinson et al., 2019). In the private sector, this is amplified by concerns to retain patient-customers.

At the same time, policy measures that restrict availability or use of certain antimicrobials (e.g., by-prescription-only policies) are also often advocated to regulate use in the human health sector. Where formal healthcare is not universally accessible (or affordable), such restrictions can push antimicrobial drugs—critical health resources in settings beset by high burdens of infectious disease—beyond the reach of people who desperately need them. Indeed, a recent study showed lack of access to antibiotics still results in more deaths than does resistance itself (Laxminarayan et al., 2016). There are also challenges in implementing regulations in such settings; 'unofficial' practices can occur under the radar, making them hard to address. Furthermore, the vast majority of workers in LMICs including Bangladesh, engage in informal work without benefits like decent pay or sick leave, and may even lose their jobs by missing a day of work (ADB and BBS, 2010). For these workers, antimicrobials are a crucial means to maintain their ability to meet their basic needs through quick recovery from illness (Denyer Willis and Chandler, 2019). This is often achieved through incomplete dosing that can contribute to AMR (Sutradhar et al., 2014).

By recognizing these alternative problem framings foregrounding the realities of differently placed individuals, their decisions to recommend or take antimicrobials can be reframed from 'irrational' to the only rational choice available to ensure survival. Through this lens, antimicrobials can be seen as a form of 'infrastructure' upholding entire economies and lives (Chandler, 2019). Restricting access thus has serious implications for health equity, particularly in the absence of broader social safety nets. A key challenge for AMR governance is thus to integrate these and other diverse framings, perspectives, interests, and needs. In the following sections, we present examples from Bangladesh which illustrate how local realities shape AMR, as well as opportunities for addressing this problem without compromising critical access to antimicrobial drugs.

An alternative vision for governing AMR: Insights from Bangladesh

In this section, we cite four sets of examples from Bangladesh. These demonstrate the wide range of actors and their different modes of engagement required to govern production, distribution, and consumption of antimicrobials in the context of Bangladesh. The first example cites the Bangladesh National Drugs Policy (NDP) of 1982 where the national government worked with industry to promote local production to ensure access to 'essential drugs' (Chowdhury et al., 2006). Second, we discuss the ways in which actors in pluralistic health systems can promote access to essential health services while contributing to the problem of AMR, and the importance of engaging them. Third, we present examples of 'bottom-up' governance implemented in the human health sector. Finally, we examine how a One Health lens can help identify modalities and challenges associated with engaging non-health sectors in AMR governance and offer an example of a 'bottom-up' initiative in this domain.

National Drugs Policy of 1982: Expanding access and equity, but creating a path-dependency for AMR

As a recently independent country under a military leadership which was impatient to achieve economic and social progress—and against the backdrop of a reformist call for Essential Drugs List by the World Health Organization (WHO)—Bangladesh developed its landmark National Drugs Policy (NDP) in 1982. The NDP aimed to remake the foreign-dominated costly pharmaceutical sector by increasing local production of 'essential' drugs and making them easily available at stable prices (Chowdhury et al., 2006).

The NDP is accepted to have successfully limited imports of drugs with limited therapeutic value, stabilized drug prices, and increased the market share of local pharmaceutical manufacturers in Bangladesh (Reich, 1994). However, the NDP could not regulate the prescription and consumption of newly available drugs, and antimicrobials are now widely available through public and private (and as an unintended consequence, informal) sector pathways. The state has limited capacity to regulate the now flourishing pharmaceutical market. Firms also engage in aggressive marketing, and provide a critical, readily available information service for healthcare providers (especially private and informal providers and drug sellers) who may not receive regular training or information from non-commercial sources (Bloom et al., 2011).

As already suggested, conventional governance approaches tend to emphasize legal frameworks, state-led and 'top down' regulation processes, with AMR interventions focused predominantly on human health. Clearly, high-level policies can be effective, as illustrated by the NDP's role in expanding access to critical drugs. However, these 'ideal' blueprints can be hard to implement and also have many unintended consequences due in part to informality in healthcare, and livelihood and work precarity.

Bangladesh's pluralistic health system

Embedded within global AMR discourses are assumptions about health systems as cohesive, monolithic, and homogenous. While this may fairly characterize health systems in many HICs, it does not resemble the reality of LMICs. Rather, health systems in these settings, including Bangladesh, are highly fragmented and pluralistic (Ahmed et al., 2013; Bloom et al., 2015). The limited capacities of states to fund and resource robust public systems leave huge gaps into which a multiplicity of private, including informal, health actors emerge. Private, especially informal health actors are often regarded with suspicion by national governments, even actively demonized, and yet play critical roles in providing essential services the state itself cannot provide (Pinto, 2004). Indeed, despite the expanded availability of essential drugs in the wake of the NDP, regular stockouts of essential drugs in public facilities in Bangladesh, and a dearth of trained medical professionals, especially in rural areas, mean private services may be the only health services upon which many can rely.

In Bangladesh, the private health sector consists of clinics and hospitals run by for-profit and non-profit actors, as well as physicians, traditional health practitioners, and 'village doctors' (unqualified, although sometimes partially trained allopathic providers, who often also sell drugs and medicines). There are as many informal drug sellers as licensed pharmacies, although even the latter are only weakly regulated (Ahmed et al., 2017). The boundaries between public and private and formal and informal health entities and actors are also blurred. For instance, informal user fees may be demanded in ostensibly free or low-cost public clinics, while formal clinics or hospitals may prescribe medications patients are expected to purchase from private and/or informal drug sellers (Bloom et al., 2015; Lucas et al., 2019). Another important force in this system is the aggressive marketing and sale of antimicrobials by pharmaceutical companies, especially to providers of such drugs (Mohiuddin et al., 2015). In a context of lax regulation and coupled with profit incentives and patient expectations for antibiotics, this results in 44 per cent of clinical consultations resulting in their prescription in Bangladesh (Ahmed and Islam, 2012). Although informal and untrained health actors may be viewed as the key problem, multiple and incomplete dosing through prescription via qualified doctors has also been observed (Lucas et al., 2019). Thus, while the pluralistic health system in Bangladesh seem to meet critical health needs, it fails to combat rising AMR rates.

'Bottom-up governance' in human health

Given the complexity of this system, including diverse actors and incentives, norms and expectations, disease burdens and socio-economic realities—how can antimicrobial medicines be governed to mitigate AMR without compromising access, and indeed, continuing to improve health equity? While top-down governance can certainly play an important role, it cannot on its own account for or shape the myriad incentives and pathways through which antimicrobial drugs flow in this system. Furthermore, the state does not have the capacity to enforce regulations adequately. To bridge this gap, complementary forms of governance 'from below', adapted to local contexts, led by diverse stakeholders at sub-national and local levels (Nahar et al., 2017) are critical.

Below we give concrete examples of initiatives where AMR governance is advanced 'from below' both through regulation as well as dialogue at community level.

Community-based regulation

In a 2007 project led by the International Health Research Institute (icddr,b), village doctors were invited to participate in a series of training events and provided with a handbook of treatment guidelines in a rural district (Bhuiya, 2009; Bloom et al., 2011). A local professional association was established, into which the doctors were offered membership and given permission to use the association's logo for their business. To keep them accountable, a governing committee comprising local civil society representatives, health experts, and government and religious leaders was established to create the membership criteria, and to recertify or dismiss members accordingly. In this way, the model acknowledges that information alone cannot change behaviour (see also Chapter 8). Rather, incentive structures themselves need to be changed; in this case, the dynamics of a 'reputational economy' (Broom et al., 2018) are harnessed, allowing the community itself to govern the local health and drug market through demand and patronization of accredited establishments. Although this initiative had the broader aim of protecting Bangladeshis from 'incompetent medical practices and dangerous medicines' (Bloom et al., 2011: 8), concerns about antimicrobial dispensing and proper information on use could also be incorporated.

In comparison, the Bangladesh government launched a Model Pharmacy programme in 2018 to accredit informal drug shops. However the success of this top-down model may be contingent on state collaboration with and leveraging of existing community structures to hold drug shops accountable, as in the icddr,b project described above. In Uganda, Tanzania, and Liberia, a scheme called the Accredited Drug Dispensing Outlet has provided a similar, scalable model, based on cooperation between state and private actors working together to ensure accountability (Lucas et al., 2019). This 'decentred understanding of regulation recognises that states, on their own, cannot ensure the effective functioning of complete markets' (Bloom et al., 2015: 8) and flips the focus from a top-down to a bottom-up strategy. With respect to the principles for governance outlined above, in embracing the role of informal drug providers in the Model Pharmacy programme, the Bangladeshi state still demonstrates willingness to enact a more networked approach to governing medicines. Working with a diversity of local actors could further enhance this governance, including by ensuring mechanisms are adapted to local contexts and dynamics, and power aware in that access to resources, support, or accreditation is equitable and fair.

Community-based dialogue

Community-based dialogue approaches in Bangladesh have been leveraged to inform health policy in alignment with local health needs and priorities, and to support reformulation of health norms and behaviours. An example of the former, 'Health Dialogue for the People'—an initiative taken by the Directorate of General Health Services in 2016—involved citizens, health workers, managers, and policy actors to facilitate collective recognition and articulation of local health needs and shortcomings, decision-making, and establishment of community-based structures for accountability of health services (iccdr,b, 2016). While the Health Dialogue may not have explicitly considered antimicrobial use and the threat of AMR locally, it may inspire future local-level action on AMR, which can also feed local insight upwards to inform higher level policy in ways that increase its context appropriateness.

In the case of targeting health norms and behaviours, community dialogue approaches (CDA) have been explicitly applied to AMR. For instance, a pilot project based on partnerships between academics and local health system actors facilitated hundreds of CDA events in peri-urban Comilla district, to which all community members were encouraged to attend and contribute (King, 2020; King et al., 2020). While lessons learned from these events have not been substantially described, there is scope and potential for further experimentation with CDA as a form of 'governance from below' in its targeting of norms and behaviour—arguably the most invisible form of 'governance', that has profound implications for AMR. The inclusion of health providers—both formal and informal—is also critical because many, especially in rural areas or with no or limited training, remain unaware of AMR (Nahar et al., 2020). While this approach has clear limitations—it cannot alter structural conditions and incentives ultimately driving antimicrobial use—it may play an important complementary role alongside other forms of governance at different levels which can address those broader issues.

In addition to being a more networked and inclusive approach which brings a wide range of community members to the table, community-based dialogue is also inherently deliberative. If facilitated with attention to power dynamics within communities (ensuring all voices, including those of vulnerable groups, are meaningfully represented), key local insights could also emerge and flow upward to ensure higher level governance and policy remains relevant, adaptive, and effective.

Governing AMR across sectors: One Health approaches in Bangladesh

As mentioned, discourses around AMR tend to centre around human health settings and interactions. This is also the case in Bangladesh where the majority of research and policy has focused on human health (Hoque et al., 2020). However, AMR is a far more complex problem that includes resistant organisms originating from and impacting multiple animal species and economic sectors. Indeed, the vast majority of antimicrobials used globally are thought to be used within animal agriculture for both infection prevention and control and for animal growth promotion (AGP), the latter of which is frequently targeted in AMR policy, including in Bangladesh (Orubu et al., 2020).

The Ganges floodplain upon which Bangladesh is situated is said to 'support more humans and animals than any other place on earth' (FAO, 2018), and many people rely on livestock for subsistence or income. This density provides ample opportunity for pathogens and resistance genes to spread. As with human medicines, antimicrobial drugs for animal use are widely available including through informal markets in which enforcement of existing regulations is challenging (Goutard et al., 2017; Hoque et al., 2020; Orubu et al., 2020). Drug manufacturers aggressively market their products, including through deployment of dealers and industry-linked veterinarians, and exploit loopholes in regulations which have banned use of antimicrobials in animal and fish feed for growth promotion (focusing instead on products to add to water) (FAO, 2018). Furthermore, the conditions with which most ordinary people are forced to contend to raise livestock are not conducive to biosecurity, leaving them reliant on antimicrobials to keep their animals alive and healthy enough to turn even the smallest margin of profit (Chandler, 2019; Kakkar et al., 2018). Cognizant of these challenges, the Bangladeshi government has taken steps to tackle AMR through a One Health approach that seeks to extend governance to include actors across sectors. In addition to banning the use of antimicrobials for AGP, it has, along with the WHO and Food and Agriculture Organization of the United Nations (FAO), supported the establishment of the Bangladesh Antimicrobial Resistance Alliance (BARA) which brings together veterinary and medical experts to develop guidelines to address AMR in respective sectors. The guidelines are available via training programmes and an app accessible 'in the field', while a social media based 'community of practice' has been established where practitioners, including veterinarians, animal health workers, and extension officers are said to share advice and resources (Fleming Fund, 2018; IACG, 2018). The extent to which this has or can change practice on the ground (including who it may or may not reach) however is unclear, and research is needed to ascertain this. Nevertheless, through bringing together experts and stakeholders operating on the ground, it may provide opportunities for members to develop new sets of norms and knowledge to adapt practices to context. Below, we give one example of how this has been done in the case of local aquacultural production in Bangladesh.

'Bottom-up governance' of AMR through a One Health lens: An example
from aquaculture
One innovative research-cum-action project sought to transcend the limitations of conventional top-down, guideline and education-based approaches to addressing AMR in agriculture. A team of anthropologists facilitated the collaboration of stakeholders in a local system of shrimp and prawn production in Bangladesh, in which substantial antimicrobial use occurs (Hinchliffe et al., 2018). Through dialogue and mapping exercises, these 'competency groups', including farmers, suppliers, and government officials, mapped the complex, multi-layered and dynamic pressures and processes which drove their use of vast quantities of antimicrobials (see Chapters 10, 13, and 19 for examples of top-driven governance initiatives). These included the poor quality of brood stock available to hatcheries (and of antimicrobials themselves), the prohibitive costs of

disease testing and biosecurity, and increasing competition in the international market which exerted constant downward pressure. Notably, many of these factors were beyond the control of farmers themselves, the group most often targeted in conventional behavioural change interventions. In drawing on their collective experience and knowledge to map this 'social ecology of food production', the emergence, persistence, and transmission of AMR is reframed from a problem solution reducible to regulation of medicine and individual behaviour alone, to one requiring recognition of context-specificity, complexity, and multi-pronged, multi-scale, adaptive solutions.

This grassroots exercise clearly embodied the principles of governance argued for in this chapter. It was: (i) networked, in that it brought together a range of stakeholders who would not normally engage in such a way; (ii) deliberative, in that it facilitated critical understanding of the local system through dialogue and mapping; (iii) power aware in that it brought more or less powerful actors together and facilitated understanding of power within the broader systems and structures in which they were embedded; (iv) and adaptive in that it is plausible that the newfound awareness and linkages developed between actors generated through the activities could conceivably lead to dynamic shifts in local practices and opportunities for collective advocacy for change at different levels. Such initiatives could provide starting points from which local actors could begin to build pathways to address aspects of AMR emergence within their control, while identifying those aspects beyond it. If supported by and networked into governance systems at higher levels which are also power aware, deliberative, and adaptive, the capacity for change and expertise produced at this level could be leveraged, further supported, and used to adapt governance and policy at national, regional, and even global levels where key structural aspects might be addressed.

Discussion: Implementing the principles of governance from below

Governance regimes tend to be designed by those who wield the most influence or are the most visible. Alternative understandings of the problems and solutions are often excluded from decision-making processes. Yet, any attempts to govern a 'wicked problem' such as AMR requires going beyond simplistic and decontextualized solutions, to recognize and embrace the messiness, complexity, and power hierarchies involved in the AMR policy scape.

None of the examples cited above represent an idealized version of AMR governance, or 'best practices' to be exported to other settings. Indeed, the examples of governance 'from below' were small-scale pilot projects or specific academic explorations, and therefore might themselves not be easily scaled or replicated. Our purpose for identifying these examples, and those illustrating the realities of the system in Bangladesh (and many other LMICs), was to highlight the diverse sets of interests, incentives, and world views that influence how antimicrobials are used, and to illustrate how more localized forms of governance, which engage a more diverse set of actors and perspectives around AMR, can support more contextually appropriate, and thus effective, solutions.

While the NDP allowed Bangladesh to expand access to essential drugs substantially, in a way representing a more networked approach that enabled small-scale drug producers to help begin to plug critical gaps, more *networked* approaches are now necessary to address the unintended consequence of AMR. Broader sets of stakeholders and inputs to feed into mutually reinforcing governance processes from the local to national and even global level will be necessary. Such engagement can take place in formal but also non-formal platforms, such as community dialogues that provide space for critical and *deliberative* feedback and reflection. There are also opportunities for explicit linkages between national policies such as Bangladesh's Model Pharmacy programme and forms of governance from below, such as community-based regulatory models.

Not everyone enjoys the same level of agency to change their circumstances and their use of antimicrobials. Quite often, as in the case of competitive export markets for aquacultural products, structural factors determine antimicrobial use and prevent changing practices. For many informal workers, drug stock-outs and lack of access to formal healthcare may leave people with no option but to purchase antimicrobials from informal pharmacies for symptomatic relief. Decisions to regulate production, distribution, dispensation, and usage of antimicrobials will therefore need to be *power aware*, in other words to take into account the different forms of power and inequalities, and how this translates into a politics of knowledge.

Lastly, there is a need to recognize the dynamic nature of AMR and its drivers. Practices contributing to AMR in health seeking, prescription patterns, and livestock rearing are influenced by availability of providers, income levels, sources of livelihood, drug availability, demands upon livestock production, and more. These and other drivers will change with time, and in turn, influence other downstream factors contributing to AMR. Therefore, AMR strategies need to go beyond static approaches and ring-fenced objectives to promote flexibility, reflection, and *adaptation*.

For governance to be effective, the principles we have outlined—networked, deliberative, power-aware, and adaptive—apply both to more traditional top-down forms governance and to forms of governance 'from below'. However, adoption of these principles by high-level, more conventional governance institutions all but mandates that bottom-up processes are integrated, or at least recognized and supported by the former. Indeed, to be power aware and adaptive, perspectives from a widely networked range of stakeholders must be represented. This includes the least powerful actors, and those existing at the 'coalfaces' of antimicrobial production, distribution, and use, and who are subject to, and often acutely aware of, shifting structural dynamics and incentives beyond their control. And while forms of governance 'from below', particularly in LMICs but also HICs, may be able to address some local pathways of AMR emergence in context-appropriate ways (and should be supported with resources to do so), they are not a panacea when it comes to the 'wicked', transboundary problem that is AMR.

Yet, they may amount to much greater than the sum of their parts if treated as critical and integral to broader 'global governance' for AMR.

Conclusion

We have argued for the value of an approach to governance that moves beyond 'top-down' approaches emphasizing regulatory frameworks to include 'bottom-up' perspectives from a wider range of relevant stakeholders. We also contend that the dominant framing of AMR that is evident in global level plans has tended to focus on individual behaviour and has been less attentive to the contextual realities in different settings and the structural drivers of AMR. With reference to Bangladesh, we explore examples of different approaches to governance 'from below' that account for the pluralistic nature of the health system in better ways than have been available, include community dialogue and input, and foster collaboration across stakeholders and sectors. These examples, albeit drawn from smaller-scale initiatives, provide some pointers to how an alternative approach to AMR might be developed based on the four principles of networked, deliberative, power-aware, and adaptive governance. This might enable progress to address the many challenges of governance and a greater appreciation of governance from the perspective of people on the ground.

References

Adeyi, O., Baris, E., Jonas, O., Irwin, A., Berthe, F., Le Gall, F., et al. (2017). *Drug-resistant Infections: A Threat to Our Economic Future* (Washington, D.C.: World Bank Group).

Ahmed, S., Evans, T., Standing, H., and Mahmud, S. (2013). 'Harnessing Pluralism for Better Health in Bangladesh'. *The Lancet*, 382/9906, 1746–55. <https://doi.org/10.1016/S0140-6736(13)62147-9>.

Ahmed, S., and Islam, Q. (2012). 'Availability and Rational Use of Drugs in Primary Healthcare Facilities Following the National Drug Policy of 1982: Is Bangladesh on Right Track?', *Journal of Health, Population and Nutrition*, 30/1, 99–108. <https://doi.org/10.3329/jhpn.v30i1.11289>.

Ahmed, S., Naher, N., Hossain, T., and Rawal, L. (2017). 'Exploring the Status of Retail Private Drug Shops in Bangladesh and Action Points for Developing an Accredited Drug Shop Model: A Facility-based Cross-Sectional Study'. *Journal of Pharmaceutical Policy and Practice*, 10(1), 1–12. <https://doi.org/10.1186/s40545-017-0108-8>.

Asian Development Bank (ADB), and Bangladesh Bureau of Statistics (BBS). (2010). *The Informal Sector and Informal Employment in Bangladesh: Country Report 2010*. Manila: Asian Development Bank.

Bhuiya, A., ed. *Health for the Rural Masses: Insights from Chakaria* (icddr,b, 2009).

Bloom, G., Standing, H., Lucas, H., Bhuiya, A., Oladepo, O., and Peters, D. (2011). 'Making Health Markets Work Better for Poor People: The Case of Informal Providers'. *Health Policy and Planning*, 26(supplement 1), i45–i52. <https://doi.org/10.1093/heapol/czr025>.

Bloom, G., Wilkinson, A., Tomson, G., Awor, P., Zhang, X., Ahmed, S. M., et al. (2015). *Addressing Resistance to Antibiotics in Pluralist Health Systems*. Brighton: STEPS Centre.

Broom, A., Kenny, K., Kirby, E., George, N., and Chittem, M. (2018). 'Improvisation, Therapeutic Brokerage and Antibiotic (Mis)Use in India: A Qualitative Interview Study of Hyderabadi Physicians and Pharmacists'. *Critical Public Health*, 0/0, 1–12. <https://doi.org/10.1080/09581 596.2018.1516032<.

Chandler, C. (2019). 'Current Accounts of Antimicrobial Resistance: Stabilisation, Individualisation and Antibiotics as Infrastructure'. *Palgrave Communications*, 5/1, 1–13. <https://doi.org/10.1057/s41599-019-0263-4>.

Chereau, F., Opatowski, L., Tourdjman, M., and Vong, S. (2017). 'Risk Assessment for Antibiotic Resistance in South East Asia'. *British Medical Journal (Clinical Research edition)*, 358, j3393. <https://doi.org/10.1136/bmj.j3393>.

Chowdhury, F., Ahasan, H., and Rahman, M. (2006). 'National Drug Policy of Bangladesh: Some Pitfalls in Implementation'. *Journal of the College of Physicians and Surgeons–Pakistan*, 16/5, 368–70. <https://doi.org/5.2006/JCPSP.368370>.

Davies, S., and Gibbens, N. (2013). *UK Five Year Antimicrobial Resistance Strategy*. Department of Health. <https://assets.publishing.service.gov.uk/government/uploads/system/uploads/attachment_data/file/244058/20130902_UK_5_year_AMR_strategy.pdf>. (Accessed 3 March 2020).

Denyer Willis, L., and Chandler, C. (2019). 'Quick Fix for Care, Productivity, Hygiene and Inequality: Reframing the Entrenched Problem of Antibiotic Overuse'. *BMJ Global Health*, 4/4, e001590. <https://doi.org/10.1136/bmjgh-2019-001590>.

FAO. (2016). *The FAO Action Plan on Antimicrobial Resistance 2016–2020* (Geneva: FAO).

FAO. (2018). *Tackling AMR in Bangladesh—A One Health Approach*. <https://www.youtube.com/watch?v=YmOey7FGrfE>. (Accessed 1 November 2019)

Fleming Fund. (2018). *Moving from Plans to Action—Updates on the FAO's Fleming Fund Work*. Fleming Fund. <https://www.flemingfund.org/publications/moving-from-plans-to-action-updates-on-the-faos-fleming-fund-work/>. (Accessed 15 October 2019)

Goutard, F. L., Bordier, M., Calba, C., Erlacher-Vindel, E., Góchez, D., Balogh, et al. (2017). 'Antimicrobial Policy Interventions in Food Animal Production in South East Asia'. *British Medical Journal*, 358, j3544. <https://doi.org/10.1136/bmj.j3544>.

Hinchliffe, S., Butcher, A., and Rahman, M. (2018). 'The AMR Problem: Demanding Economies, Biological Margins, and Co-Producing Alternative Strategies'. *Palgrave Communications*, 4/1, 142. <https://doi.org/10.1057/s41599-018-0195-4>.

Hoque, R., Ahmed, S., Naher, N., Islam, M., Rousham, E., Islam, B., et al. (2020). 'Tackling Antimicrobial Resistance in Bangladesh: A Scoping Review of Policy and Practice in Human, Animal and Environment Sectors'. *PLoS ONE*, 15/1, e0227947. <https://doi.org/10.1371/journal.pone.0227947>.

IACG. (2018). *Meeting the Challenge of Antimicrobial Resistance: From Communication to Collective Action* [Discussion paper]. <https://cdn.who.int/media/docs/default-source/antimicrobial-resistance/ iacg-meeting-challenge-amr-communication-to-collective-action-270718.pdf>. (Accessed 23 March 2023).

iccdr, b. (2016). 'Engaging People in Health Dialogues'. *Global Health Insights*. <http://blog.icddrb.org/2016/10/31/public-engagement-health-sector-icddrb-share/>. (Accessed 3 October 2019).

Kakkar, M., Chatterjee, P., Chauhan, A. S., Grace, D., Lindahl, J., Beeche, A., et al. (2018). 'Antimicrobial Resistance in South East Asia: Time to Ask the Right Questions'. *Global Health Action*, 11/1, 1483637. <https://doi.org/10.1080/16549716.2018.1483637>. (Accessed 3 September 2019).

King, R. (2020). *Community Dialogues for Preventing and Controlling Antibiotic Resistance in Bangladesh* (Research Brief). <https://medicinehealth.leeds.ac.uk/dir-record/research-projects/986/community-dialogues-for-preventing-and-controlling-antibiotic-resistance-in-bangladesh>. (Accessed 23 October 2019)

King, R., Hicks, J., Rassi, C., Shafique, M., Barua, D., Bhowmik, P., et al. (2020). 'A Process for Developing a Sustainable and Scalable Approach to Community Engagement: Community Dialogue Approach for Addressing the Drivers of Antibiotic Resistance in Bangladesh'. *BMC Public Health*, 20/1, 950. <https://doi.org/10.1186/s12889-020-09033-5>.

Kotwani, Wattal, C., Joshi, P. C., and Holloway, K. (2012). 'Irrational Use of Antibiotics and Role of the Pharmacist: An Insight from a Qualitative Study in New Delhi, India'. *Journal of Clinical Pharmacy and Therapeutics*, 37/3, 308–12.

Laxminarayan, R., Matsoso, P., Pant, S., Brower, C., Røttingen, J.-A., Klugman, K., et al. (2016). 'Access to Effective Antimicrobials: A Worldwide Challenge'. *The Lancet*, 387/10014, 168–75. <https://doi.org/10.1016/S0140-6736(15)00474-2>.

Leach, M., Bloom, G., Ely, A., Nightingale, P., Scoones, I., Shah, E., et al. (2007). *Understanding Governance: Pathways to Sustainability* [Working paper]. Brighton: STEPS Centre. <https://steps-centre.org/publication/understanding-governance-pathways-to-sustainability/>. (Accessed 10 September 2019).

Lucas, P., Uddin, M., Khisa, N., Akter, S., Unicomb, L., Nahar, P., et al. (2019). 'Pathways to Antibiotics in Bangladesh: A Qualitative Study Investigating How and When Households Access Medicine Including Antibiotics for Humans or Animals When They Are Ill'. *PLoS ONE*, 14/11, e0225270. <https://doi.org/10.1371/journal.pone.0225270>.

Mohiuddin, M., Rashid, S., Shuvro, M., Nahar, N., and Ahmed, S. (2015). 'Qualitative Insights into Promotion of Pharmaceutical Products in Bangladesh: How Ethical Are the Practices?', *BMC Medical Ethics*, 16/1, 80. <https://doi.org/10.1186/s12910-015-0075-z>.

Nahar, P., Kannuri, N. K., Mikkilineni, S., Murthy, G., and Phillimore, P. (2017). 'At the Margins of Biomedicine: The Ambiguous Position of "Registered Medical Practitioners" in Rural Indian Healthcare'. *Sociology of Health and Illness*, 39/4, 614–28. <https://doi.org/10.1111/1467-9566.12521>.

Nahar, P., Unicomb, L., Lucas, P., Uddin, M., Islam, M., Nizame, F., et al. (2020). 'What Contributes to Inappropriate Antibiotic Dispensing Among Qualified and Unqualified Healthcare Providers in Bangladesh? A Qualitative Study'. *BMC Health Services Research*, 20/1, 656. <https://doi.org/10.1186/s12913-020-05512-y>.

OIE. (2016). *The OIE Strategy on Antimicrobial Resistance and the Prudent Use of Antimicrobials* (Paris: OIE). <https://www.oie.int/fileadmin/Home/eng/Media_Center/docs/pdf/PortailAMR/EN_OIE-AMRstrategy.pdf>. (Accessed 24 March 2020).

O'Neill, J. (2016). *Tackling Drug-resistant Infections Globally: Final Report and Recommendations*. <https://wellcomecollection.org/works/thvwsuba/items> (Accessed 23 March 2023).

Orubu, E. S. F., Zaman, M. H., Rahman, M. T., and Wirtz, V. J. (2020). 'Veterinary Antimicrobial Resistance Containment in Bangladesh: Evaluating the National Action Plan and Scoping the Evidence on Implementation'. *Journal of Global Antimicrobial Resistance*, 21, 105–15. <https://doi.org/10.1016/j.jgar.2019.09.020>.

Pinto, S. (2004). 'Development without Institutions: Ersatz Medicine and the Politics of Everyday Life in Rural North India'. *Cultural Anthropology*, 19/3, 337–64. <https://anthrosource.onlinelibrary.wiley.com/doi/abs/10.1525/can.2004.19.3.337>. (Accessed 23 March 2023).

Reich, M. (1994). 'Bangladesh Pharmaceutical Policy and Politics'. *Health Policy and Planning*, 9/2, 130–43. <https://doi.org/10.1093/heapol/9.2.130>.

Sutradhar, K., Saha, A., Huda, N., and Uddin, R. (2014). 'Irrational Use of Antibiotics and Antibiotic Resistance in Southern Rural Bangladesh: Perspectives from Both the Physicians and Patients'. *Annual Research & Review in Biology*, 4/9, 1421–30.

Wernli, D., Jørgensen, P., Morel, C., Carroll, S., Harbarth, S., Levrat, N., et al. (2017). 'Mapping Global Policy Discourse on Antimicrobial Resistance'. *BMJ Global Health*, 2/2, e000378. <https://doi.org/10.1136/bmjgh-2017-000378>.

WHO. (2015). *WHO Global Action Plan on Antimicrobial Resistance* (Geneva: WHO). <https://www.who.int/antimicrobial-resistance/global-action-plan/en/>. (Accessed 12 September 2019).

Wilkinson, A., Ebata, A., and MacGregor, H. (2019). 'Interventions to Reduce Antibiotic Prescribing in LMICs: A Scoping Review of Evidence from Human and Animal Health Systems', *Antibiotics*, 8/1, 2. <https://doi.org/10.3390/antibiotics8010002>.

10

A Sociological Look beyond the Surface of the National Action Plans against AMR

How State Professionals Adjust to Global Governance

Muriel Surdez

Introduction

The global governance of antimicrobial resistance (AMR) has reached a new stage in recent years. The recommendations issued by international organizations—the World Health Organization (WHO), the Food and Agriculture Organization (FAO), and the World Organization for Animal Health (OIE)—have taken the form of a Global Action Plan which has been turned into numerous national action plans (Munkholm and Rubin, 2020).[1] These plans are central instruments for implementing at national level the objectives and action programmes drawn up at the international level. The future of global governance thus depends not only on international institutions but also on the ways national administrations and bureaucrats adapt the goals and tools of international policy against AMR to their own perspective, constraints, and interests. This is particularly true for the One Health approach, which is a cornerstone of global governance aimed at promoting collaboration between different fields: animal and human health, agriculture, and the environment (see Chapters 11, 12, and 13). From this perspective, misalignments or discrepancies between international goals and national plans should not only be measured (Chua et al., 2021; Frumence et al., 2021; Munkholm and Rubin, 2020) but also contribute to improved understanding of why and through which actors they occur, because it is not just a question of compliance or resources (Bordier et al., 2018; Stangborli and Veggeland, 2020).

Adopting the theoretical framework of the sociology of professions and based on a qualitative study on the Swiss case, this chapter has a dual purpose.

First, it will show that state bureaucrats in charge of the national strategy against AMR are actors with professional characteristics who deserves more attention, in any case in the Global North where administrations play a central role. In fact, they are designing national plans, which means organizing the programme of action, selecting

---

[1] In May 2021, 144 countries are recorded as having finalized plans, and forty-two as being in the process of preparing them (<https://www.who.int/activities/monitoring-progress-antimicrobial-resistance> accessed 17 August 2021.

Muriel Surdez, *A Sociological Look beyond the Surface of the National Action Plans against AMR* In: *Steering against Superbugs*. Edited by: Olivier Rubin, Erik Baekkeskov, and Louise Munkholm, Oxford University Press. © Oxford University Press 2023. DOI: 10.1093/oso/9780192899477.003.0010

public policy tools, and involving other stakeholders. But they also face constraints, including limited financial and organizational resources, as well as competition between units for prestige and skills. This line of research is often overlooked in the literature on AMR governance (Jensen et al., 2018). The focus on bureaucrats and the competitive processes in which they are embedded helps to explain why the One Health approach, a key piece of global governance involving collaboration between specialized entities within the administration, is so difficult to implement, as most studies on the national plans have found (Bordier et al., 2018: 5; Chua et al., 2021).

Second, the chapter will draw on Switzerland's experience in implementing its national plan against AMR to document the challenges faced in this matter by state bureaucrats from high-income countries with decentralized administrative structures. The state bureaucrats who in 2015 elaborated the first Swiss national plan against AMR, called the *Swiss National Strategy against Antibiotic Resistance* (*StAR*), dealt with the crucial issue of strengthening the capacity of the federal administration to act while mobilizing the regional administrative entities. They did so in a context of previous administrative restructuring which particularly affected the food safety units in charge of animal health policy from the 2010s (Sager et al., 2014). Still ongoing, the implementation of the *StAR* insists on the importance of combining human and animal health measures at the national level. However, it leads to a separated governance of AMR between human medicine on the one hand and animal health medicine handled by the veterinarian professionals on the other. The views of the latter are thus worth studying, especially since they are less investigated than the bureaucrats in charge with human health.

This chapter contributes to the analysis of AMR's global governance by showing that effective global governance is dependent on local/national administrative structures and on state professionals working within them.

Theoretical framework

The sociology of professions applied to the study of public policies aims at understanding which kinds of professional groups are involved in/excluded from the shaping of objectives and tools in a given policy area (Abbott, 2005; Evetts, 2011; Freidson, 2001). Times of crisis and reforms are therefore configurations in which the relationships between existing or new professional groups or specialties can change. It was the case in several Eurpean countries during and after the mad cow crisis where state veterinarians were critized for being too close to farmers (Alam, 2009). State institutions can also be viewed through the prism of professional groups on two dimensions. First, the various administrative structures (ministries, administrations, working groups, and so on) are more or less closely linked to different professional sectors and professional groups (Abbott, 2005; Demazière, 2018). This explains why it is important to understand who is in charge of the implementation of a particular policy or tool; in our case, measures to combat AMR (for other infection diseases see De Seze, 2020; Jerolmack,

2013). Secondly, people working in these administrations may (i) have a professional career as a generalist civil servant and thus belong to the professional group of bureaucrats; (ii) have first been educated and then practised as a professional outside the state before entering a state career; these are the ones designated as professional bureaucrats (Noordegraaf, 2013). The proportion of these two types of bureaucrats vary among public policy sectors (the more technical or scientific sectors tend to employ more professional bureaucrats) and countries with different traditions and recruitment patterns.

This conceptual framework leads us to consider the following questions to study the implementation of national plans and policies against antimicrobial resistance:

- Does the implementation of the plan against AMR change existing routines and hierarchies among the responsible professional bureaucrats? If so, is this at the level of the central or regional administrations?
- What room for manoeuvre do these professional bureaucrats have in their efforts to reform antibiotic use? What are their relationships internally within administrative bodies and externally with practitioners and their representative organizations?

Case study and methodology

This chapter is based on a research project conducted between 2015 and 2017[2] whose primary objective was to study the reforms of food safety policy and administration in Switzerland compared with other EU countries. In Switzerland, regional administrative authorities had until the 2000s a broad responsibility for organization and action in this area compared to that of the central administration. The centralization and professionalization of animal health services were therefore the main objectives of the reforms, as was the establishment of evaluation procedures. During the investigation, in 2015 the state bureaucrats published the official report titled 'Swiss Strategy against Antibiotic Resistance' (Federal Council, *Strategy on Antibiotic Resistance Switzerland*, 2015), which gave the opportunity to examine how these professionals deal with the problem of AMR. This strategy, developed by the Federal Office of Public Health (FOPH) and the Federal Food Safety and Veterinary Office (FFSVO),[3] takes the form of an action plan, which has so far been broken down into different documents (brochures, guidelines on specific issues, annual reports) as the implementation of the measures progresses without being revised itself. These documents were collected as support to understand the professionals' work but have not been subject to quantitative

[2] The project 'Cooperation and concurrence between professional bureaucrats. The case of food safety reforms in Switzerland', was financed by the Swiss National Science Foundation (No. 10001A_159308). The team consisted of a PhD student, Lorène Piquerez, and a post-doc, Jérôme Debons, who contributed to the data collection and analysis. They did not participate in the writing of this chapter.
    [3] Even if mentioned as signatories, the Federal Office for Agriculture (Department of Economics) and the Federal Office for Environment (Department of Environment, Transport, Energy, Communication) were not key players at this first stage.

content analysis. The reform of food safety governance and the management of anti-biotic resistance go hand in hand. Both emphasize the One Health approach and raise the challenge of collaboration between bureaucrats who were previously close but not used to working together.

The research adopts a qualitative approach focused on administrative actors and their networks as advocated by Chua et al. (2021: 21) as a promising research avenue to study AMR governance. About fifty qualitative interviews were conducted with actors involved in AMR strategy: with public veterinarians (twenty-six), chemical engineers (nine); food safety engineers (six), chemical laboratory technicians (seven), and six other specialists (doctors, biologists, lawyers). The selection criteria were (i) the home administration: different Offices at the national administration in Bern (see below) and four regional food safety departments (Cantons 1, 2, 3, 4), selected because they organize cooperative work differently (merging or not of units); (ii) the hierarchical status (heads of departments, units, or laboratories; employees or retired) and the length of employment in the administration as this may influence the way professionals view their collaborative role. The face-to-face interviews lasted between two and three hours. They were structured in three blocks of questions: (i) career path, with a focus on when and why the bureaucrats joined the public administration;[4] (ii) tasks within the administrative entity, evolution of the latter, and views on reforms; (iii) role in the *StAR*, collaborations implemented or not, and perceptions of the antibiotic resistance as a problem. A textual analysis of the interview transcripts was carried out using Atlas. ti software to examine which items were associated with 'AMR', 'cooperation', 'control', 'data gathering', 'misuses of antibiotics' by each type of professionals.

After 2017, we conducted a few additional interviews with professionals involved in the *StAR*'s follow up—a federal veterinarian in charge of the database on veterinary drugs prescription, three veterinarians of the Swiss Veterinary Society, who participated in the development of a federal booklet on good antibiotic use (FFSVO, 2016), and three agricultural engineers of the Federal Office for Agriculture.

Results

The Swiss strategy in context: The challenges of spatial-sectoral cooperation in a federalist administration

As the number of national plans against antibiotic resistance increases in line with the work invested by the WHO, social science work is beginning to investigate these plans. Several papers examine to what extent and on what governance axes (Frumence et al, 2021) various national plans, within different regional spaces (Bordier et al., 2018; Chua et al., 2021; Stangborli and Veggeland, 2020), comply with the Golbal Action Plan

---

[4] The socio-professional characteristics were analysed with the software Statistical Package for the Social Sciences but are not used here.

against AMR established by the WHO (Munkholm and Rubin, 2020). Producing an important content analysis of these documents, they highlight national particularities in terms of priorities (Stangborli and Veggeland, 2020), progress made, or dimensions to be developed. They also show a tendency to adopt the objectives of international organizations (mimicry process) formally, especially in low- and middle-income countries, without this leading to a consistent commitment to the problem (Munkholm and Rubin, 2020).

From a comparative perspective, the Swiss action plan elaborated in 2015 was developed relatively late due to the lack of legal powers of central authorities to take binding measures towards regional authorities in the field of epidemics (see below and Surdez et al, 2021). It comprises eight fields of activity formally corresponding to international recommendations: monitoring, prevention, appropriate use of antibiotics, resistance control, research and development, cooperation, informationand education and lastly general conditions[5] (Federal Council, *Strategy on Antibiotic Resistance Switzerland*, 2015: 6).[6] The One Health dimension is transversal to each field: three small images (a human figure, a cow's head, a plant) indicates if the field involves human health, animal health, or environmental/agricultural dimension.

However, this graphic representation does not specify to what extent the administrative units concerned should work together. The establishment of an intersectoral committee is planned for managing this issue (Federal Council, *Strategy on Antibiotic Resistance Switzerland*, 2015: 46). Moreover, the action plan defines the cooperation axis in a very broad way, stating that 'interdisciplinary and intersectoral coordination in the effort to control antibiotic resistance is essential so that technical and strategic synergies can be used. If political, scientific, and economic cooperation between the groups involved is still inadequate, it must be actively encouraged' (Federal Council, *Strategy on Antibiotic Resistance Switzerland*, 2015: 6).[7]

It may be added that no allocation of resources is specified, especially as regards cooperation between sectors or between central and regional authorities. Instead, the costs must respect the existing financial distributions: 'The remaining costs of individual measures will be allocated among the Confederation, the cantons and CHIF (Compulsory health insurance funds) in accordance with the existing distribution of responsibilities between the two levels of government. Any shift in the burden between the Confederation and the cantons is to be avoided' (Federal Council, *Strategy on Antibiotic Resistance Switzerland*, 2015: 61).

---

[5] General conditions are defined as follows: 'The general conditions for the groups involved must be such as to ensure that effective antibiotics will continue to be available and that they will be used responsibly. At the same time there is a need to ensure that there are no political, legal or financial incentives or market mechanisms that would stand in the way of achieving the objective' (Federal Council, *Strategy on Antibiotic Resistance Switzerland*, 2015: 6).

[6] These fields of activity guide the follow up of the plan, as shown on the FFSVO's website (<https://www.blv.admin.ch/blv/en/home/das-blv/strategien/nationale-strategie-antibiotikaresistenzen.html> accessed 18 August 2021.

[7] The cooperation axis also includes relations with the EU or other countries.

Following Stangborli and Veggeland (2020), who studied the Norwegian and Swedish plans from a neo-institutionalist perspective to confirm the path dependency hypothesis, we affirm that these general formulations show that in Switzerland, as in most countries, the plans against AMR are carried out within the framework of existing administrative structures, even if coordination mechanisms were added to fit One Health discourse and tools without being consistently adopted (for similar process with cost-effectiveness tools see Walker, 2019). This is a main issue for global governance to consider these administrative specificities.

A test for the federal authority

In Switzerland, it was managers and staff from the FOPH as well as the FFSVO who made AMR a priority. Assuming responsibility for it was a kind of test of their practical and symbolic legitimacy, as part of a longer process of controversial changes in health governance. As indicated above, the Federal Law on epidemics, adopted in 2016, was disputed for several years because it gives more decision-making power to the central government and administration. It causd reluctance on the part of the cantonal authorities, allied to groups opposed to increased surveillance of herds or compulsory vaccination. In parallel, the reform of food safety governance led to the merger of the previously separate veterinary and food safety entities at federal level and to giving more prerogatives to the FFSVO. It introduces the assessment of cantonal surveillance systems, the increased training requirements for state veterinarians, as well as revision of the law on veterinary medicines (see below).

The *StaR* is part of this context. This explains why the head and staff of both the FOPH and the FFSVO took on the role of bureaucrats who could take leading responsibility for anticipating crises, demonstrating management and planning skills. The Communicable Diseases Division, specialist in human health prevention campaigns within the FOPH, coordinated the various measures planned by the *StAR*. It was an opportunity to strengthen its position in relation to the other Offices by promoting a cross-cutting approach:

> OK, so this is a very important activity for which we have also received quite substantial new resources. We are the ones who started this project or who initiated the joint strategy project with the other departments. (M1, doctor, FOPH, Bern, 2 November 2015)

This leadership was used to convince the veterinarians of the FFSVO, to develop a common strategy that built on prevention to reduce antibiotics (mis)uses. For the FFSVO, the challenge was to institute systems for monitoring veterinary medicinal products, primarily antibiotics, on a national scale by enlisting public veterinarians at cantonal level. The aim was to demonstrate that the veterinary profession was capable of self-regulating its use of antibiotics, so that, practically, a broad variety of antibiotics remained available. As a representative of the FFSVO in a senior position told us, antibiotic resistance was an opportunity to move the profession towards a more prevention-oriented veterinary medicine: 'The aim is to have an overview of who, when and what quantity of antibiotics are used. That is our goal, that is my goal' (VET7, veterinarian, FFSVO, Bern, 2 February 2016).

Professional bureaucrats facing internal and external collaboration

While a majority of the professional bureaucrats we met agree in principle that a cross-sectoral approach is important to addressing AMR, this good will is being challenged by previous work routines and working relationships which are forged by both individual and workplace socialization.

Being trained as specialists in their field of activity,[8] the professional bureaucrats of the different federal Offices have rarely experienced collaborative work. Instead, they have internalized throughout their career the sectoral boundaries and hierarchies that have until recently divided the departments or administrative units in which they work (see Chapter 13 for further discussion). From a sociological point of view, coordination meetings, a privileged instrument to implement a One Health approach, may not be sufficient (for a more positive view of cross-sectoral meetings, see Humboldt-Dachroeden, 2021; see also Chapter 9). Some of our interviewees even considered that it might be more efficient to leave the responsibility to each sector because the explanation of sectoral specificities takes too much time compared to the assessment of the progress of the plan (see also Bordier et al., 2018: 7–10). Let's take three examples of these inter-professional relationships to highlight the barriers to more intensive collaboration between specialized professionals.

The first concerns the designers of the strategy who have deliberately chosen to divide the work for the further implementation stages. One of the doctors preferred to divide the responsibilities between human health and animal health so that 'each one could put his house in order' after he discovered that the monitoring of resistance did not at all cover the same issues in both sectors. On the human health side, a network of laboratories (called 'Anresis') linked to universities and hospitals is responsible for detecting various resistant bacteria in patient samples, while monitoring is largely absent from private medicine. In veterinary medicine, a monitoring decentralized in numerous slaughterhouses (to ensure meat consumption) focused on dead animals rather than on living animals, for cost reasons as our interlocutor notes: 'The veterinarians have a lot more trouble carrying out real monitoring of animal pathogens. Because ... it costs money [smiles]. It costs the farmer money, and it's simpler and cheaper for the farmer to pay for the antibiotic, without analyses, without detailed diagnosis of antibiotic resistance' (M1, doctor, FOPH, Bern, 2 November 2015). As the monitoring of resistance is not only organized differently but also does not have the same meaning

---

[8] The majority of our interviewees had not heard much about antibiotics resistance during their initial or on-the-job training, with little difference between specializations or generations.

and priority for the human health and for the animal health professionals, our inter-locutor finds it more appropriate to let the state veterinarians improve it on their own.

The second example reminds us that the members of the different offices involved do not have an equal voice; as a result, they do not necessarily feel they are legitimate to give their opinion or to collaborate with colleagues. In the Swiss case, this has been reflected in the second-tier position of the Federal Office for Agriculture in the *StAR*. Indeed, within the Federal Office for Agriculture, there are very few staff specialized in the field of medicated feed and animal nutrition, an issue that is directly related to the control of antibiotic administration. They are accustomed to delegating complex animal health issues to their colleagues in the veterinary office, not allowing themselves to challenge the competence of the latter: 'It is mainly the FFSVO, because for every-thing that concerns animal health, for us, the FFSVO is certainly the reference' (ENG8, agricultural engineer, Bern, 12 July 2018).

The third situation concerns the maintenance of specific areas of competence within the food safety entities, between the two main types of professionals that comprise them in Switzerland, veterinarians and chemical engineers. The fight against AMR shows that even after staff were brought together in merged administrative units, they main-tain autonomous ways of conceiving their priority tasks. Although they did not deny the issues around AMR, the chemists associated it with two main items: 'we are in the background' and 'veterinarians'. They framed AMR as a specifically human and animal health issue and not as a food safety issue as this chemist expressed it: 'Yes, yes, legally it is not relevant whether bacteria are resistant or not. It is a public health problem be-cause antibiotics are no longer effective. It is not primarily a food safety problem, but a medical problem' (CHEM6, cantonal chemical engineer, canton 5, 30 September 2016). They also see the risk that too much working time will be allocated to AMR, to the detriment of other tasks relating to environmental protection and food safety, such as researching pesticides, polychlorinated biphenyls (PCBs), genetically modified organ-isms (GMOs), or nanoparticles.

The sociology of professions emphasizes that the compartmentalization of profes-sional practices and skills has to do with the historical mode of constitution of expertise and power (Freidson, 2001). The three examples show how and why this compartmen-talization within the administration makes it difficult to implement an intersectoral approach to AMR rapidly. Moreover, for a majority of state bureaucrats in various countries, AMR is often a supplementary task for the teams (Bordier et al., 2018), without many additional resources. This also explains some reluctance to get involved. Referring to this analytical framework, it can be argued that international organiza-tions that promote the coordination of actions between sectors as a general objective of AMR governance do not sufficiently take into account the practical conditions for collaborative work within public administrations. Conversely, it might be useful to find pragmatic incentives for collaboration, including examples that offer short-term bene-fits for the implementation of measures. In one of the investigated cantons, a chemist and a veterinarian set up a pilot project to improve control of antibiotic residues in milk after antibiotics had been prescribed. While this measure is not innovative, it aims to restrict the quasi-automatic use of antibiotics by more strictly examining compliance with waiting periods between prescription and disposal.

Relationships between professional bureaucrats and targeted professional groups: A forgotten governance issue?

This section will show that due to their training and identity the professional bureaucrats have privileged contacts with their original professional group. Focusing on veterinarians, it asks what implications these relationships have for the implementation of the *StAR* that gives an important role to private stakeholders (see section 2.1).

In all countries, AMR represents a real change in relation to the widespread prescription of antibiotics, a practice that was long considered to be obvious by the whole veterinary profession. Therefore, public veterinarians working in the central administration are convinced that an increased control over private practitioners is required. They have to persuade this target group which, to say the least, is not immediately happy about having to change its prescribing patterns, the definition of which is considered a core competence of the profession rather as one of the state. This complex interplay affects two main aims of the *StAR*: the control of pharmacies and the monitoring of antibiotics use both at individual level of the veterinary practitioners.

The control of veterinary pharmacies was an issue before the launch of the national strategy: this has paved the way for and impacted on the types of controls that can be implemented. The revision of the federal law on veterinary medicinal products completed in 2004 establishes the compulsory inspection of pharmacies by cantonal public veterinarians (Sager et al., 2014). This measure was enacted following tough negotiations between the federal and cantonal authorities on the one side and the representative organization of the veterinary profession on the other side. Indeed, in the Swiss political context, draft laws are usually negotiated with the parties concerned because of the possibility of a referendum. In addition, many animal health policy objectives cannot be achieved without the active participation and support of the veterinary profession, which must therefore be convinced rather than coerced. In this negotiation process, the Swiss Veterinary Society (SVS) ultimately agree to the pharmacies' control to keep the monopoly of selling medicines, including antibiotics. The representative organization did not want to compromise this arrangement as long as other methods of remuneration were not introduced. The cantonal veterinarians then agreed to carry out inspections, but with great reluctance in several cantons, fearing the reactions of those inspected, as a cantonal veterinarian remembers:

> It is clear most veterinary practitioners are not happy when we arrive. But most of them think 'Well, if we have to do it, then let's do it'. And there are a few who are against it and get angry. We have to live with it. (VET17, employee, canton 3, 3 February 2017)

Because of the decentralized administrative structures in Switzerland, cantonal state veterinarians are used as to relay the arrangements negotiated at federal level. This puts them in the difficult position of having to carry out face-to-face controls on the prescribing practices of colleagues with whom they are in daily contact and for whom they know that the transition to new prescribing methods is not obvious, particularly for economic reasons.

The *StAR* reinforces this control over pharmacies by attempting to extend it to the systematic monitoring of the types of antibiotics prescribed by each private veterinary practitioner. New negotiations were opened between the federal veterinarians who manage the plan, the assembly of cantonal veterinarians, and the SVS (Surdez et al., 2021). As the cantonal veterinary offices do not have the tools to implement this kind of monitoring and the SVS seeks to retain control of it, the following solution was found: the FFSVO organized a database in which private practices have to enter the following data: when, with which dose, for how long, and for which animal a certain antibiotic was distributed.[9] IT support went live in 2019 but important issues related to these data (whether the database would be available to the public; measures in case of high use of certain categories of antibiotics) are still under discussion.

This section shows that the monitoring of antibiotic use can only be implemented through negotiations and accommodations between professional bureaucrats and private non-state actors, in our case representatives of the veterinary profession. At the heart of the global governance promoted by international organizations, the goal of generalizing a monitoring of antibiotic use is broken down into arrangements and stakeholder coalitions specific to each national context. The way in which this is done cannot be standardized.[10] The contribution of the sociology of professions to the understanding of AMR governance is therefore to identify which professional actors are predominant in each context and what the consequences are for the type of surveillance put in place.

The sociology of professional bureaucrats also shows that they are not always able to implement the public policy tools that they would consider most effective in achieving the objectives of One Health governance. In addition to monitoring, Swiss federal bureaucrats would like to have policy tools that support remuneration for preventive acts, as one manager of the FFSVO expressed:

It means this: if you are a farmer and I can advise you on how you can fatten your calves without using antibiotics, and if it takes me hours to explain this to you, I should be able to earn my money with this advice, and not by selling you medicinal products. (VET7, FSVO, Bern, 3 February 2016)

---

[9] In addition, a brochure summarizing good prescribing practice was produced jointly by the FFSVO and the SVS (2016). This tool was presented as a means of updating the scientific expertise of the profession rather than as a standardized guide.

[10] In several countries, the monitoring of antibiotic use in veterinary medicine relies on companies selling veterinary medicines and not on veterinary practices and clinics (Bordier et al., 2018).

However, this shift to a preventive paradigm is difficult to implement in Switzerland because it is particularly geared towards surveillance of large herds (Fortané, 2021), of which are very few in Switzerland. To counter this obstacle, some actors involved in the *StAR* are considering the possibility of paying for preventive visits by veterinarians through the subsidies that livestock farmers receive for the ecological services they provide in the framework of agricultural policy. Going beyond the targets set by international recommendations, this decompartmentalization (Chien, 2013) of agricultural and animal health policies will require further difficult negotiations to convince not only the veterinarians themselves, but also livestock professionals.

Discussion

What lessons can be drawn from the qualitative study of the Swiss case for the global governance of AMR?

National plans, even if they use a very similar standardized vocabulary, adapt to very diverse national configurations. They have to fit into existing national administrative systems for human and animal health while trying to transform it. Applying the sociological framework of the sociology of the profession to the state professional bureaucrats, our analysis shows how challenging is the relationship between central and regional administrations in the implementation of the AMR strategy. As in many countries where the central administration is not endowed with significant material and symbolic resources, central bureaucrats responsible for the plans must mobilize regional bureaucrats without taking away their competences or entrusting them exclusively with the thankless tasks of control. They also have to cope with professional representatives outside the state when aiming to collect aggregate data on the evolution of antibiotics use. In this regard, our contribution indicates that the international organizations' objectives are not necessarily achievable through the implementation of centralized bodies. Future research is, however, still needed to support the current work, which establishes that the management of AMR remains very dependent on pre-existing national structures, especially in the Global North where the problem has been dealt with for a longer period of time within the organizational framework of each country.

Our approach highlighted the organizational barriers that state professionals face in establishing cross-sectoral collaboration, a pillar of AMR global governance. These barriers are not simply a lack of communication and cooperation (Humboldt-Dachroeden, 2021) that can be overcome within One Health committees. Two main aspects have been addressed. One the one hand, professional bureaucrats were previously recruited because they were specialists in either human health, animal health, agriculture, or the environment. Their expertise within the administration is mainly based on a monopoly of tasks and knowledge. They therefore view dialogue with other specialists/colleagues rather ambivalently: as useful but also risky. The injunctions to set up One Health governance practices may seem abstract to them or else emanate from new types of generalist bureaucrats too focused on so-called good governance practices (Evetts, 2011).

One the other hand, as we have shown for state veterinarians, they also have privileged relationships with their profession of origin, an emotional commitment which they may feel is essential to achieve the objectives of the *StAR* and which they may fear will be diluted within a One Health approach. The recruitment of new specialists with more training in cross-sectoral approaches could help the next steps, provided that future social sciences work addresses how to integrate them in existing teams.

Conclusion

This chapter has shown that the discrepancies between the GAP and the national plans against AMR can be explained by the relationships that the professional bureaucrats who draw up these plans have with each other and with the professionals targeted by the public action. This line of research sheds new light on the implementation of the general objectives of the fight against AMR. National bureaucrats such as public veterinarians do not have unlimited power to act: they face resistance from, for example, private veterinary practitioners; they shared with the latter ways of using antibiotics that are difficult to change overnight; finally, they cannot use all the policy tools that they would like.

From this perspective, the assessment of national strategies against AMR would benefit from not only examine the compliance with the overall objectives of the GAP. The evaluation of the implementation stages should not only occur on a formal and standardized basis. A crucial issue is to establish with the national bureaucrats concerned which aspects they can commit to work on in a binding manner (Munkholm and Rubin, 2020).

The development of action plans devoted to antibiotic resistance have forced professional bureaucrats, especially those in the food safety sector, to take the problem seriously. Making this issue an autonomous object of attention and measures ensures that it remains on the agenda, but its articulation with existing, overarching, or adjacent, policies—notably agricultural policy on the animal health side—as well with the structure of professional groups targeted by the plans needs to be explored in more details. The study of professional bureaucrats and of the professional groups enrolled in national plans opens up new avenues to explore for a better understanding of global governance.

References

Abbott, A. (2005). 'Linked Ecologies: States and Universities as Environments for Professions', *Sociological Theory*, 23/3, 245–74.

Alam, T. (2009). 'La vache folle et les vétérinaires. Récit d'une victoire inattendue et paradoxale sur le terrain de la sécurité sanitaire des aliments', *Revue d'Etudes en Agriculture et Environnement*, 90/4, 373–98.

Bordier, M., Binot, A., Pauchard, Q. et al. (2018). 'Antibiotic Resistance in Vietnam: Moving towards a One Health Surveillance System', *BMC Public Health*, 18, 1136, <https://doi.org/10.1186/s12 889-018-6022-4>.

Chien, Y.-J. (2013). 'How Did International Agencies Perceive the Avian Influenza Problem? The Adoption and Manufacture of the "One World, One Health" Framework', *Sociology of Health & Illness*, 35/2, 213–26.

Chua, A. Q., Verma, M., Hsu, L. Y., and Legido-Quigley, H. (2021). 'An Analysis of National Action Plans on Antimicrobial Resistance in Southeast Asia Using a Governance Framework Approach', *The Lancet Regional Health—Western Pacific*, 7/100084. https://doi.org/10.1016/j.lan wpc.2020.100084

Demazière, D. (2018). 'La professionnalisation dans tous ses états', in F. Bajart, B. Crunel, C. Frau, F. Nicolas, and F. Parent, eds, *Professionnalisation(s) et Etat. Une sociologie politique des groupes professionnels* (Villeneuve d'Ascq: Presses universitaires du Septentrion), 291–307.

De Seze, M. (2020). 'Hepatitis B, a Global Disease? On Some Paradoxes of the Construction of Global Health Problems', in E. Neveu and M. Surdez, eds, *Globalizing Issues, How Claims, Frames, and Problems Cross Borders* (London: Palgrave Macmillan), 49–71.

Evett, J. (2011). 'New Professionalism and New Public Management: Changes and Continuities', *Sociologie du travail/Sociology of Work*, 53/3, 334–40.

Federal Office of Public Health, with the Federal Food Safety and Veterinary Office. (2015). *Strategy on Antibiotic Resistance Switzerland (StAR)*. <https://www.blv.admin.ch/blv/en/home/das-blv/str ategien/nationale-strategie-antibiotikaresistenzen.html>. (Accessed 17 August 2021).

Federal Food Safety and Veterinary Office. (2016). *Utilisation prudente des antibiotiques: Bovins, Porcs et Petits Ruminants. Guide thérapeutique pour les vétérinaires*. <https://www.blv.admin.ch/blv/fr/ home/tiere/tierarzneimittel/antibiotika/nationale-strategie-antibiotikaresistenzen--star--/sachge maesser-antibiotikaeinsatz.html> accessed 17 August 2021 (nda: exists only in German and in French).

Fortané, N. (2021). 'Antimicrobial Resistance: Preventive Approaches to the Rescue? Professional Expertise and Business Model of French "Industrial" Veterinarians', *Review of Agricultural, Food and Environmental Studies*, 102/2, 213–38.

Freidson, E. (2001). *Professionalism: The Third Logic* (Cambridge, Polity Press).

Frumence, G., Legido Quigley, H., Sindato, C., Katale, B. Z., Kimera, S., Metta, E., et al. (2021). 'The Governance and Implementation of the National Action Plan on Antimicrobial Resistance in Tanzania: A Qualitative Study', *Antibiotics*, 10/3, 273 <https://doi.org/10.3390/antibiotics1 0030273>.

Humboldt-Dachroeden, S. (2021). 'One Health Practices across Key Agencies in Sweden: Uncovering Barriers to Cooperation, Communication and Coordination', *Scandinavian Journal of Public Health*. doi:10.1177/14034948211024483

Jensen, C. S., Beck, N. S., and Fynbo, L. (2018). *Risking Antimicrobial Resistance. A Collection of One-Health Studies of Antibiotics and its Social and Health Consequences* (London: Palgrave MacMillan).

Jerolmack, C. (2013). 'Who's Worried about Turkeys? How "Organisational Silos" Impede Zoonotic Disease Surveillance', *Sociology of Health & Illness*, 35/2, 200–12.

Munkholm, L., and Rubin, O. (2020). 'The global Governance of Antimicrobial Resistance: A Cross-Country Study of Alignment between the Global Action Plan and National Action Plans', *Globalization and Health*, 16 /109 <https://doi.org/10.1186/s12992-020-00639-3>.

Noordegraaf, M. (2013). 'Reconfiguring Professional Work: Changing Forms of Professionalism in Public Services', *Administration and Society*, 48/7, 783–810.

Sager, F., Thomann, E., Zollinger, C., Van der Heiden, N., and Mavrot, C. (2014). Street-level 'Bureaucrats and New Modes of Governance: How Conflicting Roles Affect the Implementation of the Swiss Ordinance on Veterinary Medicinal Products', *Public Management Review*, 16/4, 481–502.

Stangborli, T. M., and Veggeland, F. (2020). 'Adapting to a Global Health Challenge: Managing Antimicrobial Resistance in the Nordics', *Politics and Governance*, 8(4), 53–64. doi:10.17645/pag. v8i4.3356.

Surdez, M., Hobeika, A., and Piquerez, L. (2021). 'Torn between Responsibility and Loyalty: How the Veterinarian Profession Designs Antibiotic Resistance Policies that Shake its Foundations', *Review of Agricultural, Food and Environmental Studies*, 102/2, 191–211.

Walker, A. (2019). 'Into the Machine: Economic tools, Sovereignty and Joy in a Global Health Institution', *Medical Anthropology Quarterly*, 33/4, 539–56.

PART IV

A ONE HEALTH (OH) PERSPECTIVE ON AMR

11

One Health and AMR Governance

Laura H. Kahn and Bernadette Dunham

Introduction

Antimicrobials are the foundation of modern medicine. Without safe and effective antimicrobials, many of the therapies of modern medicine such as cancer chemotherapies, elective surgeries, and immunosuppressive treatments for autoimmune diseases become too dangerous to use because the risks for infections become too high. While antimicrobial resistance (AMR) can occur in bacteria, viruses, fungi, and parasites, most concerns involve bacterial resistance to antibiotics. In this chapter, the focus will be on bacterial antibiotic resistance which will be synonymous with AMR. Global awareness of the threat posed by AMR has increased over the years and so has the recognition that a One Health approach is the best way to address it. One Health has a number of definitions. It is about connections: collaborative, multisectoral, and transdisciplinary approaches—working at the local, regional, national, and global levels—to achieve optimal health outcomes. It recognizes the interconnections between people, animals, plants, and their shared environments and ecosystems (Centers for Disease Prevention and Control, 2018). AMR dovetails into One Health, requiring that local efforts scale up to national and international levels, involving environments and ecosystems. AMR impacts all societies reliant upon modern medicine to save lives (Kahn, 2021).

Governance is defined as overseeing the control and direction of something such as an organization or a nation (Merriam-Webster, 2021). Effective governance requires committed political leadership and support. In the case of AMR, policies, laws, and international agreements have been developed to address it, but their effectiveness depends upon the political support provided to implement and enforce them. Countries such as the United States and Denmark have implemented AMR surveillance systems of humans, animals, and food with varying levels of success. The United States and the European Union (EU) differed in their approach to curtailing growth-promoting antibiotic use in animal agriculture. The United States used antibiotic guidelines for the animal agriculture industry to follow whereas the EU implemented bans against growth-promoting antibiotic use. These examples illustrate the different policy approaches used to address AMR (see Chapters 7, 9, 16, and 17 for a discussion of policy approaches in the Global South).

Laura H. Kahn and Bernadette Dunham, *One Health and AMR Governance* In: *Steering against Superbugs*. Edited by: Olivier Rubin, Erik Baekkeskov, and Louise Munkholm, Oxford University Press. © Oxford University Press 2023. DOI: 10.1093/oso/9780192899477.003.0011

In September 2016, the United Nations General Assembly met to deliberate on AMR. It recognized the global threat posed by AMR, and it endorsed the World Health Assembly's Global Action Plan on Antimicrobial Resistance, which had been developed in the previous year. Importantly, the UN General Assembly supported a One Health approach to national and international efforts (United Nations, 2016; World Health Organization, 2015). One of the results of the UN meeting through a joint secretariat was the establishment of an Interagency Coordination Group on AMR (World Health Organization, 2017).

While everyone agreed that a One Health approach was important to address AMR, the challenge was to implement it. What has been needed has been a framework that provides users with a concise, systematic, and comprehensive approach to AMR.

One Health multidimensional matrix

The One Health matrix could serve as an important tool to be used by policy-makers to AMR policies. It could be represented as a three-dimensional cube. The first dimension would represent One Health factors: humans, animals, plants, environments, and ecosystems. Humans could be stratified by age or other relevant characteristics such as health status. Plants and animals could either be domestic, wild, or both. Environments involve the abiotic (i.e., air, water, soil, chemical) aspects and ecosystems encompass the biotic (microbes, fauna, flora) interactions within defined geographic areas, respectively. Environments and ecosystems could include indoor and outdoor settings. Outdoor settings could include urban, suburban, rural, or undeveloped areas.

The second dimension provides complexity and scale: microbial and cellular, individual, and population. This dimension would interact with the first dimension to provide a comprehensive examination of the One Health factors at different levels. Microbial and cellular levels could include invading pathogens, normal flora, their interactions as well as the interactions between microbes and human cells. The individual level could involve one human, animal, plant, environment, or ecosystem. The population level could involve populations of humans and animals. Populations of plants could include agricultural crops, forests, marshes, grasslands, or savannas. Populations of environments and ecosystems could involve multiple geographic settings.

The third dimension would involve the political, social, and economic factors which at the most basic level would examine how humans interact with each other. These factors could be divided by political borders: local and regional, national and international. Political factors could include political leadership, laws and regulations, relevant public policies, and government funding. Social factors could be either positive or negative. Positive social factors could include education, culture, and religious tolerance. Negative social factors could include corruption, bigotry, racism, misogyny, prejudice, and xenophobia—factors that adversely affect equity, diversity, and inclusion.

Economic factors could include employment rates, poverty rates, healthcare availability and access.

A fourth dimension involving time could be added, if desired. Time could involve days, months, years, or decades. Time is not visualized when using the cube representation.

With the interface of the three dimensions, the matrix tool could provide users with a comprehensive framework to examine AMR issues holistically and could put into practice the Joint Tripartite's (the Food and Agriculture Organization (FAO), the World Organization for Animal Health (WOAH), World Health Organization (WHO)) One Health High Level Expert Panel's (OHHLEP) definition of One Health (Kahn, 2021; United Nations, 2021).

In general, national and international AMR efforts focus on the surveillance of antibiotic use in humans and food animals and the surveillance of resistant bacteria in humans, food animals, and retail meats. Antibiotic use and resistance in crops are not well studied even though there are some indications that many crops receive antibiotics, particularly in low- and middle-income countries, and might serve as important factors worsening AMR (Taylor and Reeder, 2020). In addition, environments and ecosystems, which constitute a major part of AMR, have generally not been included in governmental AMR surveillance systems (D'Costa et al., 2011; see also Chapter 13). Political, social, and economic factors are major components of AMR, including lack of political will to address poor access to primary care, the availability of cheap over-the-counter antibiotics, and minimal access to basic sanitation in poor, developing countries.

National AMR efforts

1. The United States

The US Congress deliberated about AMR for decades, holding numerous hearings and taking a range of testimonies. Elected officials agreed that something should be done, but none had the political will to appropriate funds to federal agencies to collect AMR data. Without good data, it is hard to develop effective policies. In response, senior administrators in the Centers for Disease Control and Prevention (CDC), the Food and Drug Administration (FDA), and the US Department of Agriculture (USDA) acted on their own initiative to establish AMR surveillance systems (Kahn, 2016; United States Food and Drug Administration, 2021).

National Antimicrobial Resistance Monitoring System
In 1996, the National Antimicrobial Resistance Monitoring System for Enteric Bacteria (NARMS) was established. NARMS is a collaborative programme of state and local public health departments and universities, the FDA, the CDC, and the USDA (United States Food and Drug Administration, 2021). Human data are collected from public health laboratories that submit clinical specimens involving enteric organisms such

as *Campylobacter*, *E. coli 0157*, and *Salmonella* to the CDC NARMS for antimicrobial susceptibility testing. The FDA monitors retail meats such as chicken, ground beef, and pork chops from nineteen states for genetic analyses, serotyping, and antimicrobial susceptibility testing. The USDA collects samples from food-producing animals at federally inspected slaughter houses and processing plants throughout the country (Centers for Disease Control and Prevention, 2019).

In 2019, the CDC issued an AMR report with the findings that more than 2.8 million AMR infections occur and, as a result, more than 35,000 people die from them in the United States each year. These estimates were derived from over 700 geographically diverse acute-care hospitals throughout the United States. While the One Health concept was acknowledged as important, animal and environmental data were not included (Centers for Disease Prevention and Control, 2021).

In 2020, NARMS issued a Strategic Plan for 2021–2025 with the goal to adopt a One Health approach by including surveillance of AMR in animal pathogens (e.g., *E. coli* and *Staphylococcus pseudintermedius* in dogs and *Salmonella enterica* in any animal host) and in the environment. In addition, NARMS has developed a partnership with the US Environmental Protection Agency (EPA) to conduct AMR surveillance of environmental aquatic samples (United States Food and Drug Administration, 2021).

In 1983, the USDA initiated the National Animal Health Monitoring System (NAHMS) which began to collect, analyse, and disseminate data on domestic livestock populations, management, and productivity across the United States (United States Department of Agriculture, 2021). NAHMS conducts studies of swine, dairy, beef, poultry, sheep, and other food animals by collecting information from producers using questionnaires, often in-person interviews. Biological samples may be included, but they are not necessarily screened for AMR (United States Department of Agriculture, 2010). However, in 2019 NAHMS conducted a targeted study on antimicrobial use and stewardship entitled the *Antimicrobial Use and Stewardship on U.S. Feedlots, 2017 Report*. The study focused on the use of antimicrobials used in cattle feedlots with fifty or more head before FDA policy changes went into effect to reduce the use of medically important antibiotics in animal feed and water. The goal of the study was to establish a baseline for comparison to future studies. It found that overall, 87.5 per cent of feedlots gave antimicrobials in water, by injection, or in feed (United States Department of Agriculture, 2012 & 2019). In July 2021, the USDA's Animal and Plant Health Inspection Service (APHIS) petitioned NAHMS to conduct a study of antibiotic use and AMR in the US broiler chicken industry (United States Office of Management and Budget, 2021).

Presidential Advisory Council on Combating Antibiotic-Resistant Bacteria

On 18 September 2014, the Obama administration released a National Strategy for Combating Antibiotic-Resistant Bacteria accompanied by a Presidential Advisory Council on Combating Antibiotic-Resistant Bacteria (PACCARB), established under Executive Order 13676 (United States Department of Health and Human Services, 2014). PACCARB provided advice, information, and recommendations regarding programmes and policies related to combating antibiotic-resistant bacteria such as NARMS. From 2016 to January 2021, the Trump administration sought deep funding cuts for public health including efforts to address AMR which prompted a scathing editorial in the *Annals of Internal Medicine* by the leaders of the Infectious Diseases Society of America (Boucher et al., 2017). Two months after President Biden was sworn into office, his administration delegated authority to the Secretary of Health and Human Services to re-establish PACCARB. Political leadership matters. Political leaders who believe in science and scientific expertise are essential for supporting policies and programmes dedicated to controlling AMR. PACCARB illustrates the importance of the third dimension of the One Health matrix tool: the political, social, and economic factors. Countries with dysfunctional politics will not be able to address AMR.

2. Denmark

In the early 1990s, Denmark was the largest pork-producing nation in the world and relied on avoparcin, a growth-promoting antibiotic, for production (Kahn, 2017). In 1995, Danish scientists identified vancomycin-resistant Enterococcus faecium (VRE) in faecal samples from healthy pigs and chickens. This raised alarms because vancomycin was the antibiotic of last resort against *Enterococcus faecium*, and VRE was becoming a serious problem in hospitals. Avoparcin was assumed to be the cause for the emergence of this deadly microbe. Denmark banned avoparcin from use in animal agriculture. By the end of the 1990s, in response to consumer concerns, Danish food animal producers voluntarily stopped using all antibiotic growth promoters in animal production. Unfortunately, despite the cessation of avoparcin use, VRE continued to increase in Danish hospitals (Kahn, 2016).

Danish Integrated Antimicrobial Resistance Monitoring and Research Program
Since 1996, the Danish Ministries of Health and Food, Agriculture, and Fisheries have been publishing annual Danish Integrated Antimicrobial Resistance Monitoring and Research Programme (DANMAP) reports. In line with the One Health approach, the goals of DANMAP are to monitor antibiotic use in humans and food animals, monitor AMR in humans, food animals, and food of animal origins, and study the links between antibiotic use and AMR. Three categories of bacteria are monitored for AMR: human and animal pathogens, zoonotic bacteria, and indicator bacteria. Human and animal pathogens cause illnesses. Zoonotic bacteria are animal microbes that can spread to humans and cause illness. Indicator bacteria are ubiquitous in both animals and humans and generally don't cause illness but occasionally do (Statens Serum Institute, 2021).

It was not until the 2019 DANMAP report, however, that the steering committee explicitly acknowledged the importance of the environmental sector on the development and spread of AMR. In other words, they expanded on the first dimension of the One Health matrix. Further, the report recognized water contamination as an important source, but it did not include surveillance data from environmental samples. Human clinical surveillance specimens were obtained from patients with bacteraemia (blood-stream infections), gastroenteritis, and urinary tract infections. In the livestock sector, the Danish pork industry used approximately 75 per cent of all veterinary-prescribed antimicrobials. Historically, tetracyclines had been the most frequently used antibiotic in pork production, but the trend from 2016 had been downward. *Enterococci* isolated from pigs showed zero resistance to vancomycin. In humans, invasive VRE in hospitalized patients remained a worsening problem. There is evidence that companion animals, such as dogs, might serve as reservoirs for antibiotic-resistant bacteria (Pasotto et al., 2016; Wada et al., 2021). DANMAP does not conduct routine AMR surveillance of companion animals, but it does collect some data such as skin and urinary tract infections of dogs and cats. Trends of resistant *E. coli* and *Staphylococcus pseudintermedius* in pets have remained stable since 2011 (DANMAP, 2019). Companion animals share people's homes, beds, and food. Surveillance of these animals should be a priority.

International AMR efforts

Similar to national AMR efforts, international efforts focus on reducing AMR in humans, food animals, and animal-derived food products such as pork and chicken. Plants, environments, and ecosystems are typically not addressed. Political, social, and economic factors are very challenging to address at national, much less at international levels. While the One Health approach has been recognized as an essential strategy to address AMR, implementing it remains aspirational.

The following five global initiatives are testaments to both the successful advancement of the One Health agenda but also the barriers to effective implementation. These include a lack of leadership and enforcement on the global level, but some barriers are also linked to the ambiguity of the One Health concept itself. A widespread adoption of the One Health matrix tool might help to clarify the ambiguities and to further advance the concept into concrete initiatives that address the multicausal nature of AMR.

1. Global Health Security Agenda

In 2014, a group of thirty countries, non-governmental and international organizations, and corporations collaboratively established the Global Health Security Agenda. The GHSA seeks to improve countries' capacities to detect and prevent naturally occurring, accidental, or deliberate infectious disease threats while complying with the WHO's International Health Regulations, the WOAH's international standards and guidelines, UN Security Council Resolution 1540, the Biological Weapons Convention, and other relevant guidelines and frameworks designed to improve global health security (Global Health Security Agenda, 2018). GHSA's goal is to have more than 100 countries join the effort by 2024 (Global Health Security Agenda, 2020). The GHSA has made AMR one of its top priorities by keeping it on the agenda at the highest political levels ((Global

Health Security Agenda, 2021). Using the One Health matrix tool might assist the GHSA in implementing and enforcing a comprehensive One Health approach.

2. WHO—Global Action Plans, GLASS, and AWaRe

In 2015, the WHO released its Global Action Plan on Antimicrobial Resistance which recognized the need for a One Health approach that involved coordination between human and veterinary medicine, agriculture, the environment, and the financial sector. This Global Action Plan is extremely important because it includes agriculture and the environment. The plan served as a model for nations to use when developing their national action plans (World Health Organization, 2016, 2021). The action plans were based on five strategic objectives: (i) improve awareness and understanding of AMR through effective communication, education, and training; (ii) strengthen the knowledge and evidence base through surveillance and research; (iii) reduce the incidence of infection through effective sanitation, hygiene, and infection prevention measures; (iv) optimize the use of antimicrobial medicines in human and animal health; and (v) develop the economic case for sustainable investment that takes account of the needs of all countries, and increase investment in new medicines, diagnostic tools, vaccines, and other interventions (World Health Organization, 2016).

That same year, WHO also launched the Global Antimicrobial Resistance and Use Surveillance System (GLASS) which was an effort to standardize global AMR surveillance. Standardization and harmonization in the collection, analysis, and interpretation of AMR data by all member countries would improve the monitoring of global trends using clinical, epidemiological, and population-level data. The goal of GLASS was the inclusion of AMR data from humans, the food chain, and the environment (World Health Organization, 2018). Environmental surveillance focused on water bodies: market runoff, sewage, and river sites in urban areas. By May 2021, almost 110 countries and territories had enrolled in GLASS. The 2021 GLASS report provided surveillance information of high-priority resistant pathogens in humans (World Health Organization, 2021).

In October 2019, WHO released the '2019 WHO AWaRe Classification Database' which was developed on the recommendation of the WHO Expert Committee on Selection and Use of Essential Medicines. The term 'AWaRe' stands for Access, Watch, and Reserve. This system was developed for antibiotic use in humans. Forty-eight antibiotics were categorized as Access antibiotics which are considered first- or second-choice treatment options for specific infections. Watch antibiotics includes 100 compounds that have higher resistance potential and that should be prioritized as key targets of antibiotic stewardship programmes. The Reserve antibiotics include twenty-two drugs that should be used as a last resort. The system was designed as a tool for antibiotic stewardship at the local, national, and global levels (World Health Organization, 2019).

Similar to the GHSA, some of the WHO efforts circumvented the most difficult factors in addressing AMR. When applying the One Health matrix tool, these factors become evident. With the exception of GLASS, One Health, which includes surveillance of water bodies, surveillance of crops, soil environments, and microbial ecosystems are typically missing. In addition, political, social, and economic factors are missing.

3. WOAH AMR efforts

In 2016, WOAH's General Assembly unanimously adopted Resolution No. 36 mandating that the organization address AMR using a One Health approach (World Organization for Animal Health, 2016). The resolution recommended that WOAH develop standards and guidelines for the veterinary stewardship of antimicrobials, guidance on alternative antimicrobials, and for member countries to implement WOAH's strategy through national action plans (World Organization for Animal Health, 2016). Later that year, WOAH published its strategy on AMR and the prudent use of antimicrobials in animals which closely aligned with WHO's Global Action Plan on AMR (World Organization for Animal Health, 2016). The WOAH also developed a global database on antimicrobial agents intended for use in animals. The first report was issued in 2016; the second report, issued the following year, included improved methodologies for adjusting administered antimicrobial quantities based on animal biomass at regional and global scales (Gochez et al., 2019). The fifth report was issued in September 2021 with data submitted by 156 out of 182 WOAH member countries. One hundred and twelve responding countries indicated that they did not use any antimicrobials as growth-promoting agents in food animals as of 2019 (World Organization for Animal Health, 2021).

4. FAO AMR efforts

The FAO supports producers, traders, and nations to produce food. During its 39th conference in June 2015, the FAO adopted Resolution 4/2015 on AMR. The resolution prompted the FAO to develop an Action Plan on AMR focusing on four main areas: improve awareness of the threat, develop capacity for surveillance of AMR and monitoring of antimicrobial use in agriculture, strengthen governance in AMR and antibiotic use in agriculture, and promote the prudent use of antimicrobials in agriculture. The Action Plan supports the WHO's AMR Action Plan and the use of a One Health approach in animal agriculture. However, there is minimal, if any, mention of the importance of prudent antimicrobial stewardship in crop agriculture (Food and Agriculture Organization, 2015, 2016).

5. Tripartite (FAO/OIE/WHO) AMR efforts

In 2010, a formal collaborative effort known as the FAO/OIE (i.e.,WOAH)/WHO Tripartite Concept Note was established. The Tripartite used a One Health approach as a guiding principle to address complex health issues involved humans, animals, and the environment. The collaboration developed the Global Action Plan on AMR which helped precipitate the UN General Assembly's High-Level Meeting (World Health Organization, 2017). In March 2020, the Dutch and Swedish governments established an AMR Multi-Partner Trust Fund to support the ongoing Tripartite collaboration. The British government joined the original funders to launch a Call for Concept Note to address AMR priorities (World Organization for Animal Health, 2020).

In November 2020, the Tripartite invited the UN Environmental Program (UNEP) to join the tripartite cooperative, recognizing the importance of the environment in addressing AMR. By April 2021, the process of including the UNEP remained unfinished. Nevertheless, the UNEP had been collaborating with the Tripartite to create a High-Level Expert Panel on One Health which convened its first meeting in June 2021 (United Nations, 2021; World Health Organization, 2021). In a 2019 report to the UN Secretary-General, the Interagency Coordination Group on AMR recommended the establishment of such a group (World Health Organization, 2020).

Barriers to implementation

The preceding brief account of the two national examples and five international initiatives have elucidated four barriers to implementing One Health strategies against AMR. The first is the need to define exactly what a One Health approach is. While it is important to recognize that the health of humans is connected to other species as well as to ecosystems and environments, it's essential to implement a coherent One Health framework. A One Health proof of concept is still being worked out, primarily for zoonotic disease surveillance (Kelly et al., 2017).

As discussed earlier, a One Health approach using a three-dimensional matrix as a framework might be extremely useful for identifying overlooked One Health factors including plants, environments, and ecosystems as well as the political, social, and economic factors that are essential for implementing effective AMR politics. However, as with the One Health concept in general, the matrix remains to be implemented as a proof of concept (Kahn, 2021).

Second, the Tripartite effort assumes that each of the three collaborating organizations are equal. This is not the case. For a stool to be stable, the three legs must be the same length. In the case of WHO, FAO, and WOAH, the three organizations are vastly different in terms of size, resources, and funding. The WHO's budget is the largest of the three. The most recent fiscal year available, 2020–2021, WHO's budget was US$ 5.84 billion (World Health Organization, 2020). WHO has a workforce of over 8,000 people, almost 70 per cent stationed in regional and country offices around the world (World Health Organization, 2019). The FAO's fiscal year 2022–2023 budget was US$ 3.25 billion (Food and Agriculture Organization, 2021). In 2019, FAO employed over 11,000 employees, most of whom were stationed in offices worldwide (Food and Agriculture Organization, 2021). In contrast to WHO and FAO, the WOAH is not part of the UN and subsequently relies on funding from member country contributions to the WOAH World Fund. WOAH's fiscal year 2021 budget was EUR 15.96 million (approximately US$ 18.2 million) (World Organization for Animal Health, 2021). Approximately 156 people work at WOAH, all of whom are located in its Paris headquarters in France (World Organization for Animal Health, 2021). Even if WOAH's budget were doubled to US$ 36.4 million to cover two fiscal years, it is still many times smaller than the FAO and WHO budgets. With great disparities in funding and human resources, the capabilities of these three organizations are vastly different.

Thirdly, there should be improved enforcement mechanisms to encourage nations to implement and enforce AMR action plans. WHO and FAO collaborate to set standards, guidelines, and codes for safe and fair international trade of food by the Codex Alimentarius Commission (Codex) (Food and Agriculture Organization, 2021). These standards serve as models for national legislation (Food and Agriculture Organization, 2021). WOAH sets standards to facilitate international trade of animals and animal products (World Organization for Animal Health, 2021). In 1994, multilateral trade negotiations included agreements on the Application of Sanitary and Phytosanitary Measures, known as the 'SPS Agreement' (World Trade Organization, 1998). The treaty also included the establishment of the World Trade Organization (WTO) which ensures that international trade rules are followed, including the periodic scrutiny of member nations' trade policies and practices (World Trade Organization, 1995). Including AMR policies in the Codex Alimentarius has been suggested (George, 2019). This recommendation could be expanded to include AMR policies in the WOAH's SPS Agreement which is used by the WTO.

Finally, and arguably, the greatest barrier to implementing effective AMR policies is the issue of AMR itself. AMR is ancient, ubiquitous, and naturally occurring in the world's microbial ecosystems (D'Costa et al., 2011; Kim and Cha, 2021). The challenge of AMR has been compared to the challenge of climate change (see Chapters 4, 14, and 15). Both require individual short-term sacrifice from using cheap, easy-to-use conveniences for the long-term benefits of society (Harring and Krockow, 2021). The use of fossil fuels and antibiotics both harm the environment. In the case of fossil fuels, the extraction industries damage environments and ecosystems and worsen climate change. In the case of antibiotics, their continued use worsens antimicrobial resistance and alter the 'Global Resistome'. There is evidence that antibiotics damage the microbiomes of individuals contributing to chronic illnesses such as food allergies, obesity, asthma, and some cancers (Blaser, 2014). Broad spectrum antibiotics kill the good bacteria along with the bad. A potential alternative, or adjunct, to antibiotics is bacteriophage therapy which has been successfully used to cure pan-resistant infections (Strathdee and Patterson, 2019). There are challenges to developing such therapies for widespread use, but investments in such therapies should come from a public–private partnership collaborating under a One Health approach (Kahn, 2018).

Conclusion

The goal of national and international AMR efforts is to ensure the availability and access of safe and effective antimicrobials allowing modern medicine to continue. The United States and Denmark provided national examples of AMR efforts, but of course these are affluent countries with the resources to conduct extensive surveillance and data analysis. Denmark's AMR efforts have existed for decades attesting to the importance of political will, support, and public demands. While a One Health approach has been recognized as important to address AMR, implementing comprehensive programmes that encompasses humans, animals, plants, environments, and ecosystems remains aspirational at the national and international levels. Increasing WTO involvement might help with enforcement, providing financial incentives to political leaders to take AMR seriously. Ultimately, it is up to political leaders to implement and enforce One Health initiatives in their countries that will determine if safe and effective antimicrobials will continue to serve as the foundation of modern medicine.

References

Blaser, M. J. (2014). *Missing Microbes. How the Overuse of Antibiotics is Fueling Our Modern Plagues* (New York, NY: Henry Holt and Company).

Boucher, H. W., Murray, B. E., and Powderly, W. G. (2017). 'Proposed U.S. Funding Cuts Threaten Progress on Antimicrobial Resistance', *Annals of Internal Medicine*, 167/10, 738–40. <https://doi.org/10.7326/M17-1678>.

Centers for Disease Control and Prevention. (2018). *One Health Basics*. <https://www.cdc.gov/onehealth/basics/index.html> accessed 23 January 2021.

Centers for Disease Prevention and Control. (2019). *Antibiotic Resistance Threats in the United States, 2019*. <https://www.cdc.gov/drugresistance/pdf/threats-report/2019-ar-threats-report-508.pdf> accessed 23 January 2021.

Centers for Disease Control and Prevention. *National Antimicrobial Resistance Monitoring System (NARMS)*. <https://www.cdc.gov/narms/index.html>

Centers for Disease Prevention and Control. (2021). *About NARMS. Tracking Trends in Resistance*. <https://www.cdc.gov/narms/about/index.html> accessed 14 September 2021.

Danish Integrated Antimicrobial Resistance Monitoring and Research Programme (DANMAP). (2019). *Use of Antimicrobial Agents and Occurrence of Antimicrobial Resistance in Bacteria from Food Animals, Food and Humans in Denmark*. https://www.danmap.org/reports/2019 accessed 14 September 2021.

D'Costa, V. M., King, C. E., Kalan, L., Morar, M., Sung, W. W. L., Schwarz, C., et al. (2011). 'Antibiotic Resistance is Ancient', *Nature*, 477, 457–61. <https://doi.org/10.1038/nature10388>.

Gochez, D., Raicek, M., Ferreira, J. P., Jeannin, M., Moulin, G., and Erlacher-Vindel, E. (2019) 'OIE Annual Report on Antimicrobial Agents Intended for Use in Animals: Methods Used', *Frontiers in Veterinary Science*, 6, 317. <https://doi.org/10.3389/fvets.2019.00317>.

Food and Agriculture Organization. (2016). *The FAO Action Plan on Antimicrobial Resistance 2016– 2020. Supporting the Food and Agriculture Sectors in Implementing the Global Action Plan on Antimicrobial Resistance to Minimize the Impact of Antimicrobial Resistance. Rome, 2016.* <http://www.fao.org/3/i5996e/i5996e.pdf> accessed 21 September 2021.

Food and Agriculture Organization. (2021). *Office of Strategy, Programme and Budget (OSP). FAO's Budget.* <http://www.fao.org/about/strategy-programme-budget/budget/en/> accessed 21 September 2021.

Food and Agriculture Organization. (2021). *Structure and Finance.* <http://www.fao.org/about/who-we-are/en/> accessed 21 September 2021.

Food and Agriculture Organization. (2021). *Codex Alimentarius. International Food Standards. Protecting Health, Facilitating Trade.* <http://www.fao.org/fao-who-codexalimentarius/en/> accessed 21 September 2021.

Food and Agriculture Organization. (2021). *Codex Alimentarius. About Codex Alimentarius.* <http://www.fao.org/fao-who-codexalimentarius/about-codex/en/> accessed 21 September 2021.

George, A. (2019). 'Antimicrobial Resistance (AMR) in the Food Chain: Trade, One Health and Codex', *Tropical Medicine and Infectious Disease*, 4/1, 54. <https://doi.org/10.3390/tropicalmed 4010054>.

Global Health Security Agenda. (2018). *2024 Framework.* <https://ghsagenda.org/wp-content/uplo ads/2020/06/ghsa2024-framework.pdf> accessed 17 September 2021.

Global Health Security Agenda. (2020). *A Partnership against Global Health Threats.* <https://ghsage nda.org/> accessed 15 September 2021.

Global Health Security Agenda. (2021). *Antimicrobial Resistance.* <https://ghsagenda.org/antimicrob ial-resistance/> accessed 17 September 2021.

Gochez, D., Raicek, M., Ferreira, J. P., Jeannin, M., Moulin, G., and Erlacher-Vindel, E. (2019) 'OIE Annual Report on Antimicrobial Agents Intended for Use in Animals: Methods Used', *Frontiers in Veterinary Science*, 6, 317. <https://doi.org/10.3389/fvets.2019.00317>.

Harring, N., and Krockow, E. M. (2021). 'The Social Dilemmas of Climate Change and Antibiotic Resistance: An Analytic Comparison and Discussion of Policy Implications', *Humanities & Social Sciences Communications*, 8, 125. <https://doi.org/10.1057/s41599-021-00800-2>.

Kahn, L. H. (2016). *One Health and the Politics of Antimicrobial Resistance* (Baltimore, MD: Johns Hopkins University Press).

Kahn, L. H. (2017). 'Perspective: The One-Health Way', *Nature*, 543/7647, S47. <https://www.ncbi. nlm.nih.gov/pmc/articles/PMC7094977/>. doi:10.1038/543S47a.

Kahn, L. H. (2018). 'Bacteriophages: A Promising Approach to Fighting Antibiotic Resistant Bacteria', *Bulletin of the Atomic Scientists.* <https://thebulletin.org/2018/10/bacteriophages-a-promising-approach-to-fighting-antibiotic-resistant-bacteria/> accessed 21 September 2021.

Kahn, L. H. (2021). 'Developing a One Health Approach by Using a Multi-Dimensional Matrix', *One Health*, 13/100289. <https://doi.org/10.1016/j.onehlt.2021.100289>.

Kelly, T. R., Karesh, W. B., Johnson, C. K., Johnson, C. K., Gilardi, K. V. K., Anthony, S. J., et al. (2017). 'One Health Proof of Concept: Bringing a Transdisciplinary Approach to Surveillance for Zoonotic Viruses at the Human-Wild Animal Interface', *Preventive Veterinary Medicine*, 137, 112–18. <https://doi.org/10.1016/j.prevetmed.2016.11.023>.

Kim, D-W., and Cha, C-J. (2021). 'Antibiotic Resistome from the One-Health Perspective: Understanding and Controlling Antimicrobial Resistance Transmission', *Experimental & Molecular Medicine*, 53, 301–9. <https://doi.org/10.1038/s12276-021-00569-z>.

Merriam-Webster. (2021). 'Governance', *Merrian-Webster.com Dictionary.* <https://www.merriam-webster.com/dictionary/governance> accessed 13 September 2021.

Pasotto, D., Dotto, G., Menandro, M. L., Mondin, A., and Martini, M. (2016). 'Prevalence and Antimicrobial-resistance Characterization of Vancomycin Resistant Enterococci (VRE) Strains in

Healthy Household Dogs in Italy', *International Journal of Infectious Diseases*. 53S, 4–163. <https://doi.org/10.1016/j.ijid.2016.11.129>.

Statens Serum Institute. (2021). *About DANMAP*. <https://www.danmap.org/about-danmap> accessed 14 September 2021.

Strathdee, S., and Patterson, T. (2019). *The Perfect Predator* (New York, NY: Hachette Books).

Taylor, P., and Reeder, R. (2020). 'Antibiotic Use on Crops in Low and Middle-Income Countries Based on Recommendations Made by Agricultural Advisors', *CABI Agriculture and Bioscience*, 1, 1. <https://doi.org/10.1186/s43170-020-00001-y>.

United Nations. (2016). *Political Declaration of the High-Level Meeting of the General Assembly on Antimicrobial Resistance: Draft Resolution/submitted by the President of the General Assembly*. <https://digitallibrary.un.org/record/842813/?ln=en> accessed 13 September 2021.

United Nations. (2021). *United Nations Environment Programme. Agenda Item 2: Update on UNEP's engagement in the One Health collaboration*. <https://wedocs.unep.org/bitstream/handle/20.500.11822/35824/CPR%20subcom%2022%20April%20item%202%20-%20One%20Health.pdf?sequence=1&isAllowed=y> accessed 19 September 2021.

United Nations. (2021). 'Food and Agriculture Organization. Joint Tripartite (FAO, OIE, WHO) and UNEP Statement. Tripartite and UNEP Support OHHLEP's definition of "One Health"', 1 December 2021. <https://www.fao.org/3/cb7869en/cb7869en.pdf> accessed 2 December 2021.

United States Department of Agriculture. *National Antimicrobial Resistance Monitoring System (NARMS)*. <https://www.fsis.usda.gov/science-data/data-sets-visualizations/microbiology/national-antimicrobial-resistance-monitoring> accessed 23 January 2021.

United States Department of Agriculture. (2010). *National Animal Health Monitoring System. Collecting Vital Information on Animal Health*. <https://www.aphis.usda.gov/animal_health/nahms/downloads/NAHMS_brochure_1.pdf> accessed 14 September 2021.

United States Department of Agriculture. (2019). *National Animal Health Monitoring System Antimicrobial Use and Stewardship on U.S. Feedlots, 2017*. <https://www.aphis.usda.gov/animal_health/nahms/amr/downloads/amu-feedlots_1.pdf> accessed 23 January 2021.

United States Department of Agriculture. (2021). *National Animal Health Monitoring System (NAHMS)*. <https://www.aphis.usda.gov/aphis/ourfocus/animalhealth/monitoring-and-surveillance/nahms/about> accessed 23 January 2021.

United States Food and Drug Administration. (2012). *FDA Guidance for Industry #209 The Judicious Use of Medically Important Antimicrobial Drugs in Food-Producing Animals*. <https://www.fda.gov/regulatory-information/search-fda-guidance-documents/cvm-gfi-209-judicious-use-medically-important-antimicrobial-drugs-food-producing-animals> and *FDA Guidance for Industry #213 New Animal Drugs and New Animal Drug Combination Products Administered in or on Medicated Feed or Drinking Water of Food-Producing Animals: Recommendations for Drug Sponsors for Voluntarily Aligning Product Use Conditions with GFI #209*. <https://www.fda.gov/regulatory-information/search-fda-guidance-documents/cvm-gfi-213-new-animal-drugs-and-new-animal-drug-combination-products-administered-or-medicated-feed> accessed 14 September 2021.

United States Food and Drug Administration. (2021). *The National Antimicrobial Resistance Monitoring System*. <https://www.fda.gov/animal-veterinary/antimicrobial-resistance/national-antimicrobial-resistance-monitoring-system> accessed 23 January 2021.

United States Food and Drug Administration. (2021). *Timeline of FDA Action on Antimicrobial Resistance*. <https://www.fda.gov/animal-veterinary/antimicrobial-resistance/timeline-fda-action-antimicrobial-resistance> accessed 2 December 2021.

United States Department of Health and Human Services. (2014). *Presidential Advisory Council on Combating Antibiotic-Resistant Bacteria (PACCARB)*. <https://www.hhs.gov/ash/advisory-committees/paccarb/index.html> accessed 23 January 2021.

United States Office of Management and Budget. (2021). *NAHMS AMR SS Part A (20210706). Supporting Statement On-Farm Monitoring of Antimicrobial Use and Resistance in U.S. Broiler Production*. OMB Number 0579-XXXX. <https://omb.report/icr/202106-0579-011/doc/112378300> accessed 15 September 2021.

Wada, Y., Irekeola, A. A., Syafirah, E. N., Yusof, W., Huey, L. L., Muhammad, S. L., et al. (2021). 'Prevalence of Vancomycin-Resistant Enterococcus (VRE) in Companion Animals: The First

Meta-Analysis and Systematic Review', *Antibiotics*, 10/2, 138. <https://doi.org/10.3390/antibiotics1 0020138>.

World Health Organization. (2015). Sixty-Eighth World Health Assembly. *Global Action Plan on Antimicrobial Resistance*. 26 May 2015. <https://www.who.int/docs/default-source/antimicrobial-resistance/amr-spc-sel-glass/a68-r7-en.pdf?sfvrsn=fa7f3dde_2> accessed 13 September 2021.

World Health Organization. (2016). *Global Action Plan on Antimicrobial Resistance*. <https://www.who.int/publications/i/item/9789241509763> accessed 13 September 2021.

World Health Organization. (2017). 'Food and Agriculture Organization/World Organization for Animal/World Health Organization. The Tripartite's Commitment. Providing multi-sectoral, collaborative leadership in addressing health challenges. 2017'. <https://www.who.int/zoonoses/tri partite_oct2017.pdf> accessed 19 September 2021.

World Health Organization. (2017). *Global Antimicrobial Resistance and Use Surveillance System (GLASS)*. <https://www.who.int/initiatives/glass> accessed 19 September 2021.

World Health Organization. (2019). *Human Resources: Annual Report. Report by the Secretariat*. <https://apps.who.int/gb/ebwha/pdf_files/WHA72/A72_43-en.pdf> accessed 21 September 2021.

World Health Organization. (2019). *WHO releases the 2019 AWaRe Classification Antibiotics*. <https://www.who.int/news/item/01-10-2019-who-releases-the-2019-aware-classification-antibiotics> accessed 19 September 2021.

World Health Organization. (2020). *One Health Global Leaders Group on Antimicrobial Resistance. 20 July 2020*. <https://www.who.int/news-room/articles-detail/one-health-global-leaders-group-on-antimicrobial-resistance> accessed 19 September 2021.

World Health Organization. (2020). *WHO's Budget Segments*. <https://www.who.int/about/account ability/budget> accessed 21 September 2021.

World Health Organization. (2021). *Global Antimicrobial Resistance Surveillance System (GLASS) Report: 2021*. <https://www.who.int/publications/i/item/9789240027336> accessed 19 September 2021.

World Health Organization. (2021). *26 International experts to kickstart the One Health High Level Expert Panel (OHHLEP)*. <https://www.who.int/news/item/11-06-2021-26-international-experts-to-kickstart-the-joint-fao-oie-unep-who-one-health-high-level-expert-panel-(ohhlep)> accessed 19 September 2021.

World Health Organization. (2021). *Library of AMR National Action Plans*. <https://www.who.int/teams/surveillance-prevention-control-AMR/national-action-plan-monitoring-evaluation/libr ary-of-national-action-plans> accessed 13 September 2021.

World Organization for Animal Health. (2016). *Antimicrobial Resistance*. <https://www.oie.int/en/what-we-do/global-initiatives/antimicrobial-resistance/#ui-id-3> accessed 20 September 2021.

World Organization for Animal Health. (2016). *Resolution No. 36. Combating Antimicrobial Resistance through a One Health Approach: Actions and OIE Strategy*. <https://www.oie.int/filead min/Home/eng/Our_scientific_expertise/docs/pdf/AMR/A_RESO_AMR_2016.pdf> accessed 20 September 2021.

World Organization for Animal Health. (2016). *The OIE Strategy on Antimicrobial Resistance and the Prudent Use of Antimicrobials. November 2016*. <https://www.oie.int/fileadmin/Home/eng/Media _Center/docs/pdf/PortalAMR/EN_OIE-AMRstrategy.pdf> accessed 20 September 2021.

World Organization for Animal Health. (2020). *Food and Agriculture Organization/ World Organization for Animal Health/World Health Organization/ United Nations Development Multi Partner Trust Fund and resource partners kick off the allocation of funds to combat against AMR. 13 March 2020*. <https://www.oie.int/en/fao-oie-who-undp-and-resource-partners-kick-off-the-all ocation-of-funds-to-combat-against-amr/> accessed 19 September 2021.

World Organization for Animal Health. (2021). *OIE Annual Report on Antimicrobial Agents Intended for Use in Animals. Fifth Report. 13 September 2021*. <https://www.oie.int/en/docum ent/fifth-oie-annual-report-on-antimicrobial-agents-intended-for-use-in-animals/> accessed 20 September 2021.

World Organization for Animal Health. (2021). *2021 Budget Estimates and Proposed 2021 Contributions Scale*. <https://web.oie.int/downld/PROC2020/A_BUDGET2021-CONTRIB.pdf> accessed 21 September 2021.

World Organization for Animal Health. (2021). *Headquarters. OIE Headquarters Organizational Chart.* <https://www.oie.int/en/who-we-are/structure/headquarters/> accessed 21 September 2021.

World Organization for Animal Health. (2021). *Standards. OIE International Standards.* <https://www.oie.int/en/what-we-do/standards/> accessed 21 September 2021.

World Trade Organization. (1995). *Understanding the WTO. What We Do.* <https://www.wto.org/english/thewto_e/whatis_e/what_we_do_e.htm> accessed 21 September 2021.

World Trade Organization. (1998). *Understanding the WTO Agreement on Sanitary and Phytosanitary Measures.* <https://www.wto.org/english/tratop_e/sps_e/spsund_e.htm> accessed 21 September 2021.

12

From Policy to Practice

Challenges and Opportunities for Cross-Sectoral AMR Mitigation and Response Efforts

Jessica Craig, Jyoti Joshi, and Isabel Frost

Introduction

Antimicrobial resistance (AMR) is emerging as one of the most complex global public health challenges of the twenty-first century. Since the discovery of penicillin in 1928, the widespread use of antimicrobials, alongside improvements in access to clean water, sanitation, and vaccines, has helped eliminate infectious diseases as a leading cause of death in most developed countries and increased the average human life-span (Gottfried, 2005). But today, the efficacy of many antimicrobial agents is under threat as micro-organisms are increasingly becoming resistant to commonly available antimicrobials (Center for Disease Dynamics, Economic & Policy, 2021; World Health Organization, 2019). The US Centers for Disease Control and Prevention (CDC) estimate that more than 2.8 million Americans acquired antibiotic-resistant infections each year and more than 35,000 people die from those infections (Centers for Disease Control and Prevention, 2019). Globally, the World Health Organization (WHO) estimates that 700,000 people die each year from drug-resistant diseases (World Health Organization, 2019). Beyond direct morbidity and mortality from drug-resistant infections, AMR also compromises our ability to treat other diseases including cancer, HIV, and diabetes, and to manage common and life-saving clinical procedures such as surgery, organ transplant, and intensive care.

Though AMR is a naturally occurring consequence of evolution, there are several factors—such as high antimicrobial use (AMU) and consumption (AMC) including their misuse and overuse in the human health, animal health, and agricultural sectors and pharmaceutical pollution in the environment—that exacerbate the emergence and spread of AMR (Willis and Chandler, 2019). Moreover, drug-resistant microbes do not need visas to travel. In an increasingly globalized world, resistant microbes and genes that confer resistance are often found causing resistant infections far from the sites of their original discovery. Hence, AMR is a truly global challenge that requires international collaboration and investment.

In this chapter, we will explore key challenges to and opportunities for AMR mitigation and policy implementation efforts with a specific focus on low- and middle-income

Jessica Craig, Jyoti Joshi, and Isabel Frost, *From Policy to Practice* In: *Steering against Superbugs*. Edited by: Olivier Rubin, Erik Baekkeskov, and Louise Munkholm, Oxford University Press. © Oxford University Press 2023. DOI: 10.1093/oso/9780192899477.003.0012

countries (LMICs) (see Chapter 7 for further discussion of LMIC challenges). We will begin by looking at barriers to moving national action plans and policies from paper to practice and challenges in realizing the One Health approach set forth at the policy level. We will discuss specific challenges in implementing routine AMR surveillance and will then describe the importance of synergizing AMR mitigation efforts with existing public health efforts, namely infection prevention and control (IPC), water, sanitation, and hygiene (WASH), and vaccination. Throughout, we will present examples from various countries to illustrate implementation successes and barriers. We close with a summary of key policy recommendations to accelerate AMR mitigation and response efforts in LMICs.

From paper to practice: Implementing AMR action plans, policies, and the One Health approach

In 2015, United Nations' member countries endorsed the WHO's Global Action Plan on Antimicrobial Resistance (GAP on AMR) at the World Health Assembly solidifying international recognition of AMR as a global public health challenge and a threat to modern medicine (World Health Organization, 2015). The GAP on AMR provided a framework for addressing AMR and outlined five strategic objectives to improve awareness and understanding of AMR, strengthen knowledge through surveillance and research, reduce the incidence of infection, optimize AMU, and ensure sustainable investment in countering AMR. The GAP on AMR spurred momentum to address AMR at the national level as individual countries enhanced their commitment to addressing AMR by developing and introducing national action plans and other national and sub-national policy and regulatory changes. Just two years after the GAP on AMR was endorsed, 100 countries had developed and published national actions plans and other national policies, regulations, and calls-to-action around AMR prevention and response (World Health Organization 2020). These action plans and policies outlined specific national priorities, introduced avenues for AMR prevention and response, and represented an important step forward in putting AMR on the national and global public health agendas.

Yet despite widespread recognition and support for AMR at the policy level, the implementation of national action plans and policies has faced practical challenges particularly in LMICs and other resource-constrained settings. Prioritization of AMR activities within broader national development agendas has proven difficult to overcome, and domestic financial investment for AMR activities is lacking. Consequently, national action plans and policies for AMR have become orphaned documents in many LMICs. In 2019, only twenty-seven of 115 countries (19.9 per cent) who provided data on their AMR national action plan development and implementation status to the WHO reported that their plans and policies were accompanied by identified funding sources (World Health Organization, 2020). This is driven, in part, by the continued lack of awareness and understanding of AMR outside of medical, scientific, and public health stakeholder groups.

In addition, there is an increasing number of competing health and other national priority investment areas. For instance, in the human health sector, LMICs continue to face a high burden of infectious diseases including TB, HIV/AIDS, neglected tropical diseases, and several new and emerging diseases. While the impact of the SARS-CoV-2 (COVID-19) pandemic on AMR policy implementation and mitigation efforts (and other longer term public health challenges) has not yet been fully characterized, pandemic response has strained national economies and health systems forcing significant financial and human resources earmarked for AMR to be diverted to pandemic response (Huttner et al., 2020; Rawson et al., 2020). At the same time, non-communicable diseases such as heart disease, hypertension, and cancer are becoming more prevalent (Ndubuisi, 2021). Consequently, LMICs face a dual burden of disease with implications for budgetary allocation, health spending, and reliance on donor funds for vertical disease control programmes. Moreover, financial support for health does not always take priority amid other competing issues such as national security, food security, and livelihoods.

Moreover, AMR is a truly 'One Health' challenge. Its drivers and solutions fall across the human, animal, plant, and environmental health sectors including the agricultural and food-producing, food safety, and pharmaceutical sectors. Antimicrobials are used to prevent, treat, and control infectious diseases in humans and animals and to enhance and promote growth in farm animals. Antimicrobials are used as pesticides and sprayed on crops to control pests in agriculture. Antimicrobial residues from human, animal, and plant sector consumption and use and pharmaceutical manufacturing enter soil and water ecosystems where pathogenic and non-pathogenic genes that impart resistance are widely shared across species of micro-organisms. Drug-resistant microbes can be transmitted between humans, animals, and the environment either directly or through contaminated food and water sources. Since humans and animals are infected by the same bacteria and share a common ecosystem, actions taken in one sector directly affect the other.

As such, there is a need to coordinate actions across sectors using a One Health approach defined by the WHO as a strategy to design and implement programmes, policies, legislation, and research so that multiple sectors communicate and work together to achieve better public health outcomes. A One Health approach to AMR requires multisectoral coordination and active engagement with all relevant stakeholders including nurses, physicians, and other healthcare workers; researchers and academics; pharmacists and laboratory technicians; farmers and veterinarians; industry and private sector groups including pharmaceutical companies, manufacturers, and those involved in food supply chains; policy-makers, legislators, and regulators; and the public, who consume both antimicrobial medicines and food products produced using antimicrobials.

Several international partnerships for AMR solutions have emerged. For example, the United Nations has brought together three key animal and human health agencies—the

Food and Agriculture Organization (FAO), the World Organization for Animal Health (OIE), and the WHO—in a Tripartite partnership to coordinate global one-health activities (FAO, OIE, WHO, 2021). At the national level, AMR action plans and policies incorporate the One Health approach to varying degrees. Often, a multisectoral group of stakeholders representing key sectors are involved in the development of such policy documents; however, the implementation and coordination of a One Health response is often lacking. As a result, cross-sectoral coordination and collaboration is largely unrealized in most countries, particularly LMICs where the human and animal health sectors are in different levels of maturity with varied capabilities for key mitigation activities such as awareness and education, surveillance, and stewardship.

Although a comprehensive analysis assessing whether the One Health approach has been achieved at the global or national levels has not yet been conducted, the authors' previous and ongoing work with international and national stakeholders across Asia and Africa indicates that it has not. Generally, AMR-relevant capacities and activities are most active and developed in the human health sector followed by the animal health sector; AMR mitigation efforts in the environmental health sector are altogether largely unrealized.

To illustrate the challenges in translating AMR policy documents from paper to practice and in achieving a true One Health approach, we will present an example from Burkina Faso, where the authors have worked extensively.

Burkina Faso, a low-income country in western Africa, published a national action plan for AMR which outlined national priorities and activities to take place between 2017 and 2020 (Kalanxhi et al., 2022). The Ministry of Health spearheaded the plan's development in collaboration with other relevant government ministries for animal health, livestock/agriculture, and environment and with technical and financial support from the WHO and a US non-profit organization. Burkina Faso's national action plan outlined key goals and overall activities for AMR mitigation and was aligned well with the GAP on AMR. However, the plan did not include a timeline for implementation, budget, or a monitoring and evaluation framework which left gaps in stakeholder accountability and in assessing progress in implementation.

Although the national action plan became publicly available in 2016, it was never approved nor formally implemented by the national government in the period that the plan covered. The lack of a clear legislative agreement on the national action plan meant that a broadly framed finance law provided a provision for a budget line for the management of epidemics but did not specifically cover resources for AMR. This highlights the need for advocacy at the top level of political leadership and finance ministry to mobilize resources and ensure sustainable funding for NAP activities (see Chapter 14 for a further discussion of the advocacy ecology). A 2019 interministerial decree established a One Health AMR committee to oversee decision-making and regulation for AMR strategies in Burkina Faso. The committee includes representatives from the human, animal, and environmental health sectors and meets regularly; however, the lack of domestic and donor funding is a major barrier to further policy implementation. Previous and ongoing donor support is limited and is skewed towards the human health sector which has caused key AMR capacities in the animal health sector to lag those in the human health one. For example, as of 2018, there were fifteen laboratories that reported AMR data to the national surveillance system. Of those, fourteen dealt with the human health sector and only one with the animal health sector. Of fifty-three total laboratories capable of isolating and testing for drug resistance, there is only one national livestock laboratory and six non-operational regional livestock laboratories.

AMR surveillance for evidence, policy, and change

To detect, respond, and prevent drug-resistant infections at the clinical, public health, and policy levels, researchers and policy-makers must have a robust evidence base. Surveillance is a critical lynchpin in understanding the burden of AMR, monitoring and elucidating trends and epidemiological patterns, and assessing the impact of AMS interventions, policies, and other mitigation efforts.

In the context of AMR, surveillance encompasses community- and hospital-acquired (nosocomial) infectious diseases, drug resistance, and AMC and/or AMU. Generally, AMC and AMU surveillance has lagged AMR surveillance which has lagged surveillance efforts for other diseases and health challenges such as HIV, TB, and malnutrition. Given the complexity of AMR and the status of AMR among other health and investment priorities, there are a number of implementation challenges for AMR surveillance which thus far have hindered robust data collection and have prevented available evidence from widely informing emerging interventions and policies.

Since 2015, numerous regional and international surveillance systems have been developed and implemented including the WHO's Global Antimicrobial Resistance and Use Surveillance System (GLASS) which now has AMR and AMC surveillance components, the Central Asian and European Surveillance of Antimicrobial Resistance (CAESAR), the European Antimicrobial Resistance Surveillance Network (EARS-Net), and the Latin American Network for Antimicrobial Resistance Surveillance (ReLAVRA) (Frost et al., 2021). In addition, there are industry-funded surveillance systems and other independent surveillance efforts ongoing around the world. Most regional AMC surveillance networks are confined to Europe and include European Surveillance of Antimicrobial Consumption Network, Antimicrobial Medicines Consumption Network (run by the WHO Regional Office for Europe), Western Pacific Regional Antimicrobial Consumption Surveillance System (run by the WHO Regional Office for the Western Pacific).

Despite these efforts, there are still significant gaps and challenges in global AMR surveillance and reporting capacity. For one, international and regional surveillance systems capture data from only a fraction of countries, limited by surveillance capacities within each country and even in each facility collecting AMR and AMC data. The 2021 GLASS report, for example, captured AMR data from only seventy countries, thirty-seven of which were LMICs, and AMC data from only nineteen countries, seventeen of which were LMICs (WHO, 2021). Ten countries in Africa that were enrolled in GLASS did not report data in 2021 demonstrating challenges in consistent data collection and reportage from the national to international levels. Even in facilities or countries where AMR surveillance is active, there are severe inconsistencies and limitations in data collection methodologies and data quality which makes it challenging, at present, to elucidate meaningful conclusions from available surveillance data or to compare AMR burdens across countries or regions (Frost et al., 2021). Many of the barriers to robust AMR surveillance reflect wider health systems challenges such as the lack of funding, human resources, and technological and laboratory capacity required for accurate surveillance (see Chapter 7 for a further discussion).

The best surveillance systems are those that consistently and systematically collect, analyse, and report data. There are two broad types of health surveillance: passive and active (Nsubuga et al., 2006). In passive surveillance systems, individual healthcare facilities are responsible for reporting data to a central body, such as district hospitals reporting AMR data to the national government. In these systems, methodologies and data quality can vary across facilities which may have different standards or requirements for when to report data and across individual healthcare workers tasked with inputting patient and health data. Active surveillance systems employ staff who collect data from health facilities thereby alleviating burden on healthcare facilities and eliminating data quality and methodological variance issues. However, high operational costs and a lack of human resources are drawbacks of active surveillance systems. Surveillance systems also come in a variety of paper-based, SMS-based, or other electronic formats, each with a varying ease of utility that may impact data quantity and quality. Taken together, different surveillance platforms and strategies may allow for far more robust and consistent data collection which better reflect reality. As different facilities and countries have implemented different strategies and platforms, the resulting data streams are difficult to assess for comparability.

Regardless of the type and format of data collection, analysis, and reporting, two critical questions are those of sustainability and interlinkage across health areas. Historically the approach to surveillance is disease specific. HIV surveillance is independent from malaria surveillance which is independent from emerging AMR surveillance. The separation of such efforts may reflect disease-specific funding streams. At the implementation level, independent, disease-specific surveillance systems allow each system to be tailored to each disease; however, these parallel efforts are costly and often cannot be interlinked. Overall, this increases the burden on already strained health systems, particularly in LMICs, which threatens long-term viability of all surveillance efforts which often begin with foreign donor support. Importantly, the lack of interlinkage between systems may also prevent cross-systems analyses, critical to such a complex challenge as AMR, and may therefore lead to missed opportunities to identify epidemiological trends, priority areas for intervention, or novel cross-cutting solutions. Moreover, AMR surveillance needs to go beyond individual diseases in humans to include the animal and environmental health sectors. Thus, effective AMR surveillance systems need to adapt and expand on traditional disease surveillance mechanisms to adequately match the complexity of AMR.

Other challenges in current AMR surveillance include the lack of standardization in data collection, analysis, and reporting methodologies including variations in units of measurement, data points collected, and volume and detail of information reported. In addition, AMR surveillance is often limited to results of antimicrobial susceptibility testing (AST) data; however, in order to better understand the patient- and population-level drivers of AMR, surveillance systems must also collect and link patient- and facility-level clinical and sociodemographic information such as clinical diagnosis, prescribed antimicrobial treatment, adherence to prescribed treatment, previous exposure to antimicrobials, access to improved water and sanitation facilities, or length of hospital stay for admitted patients. However, in many LMICs there are wide-sweeping evidence gaps across these key clinical and sociodemographic areas.

The ability to generate AMR data hinges on the availability and utilization of certain clinical and laboratory capacities. Testing for drug resistance requires a series of clinical and microbiological tests and capacities including patient specimen collection, culturing micro-organisms, and conducting AST. This, in turn, means that specialized equipment, reagents and antimicrobial disks (for AST), and trained laboratory technicians must be consistently available and accessible for accurate surveillance data.

In many LMICs, it is often not feasible to have these capacities available at every healthcare facility given the lack of human resources and equipment and frequent stock-outs of reagents and antimicrobial disks at both the facility and national levels. Moreover, it is often not feasible to sustain an inter-facility specimen transport mechanism given logistical, infrastructure, human resources, or even security challenges. Consequently, the ability to isolate, detect, and identify drug-resistant organisms and contribute AMR data to a surveillance platform is limited to national referral hospitals and a small fraction of other facilities. Limiting AMR surveillance to national referral or regional hospitals may lead to an overestimation of the true AMR burden or other biases as most patients who seek healthcare services at tertiary healthcare facilities represent the sickest patients, those of higher socio-economic status, or those who live nearer to national or regional referral hospitals, often located in urban centres.

The Center for Disease Dynamics, Economics & Policy's Resistance Map is a platform that collates AMR data from all available international, regional, national, and subnational surveillance systems. Across these systems, AMR and/or AMU data is available for only twelve of fifty-five Africa Union Member States (Center for Disease Dynamics, Economics & Policy, 2021). Of those twelve countries, Malawi has the most robust AMR surveillance data available dating back to 1998 for select antibiotic–organism combinations. Therefore, we will take Malawi as an illustrative example of surveillance implementation challenges common, in many ways, to LMICs around the world.

Malawi first introduced a national action plan for AMR in 2017 (Government of the Republic of Malawi, 2017). The plan estimates that all AMR-related implementation activities ranging from awareness and education to laboratory capacity building and surveillance efforts will cost about US$ 1 million. Since the 2017/2018 fiscal year, the national government has allocated approximately $US 24,000 for AMR (Craig et al.,

2021). Malawi's national AMR surveillance system was quickly established to include fifteen district-level laboratories, representing 40 per cent of the country's healthcare facilities. Progress to incorporate additional laboratories into its national AMR surveillance system has since stalled due to a lack of financial resources to purchase equipment and reagents and to hire and train staff (Craig et al., 2021). However, although fifteen laboratories regularly collect and report AMR surveillance data to the national surveillance platform, the country only reports data from two surveillance sites to GLASS. Moreover, even at facilities where the clinical and laboratory capacity to generate AMR data is available, healthcare workers rarely request that patient specimens be collected and tested for resistance preferring instead to treat patients empirically, according to Ministry of Health staff (Craig et al., 2021).

According to available AMR surveillance data from Malawi, rates of resistance of common pathogens to most antimicrobials has increased since the early 2000s. For example, *Escherichia coli* resistance to third-generation cephalosporins rose from 0 per cent (Confidence interval (CI): 0–7 per cent for 43 isolates tested) in 2003 to 72 per cent (CI: 69–75 per cent of 1,125 isolates tested) in 2017, and resistance to fluoroquinolones rose from 0 per cent (CI: 0–2 per cent of 131 isolates tested) in 2001 to 21 per cent (CI: 14–29 per cent of 107 isolates tested) in 2014 (Center for Disease Dynamics, Economics & Policy, 2021). Critical information such as on data quality, data collection methods, or stock-outs that impacted AST are not reported alongside these data.

Given the limitations just described of Malawi's AMR surveillance system, it is unclear how to interpret this available AMR data and how to utilize it to inform policy and practice. The case of Malawi demonstrates the various implementation challenges and other barriers that prevent robust AMR surveillance globally. Resolving these challenges and minimizing barriers to accurate AMR surveillance will include system-wide investments and capacity building. Epidemiological research that assesses how to reach representative population-based surveillance with the fewest resources required may help focus efforts as will international consensus on how to interpret and utilize AMR surveillance data (i.e., at what level do national resistance rates need to reach to warrant certain interventions?). Of course, the challenges outlined here only explore the human health sector. At present, there is no international equivalent for AMR or AMC surveillance in the animal or environmental health sectors. Surveillance efforts in these sectors generally lag that of the human health sector. For example, in Malawi, there are only two facilities that collect and report data on AMR in animals.

Synergizing AMR mitigation efforts with existing public health efforts: The role of IPC, WASH, and vaccination

Improvements in infection prevention and control (IPC), provision of safe water, hygiene, and sanitation (WASH) and preventive vaccines all contribute to reducing the burden of infectious diseases and, therefore, the need for clinical treatment with antimicrobials. With a declining antibiotic development pipeline, increased investment in improving IPC, vaccine roll out and development, and provision of WASH infrastructure are essential to improve health system preparedness while also addressing AMR.

It is estimated that vaccines avert 4 to 5 million deaths from diphtheria, tetanus, pertussis (whooping cough), and measles (WHO, 2019). Approximately 1.5 million deaths could be averted by improving global vaccination coverage (WHO, 2019). The mechanisms by which vaccines reduce AMR are complex but can be simplified into two main pathways: By reducing the burden of both resistant and susceptible infections, and by reducing the selection pressure for AMR, as AMU falls with the number of total infections (Sriram et al., 2021). Ultimately, this reduction in resistant cases will lead to fewer untreatable infections and save lives. Several vaccines including those against pneumococcal disease, seasonal influenza, typhoid, and rotavirus which are already available on the market and included in many national immunization programs have been shown to have an impact on AMU, or the occurrence of resistant pathogens, or both. There are several other vaccines in the pipeline, such as those for Tuberculosis, shigella, and gram-negative bacteria that may have a substantial impact in reducing the AMR burden.

Over the past few years, efforts to better quantify the impact of vaccination on the current and future AMR burden have been made. A recent global study reported that the pneumococcal conjugate vaccines and live-attenuated rotavirus vaccines confer 19.7 per cent (3.4–43.4 per cent) and 11.4 per cent (4.0–18.6 per cent) protection against antibiotic-treated episodes of acute respiratory infection and diarrhoea, respectively, in age groups with the greatest disease burden attributable to the vaccine-targeted pathogens (Lewnard et al., 2020). Studies have estimated that even with limited use, pneumococcal and rotavirus vaccines prevent 23.8 million and 13.6 million antibiotic-treatable illness episodes, respectively, among children under five in LMICs (Atkins and Flasche, 2018). However, by achieving universal coverage with these two vaccines, an additional 40 million episodes of antibiotic-treated illness can easily be prevented.

Although the impact has not yet been quantified, improving IPC and WASH in the community and healthcare settings are similarly recognized pathways to reduce the total infectious disease and AMR burden; however, building IPC and WASH capacity and infrastructure requires significantly more time and financial investment than increasing vaccine coverage.

Global attention and investment for improving vaccine coverage, IPC, and WASH has a significantly longer lifespan than the global focus on AMR, and great strides have been made in these areas. However, implementation challenges—some historic, some emerging—in vaccination, IPC, and WASH persist, and progress is beginning to stall. Global coverage for all internationally recommended vaccines, for example, has stagnated at around 86 per cent, below the global herd immunity target of 95 per cent (UNICEF, 2019). More than 2 billion people worldwide do not have access to basic sanitation facilities and more than 3 billion do not have access to hand-washing facilities in their households (Centers for Disease Control and Prevention, 2021). The Centers for Disease Control and Prevention estimates that more than 800,000 people die each from diarrhoea from a vaccine-preventable disease or from unsafe drinking water, lack of sanitation, or poor hand hygiene practices (Centers for Disease Control and Prevention, 2015). An estimated 50 per cent of healthcare facilities in LMICs lack access to piped water and nearly 40 per cent do not have soap or alcohol-based sanitizer for handwashing (Centers for Disease Control and Prevention, 2020). An assessment of IPC in over 16,000 healthcare facilities across eighteen countries in sub-Saharan Africa found that only 17 per cent had standard operating procedures for IPC (Kanyangarara et al., 2021).

Barriers to improving IPC and WASH in LMICs include insufficient data collection and evaluation of current capacities, lack of domestic and donor funding, lack of political will, and economic and socio-political marginalization of those with the least degree of access to community-based WASH (Kmentt et al., 2021; Sinharoy et al., 2019). Globally, drivers of vaccine coverage stagnation and/or decline vary. Vaccine hesitancy driven by complacency, misinformation, disinformation, or religious and political beliefs is cited as a driver for lower vaccine coverage or uptake rates in both developed and developing countries (Larson et al., 2019; Vinck et al., 2019). Anti-vaccinations movements have emerged and gained traction in North America and parts of Europe; the 'anti-vax phenomenon' is now recognized as one of the top ten global public health threats (Martin et al., 2019). There has also been an overall decline in foreign or international investment for vaccines globally perhaps fuelled by complacency regarding vaccine-preventable diseases and shifting political priorities (Loharikar et al., 2016). In LMICs, the lack of healthcare workers, long distances to healthcare facilities, and frequent stock-outs of vaccines, particularly in rural areas, are continued barriers to vaccination. At the same time, humanitarian crises ranging from war and conflict to natural disasters has resulted in an unprecedented number of displaced persons globally which has impeded vaccination and other public health efforts (UNICEF, 2019; Internal Displacement Monitoring Centre, 2021).

In recent years, Zimbabwe has experienced recurrent and increasingly frequent outbreaks of drug-resistant typhoid and cholera. Between October 2017 and February 2018, an outbreak of ciprofloxacin-resistant typhoid resulted in more than 3,000 suspected cases, according to the WHO (World Health Organization, 2021). Between September 2018 and March 2019, there was an outbreak of cholera that was resistant to nearly all antibiotics. In response, the Zimbabwean government improved WASH, conducted AMU education sessions, and carried out mass vaccination campaigns in the communities affected by the outbreaks. Zimbabwean Ministry of Health staff noted that while WASH and IPC are important in reducing and preventing infectious diseases transmission, this infrastructure requires time and significant financial investments to implement and sustain; therefore, vaccination became key to preventing future outbreaks of drug-resistant typhoid and cholera.

The potential of vaccination to reduce inappropriate AMC and reduce the burden of infectious disease requires large-scale investments in childhood vaccination. Research is needed to understand how the use of vaccines can be optimized to combat AMR and to quantify the value of vaccines in terms of their impact on AMR. This would encourage further investment in the roll-out and uptake of licensed vaccines known to have an impact on AMR and enable the prioritization of research activities on novel vaccines against resistant pathogens.

Key policy recommendations to accelerate AMR mitigation and response efforts in LMICs

AMR is an emerging global public health threat, perhaps unprecedented in its potential scale and complexity. To meet this challenge, international and national actors must move beyond recognizing the threat of AMR at the policy level and begin to put mitigation and response efforts into practice. This will require national governments to prioritize AMR and to increase domestic financing for AMR-specific activities.

However, recognizing that this may not be feasible in the context of many competing health and national priorities, national and international stakeholders should identify and invest in cross-cutting areas such as IPC, WASH, and vaccines which will not only slow and prevent AMR but will also reduce the overall infectious disease burden, improve the quality of life and healthcare, and reduce economic losses from lost wages and costs due to outbreak response.

While financial and human resource allocations for AMR surveillance, including for the clinical and laboratory infrastructure required to generate AMR data, may not result in an immediate and tangible return on investment, surveillance is critical for generating an evidence base on the AMR burden which will help ensure that future policies and mitigation efforts will be effective. Opportunities to piggyback AMR surveillance activities on existing disease surveillance systems should be explored and exploited whenever possible, as should surveillance efforts across the human, animal, and environmental health sectors. In summary, tackling AMR can seem like an overwhelming challenge akin to combatting climate change or alleviating global poverty. However, small but strategic investments and interventions that move policy to practice can help turn the tide.

References

Atkins, K. E., and Flasche, S. (2018). 'Vaccination to Reduce Antimicrobial Resistance', *Lancet Global Health*, 6/3, e252. doi:10.1016/S2214-109X(18)30043-3. Accessed 29 March 2023.

Centers for Disease Control and Prevention 2019. (2019). Antibiotic Resistance Threats in the United States. https://www.cdc.gov/drugresistance/pdf/threats-report/2019-ar-threats-report-508.pdf. US CDC: Atlanta, Georgia. Accessed 29 March 2023.

Centers for Disease Control and Prevention. (2020). *Global Water, Sanitation, & Hygiene (WASH)-WASH in Healthcare Facilities.* <https://www.cdc.gov/healthywater/global/healthcare-facilities/overview.html>. US Department of Health and Human Services. Atlanta, Georgia, USA. Accessed 29 March 2023.

Centers for Disease Control and Prevention. (2021). *Global Water, Sanitation, & Hygiene (WASH)—Fast Facts.* <https://www.cdc.gov/healthywater/global/wash_statistics.html#:~:text=More%20than%202%20billion%20people,%25%20of%20the%20world's%20population).&text=About%203%20billion%20people%20worldwide,wash%20their%20hands%20at%20home>. US Department of Health and Human Services. Atlanta, Georgia, USA. Accessed 29 March 2023

Centers for Disease Control and Prevention. (2015). *Global Water, Sanitation, & Hygiene (WASH)—Global Diarrhea Burden.* <https://www.cdc.gov/healthywater/global/diarrhea-burden.html>. US Department of Health and Human Services. Atlanta, Georgia, USA. Accessed 29 March 2023.

Craig, J., Kalanxhi, E., van Wijk, M., Naing, S. Y., Nyasulu, I., Fuller, W., et al. (2022). *Malawi National Action Plan on Antimicrobial Resistance—Review of Progress in the Human Health Sector.* Antimicrobial Resistance Policy Information and Action Brief Series 2022. Geneva, Switzerland: World Health Organization.

FAO, OIE, WHO. (2021). Antimicrobial Resistance Multi-Partner Trust Fund: Forging Tripartite collaboration for urgent global and country action against antimicrobial resistance (AMR). FAO, OIE, WHO: Geneva, Switzerland. https://www.fao.org/documents/card/en/c/cb5222en. Accessed 29 March 2023.

Frost, I., Kapoor, G., Craig, J., Liu, D., and Laxminarayan, R. (2021). 'Status, Challenges and Gaps in Antimicrobial Resistance Surveillance around the World', *Journal of Global Antimicrobial Resistance*, 25, 222–26. doi:10.1016/j.jgar.2021.03.016.

Government of the Republic of Malawi. (2017). *Antimicrobial Resistance Strategy, 2017–2022.* <https://www.who.int/publications/m/item/malawi-antimicrobial-resistance-strategy-2017-2022>. Accessed 29 March 2023.

Huttner, B. D., Catho, G., Pano-Pardo, J. R., Pulcini, C., and Schouten, J. (2020). 'COVID-19: Don't Neglect Antimicrobial Stewardship Principles!', *Clinical Microbial Infections*, 26/7, 808–10. doi:10.1016/j.cmi.2020.04.024. Accessed 29 March 2023.

Internal Displacement Monitoring Centre and Norwegian Refugee Council. 2021. *Global Report on Internal Displacement.* <https://www.internal-displacement.org/sites/default/files/publications/documents/grid2021_idmc.pdf>. Accessed 29 March 2023.

Kalanxhi, E., Craig, J., Joshi, J., van Wijk, M., Naing, S. Y., Balachandran, A., et al. (2022). *Burkina Faso National Action Plan on Antimicrobial Resistance—Review of Progress in the Human Health Sector.* Antimicrobial Resistance Policy Information and Action Brief Series 2022. Geneva, Switzerland: World Health Organization.

Kanyangarara, M., Allen, S., Jiwani, S. S., and Fuente, D. (2021). 'Access to Water, Sanitation and Hygiene Services in Health Facilities in Sub-Saharan Africa 2013–2018: Results of Health Facility Surveys and Implications for COVID-19 Transmission', *BMC Health Services Research*, 21. doi:https://doi.org/10.1186/s12913-021-06515-z. Accessed 29 March 2023.

Kmentt, L., Cronk, R., Tidwell, J. B., and Rogers, E. (2021). 'Water, Sanitation, and Hygiene (WASH) in Healthcare Facilities of 14 Low- and Middle-Income Countries: To What Extent is WASH Implemented and What Are the "Drivers" of Improvement in Their Service levels?', *H2 Open Journal*, 4/1, 129–37. doi:https://doi.org/10.2166/h2oj.2021.095.

Larson, H. J., and Schulz, W. S. (2019). 'Reverse Global Vaccine Dissent', *Science*, 364/6436, 105. doi:10.1126/science.aax6172.

Lewnard, J. A., Lo, N. C., Arinaminpathy, N., Frost, I., and Laxminarayan, R. (2020). 'Childhood Vaccines and Antibiotic use in Low- and Middle-Income Countries', *Nature*, 581/7806, 94–9. https://doi.org/10.1038/S41586-020-2238-4

Loharikar, A., Dumolard, L., Chu, S., et al. (2016). Status of New Vaccine Introduction—Worldwide, September 2016. *MMWR Morb Mortal Wkly Rep*, 65/41, 1136–40. doi:10.15585/mmwr.mm6541a3. Accessed 29 March 2023.

Martin, W., Taylor, N., Gough, A., Chambers, D., and Jessop, M. (2019). 'The Anti-vax Phenomenon', *The Veterinary Record*, 184/24:744. doi:10.1136/vr.l4027.

Ndubuisi, N. E. (2021). 'Noncommunicable Diseases Prevention in Low- and Middle-Income Countries: An Overview of Health in All Policies (HiAP)', *Inquiry*, 58. doi:10.1177/0046958020927885.

Nsubuga, P., White, M. E., Thacker, S. B., Anderson, M. A., Blount, S. B., Broome, C. V., et al. (2006). *Public Health Surveillance: A Tool for Targeting and Monitoring Interventions. Disease Control Priorities in Developing Countries* (2nd edn, Washington, DC: The International Bank for Reconstruction and Development).

Rawson, T. M., Ming, D., Ahmad, R., Moore, L. S. P., and Holmes, A. H. (2020). 'Antimicrobial Use, Drug-resistant Infections and COVID-19', *Nature Reviews Microbiology*, 18, 409–10. doi:10.1038/s41579-020-0395-y. Accessed 29 March 2023.

Sinharoy, S. S., Pittluck, R., and Clasen, T. (2019). 'Review of Drivers and Barriers of Water and Sanitation Policies for Urban Informal Settlements in Low-Income and Middle-Income Countries', *Utility Policy*, 2019/60:100957. doi:10.1016/j.jup.2019.100957. Accessed 29 March 2023.

Sriram, A., Kalanxhi, E., Kapoor, G., Craig, J., et al. (2021). The State of the World's Antibiotics 2021. https://onehealthtrust.org/wp-content/uploads/2021/02/The-State-of-the-Worlds-Antibiotics-in-2021.pdf. Washington, DC: Center for Disease Dynamics, Economics & Policy. Accessed 29 March 2023.

UNICEF. (2019). 20 million children missed out on lifesaving measles, diphtheria and tetanus vaccines in 2018. <https://www.unicef.org/press-releases/20-million-children-missed-out-lifesaving-measles-diphtheria-and-tetanus-vaccines>. Accessed 29 March 2023.

Vinck, P., Pham, P. N., Bindu, K. K., Bedford, J., and Nilles, E. J. (2019). 'Institutional Trust and Misinformation in the Response to the 2018–19 Ebola Outbreak in North Kivu, DR Congo: a Population-based Survey', *The Lancet Infectious Diseases*, 19/5, 529–36. doi:https://doi.org/10.1016/S1473-3099(19)30063-5.

Willis, L. D., and Chandler, C. (2019). 'Quick Fix for Care, Productivity, Hygiene and Inequality: Reframing the Entrenched Problem of Antibiotic Overuse', *BMJ Global Health*, 4, e001590. https://gh.bmj.com/content/4/4/e001590.info. Accessed 29 March 2023

World Health Organization. (2015). Global Action Plan on Antimicrobial Resistance. World Health Organization: Geneva, Switzerland. https://www.emro.who.int/health-topics/drug-resistance/global-action-plan.html. Accessed 29 March 2023

World Health Organization. (2019). New report calls for urgent action to avert antimicrobial resistance crisis. https://www.who.int/news/item/29-04-2019-new-report-calls-for-urgent-action-to-avert-antimicrobial-resistance-crisis. World Health Organization: Geneva. Accessed 29 March 2023.

World Health Organization. (2020). *Monitoring Global Progress on Antimicrobial Resistance: Tripartite AMR Country Self-Assessment Survey (TRACSS) 2019–2020.* <https://apps.who.int/iris/bitstream/handle/10665/340236/9789240019744-eng.pdf?sequence=1&isAllowed=y>.

World Health Organization. (2021). *Global Antimicrobial Resistance and Use Surveillance System (GLASS) Report: 2021.* <https://www.who.int/publications/i/item/9789240027336>.

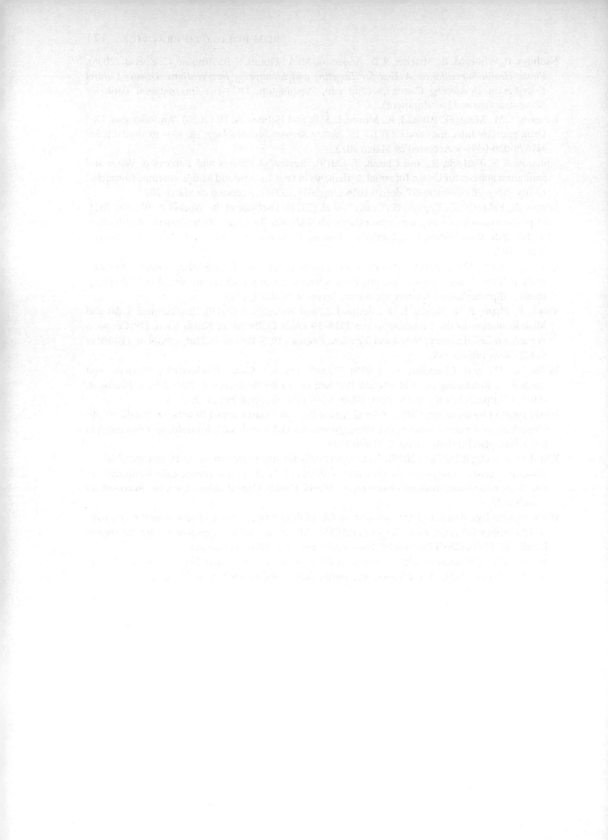

Nicholas, P., Wang, H., Baker, R., Anderson, W. A., Fischer, S. & Brosius, J., et al. (2009). "Frame Choices, Framing Effects, and Manipulating and Manipulation Attempts", United Nations Framework Convention on Climate Change (New York and Geneva, Washington, DC): the International Bank for Economic and Financial Development).

Johnson, C. M., Marques, J. F., Zhao, L. B., Marotta, S. R., and Hulme, M. N. (1830) "An Interaction That Drug vaccine risks does an COVID-19", *Nature Reviews Microbiology*, 18: 405–10 (June 2010).
    doi: 10.1038/s41586-9. Accessed 28 March 2021.

Williams, K. S., Perlman, R. and Cheard, C. (2019), 'Barriers to Uptake and Barriers to Water and Sanitation Policies for Household Sanitation in a Frame in a Low- and Middle-Income Countries', *PLOS Medicine*, 16(10) e100XXXX. doi: 10.1371/journal.

Wilson, A., Salter, C. K., Kopp, J. & Zurita, S. et al. (2020) 'Introduction to Weekly', 20: 291–301.
    'An overview of environmental communication about SARS-CoV-2' the Frame. Environmental Science & Health, 27(4), Elsevier Ltd.

13

Joint Action against AMR with a One Health Perspective

Sarah Humboldt-Dachroeden and Chris Degeling

Introduction

One Health and antimicrobial resistance (AMR)

This section defines the One Health approach and describes it in relation to antimicrobial resistance (AMR). It elaborates on the methods used for this chapter.

The One Health approach can be a crucial tool to enhance measures taken to tackle AMR. A key aspect a One Health is that drivers and outbreaks cannot be managed through disciplinary or sectoral isolation. Instead, the effective mitigation of AMR risks requires coordinated and complementary actions at the human-animal-environment interface. To establish, maintain, and optimizes interventions for AMR in a One Health context, cross-sectoral collaboration at local, national, and international levels must be achieved. It is important that all implicated sectors and relevant actors engage as AMR has consequences for maintaining human, animal, and environmental health from local to global settings.

Based on an analysis of policy initiatives and a survey of relevant policy actors on One Health governance, this chapter describes some of the key approaches taken to control and prevent AMR in Europe. Drawing on this research, potential further actions that can be introduced to enhance effective AMR governance in Europe, and potentially facilitate investigations in similar countries and contexts. The policy actor survey was open from March to July 2021 and completed by 104 experts from twenty-three European countries (see Table 13.1.

The survey respondents work at national agencies or institutes, universities, European Union (EU) agencies like the European Food and Safety Authority (EFSA), the European Environment Agency (EEA), and non-governmental organizations like the World Health Organization (WHO), and the World Organisation for Animal Health (WOAH, formerly known as OIE).

This chapter addresses the engagement of these experts in advocating for greater efforts towards AMR mitigation, their perceptions on multi-stakeholder engagements focusing on AMR, as well as their understanding of how AMR-related responsibilities are distributed across their national ministries and institutes.

Sarah Humboldt-Dachroeden and Chris Degeling, *Joint Action against AMR with a One Health Perspective* In: *Steering against Superbugs*. Edited by: Olivier Rubin, Erik Baekkeskov, and Louise Munkholm, Oxford University Press. © Oxford University Press 2023.
DOI: 10.1093/oso/9780192899477.003.0013

Table 13.1 Characteristics of study population

Countries	[n]	Workplace	[n]
Sweden	10	Veterinary institute	18
United Kingdom	10	Public health institute	17
Germany	9	University	12
Italy	9	Food institute	12
Denmark	8	Ministry (Ministries of Agriculture; Health; Education and Research)	7
France	8	NGO (WHO, WOAH, ICARS*)	5
The Netherlands	7	Interdisciplinary research institutes:	

Vet	Food	Env	Agric	[n]
x	x			4
	x	x	x	4
x	x	x		4**
x	x	x	x	3
x			x	2
			x	2

Countries	[n]	Workplace	[n]
Portugal	6	EU agency (EFSA, EMA, EEA)	4
Belgium	5	Funding institute	1
Austria	4	Museum (Natural history)	1
Finland	3	N/A	8
Norway	3		
Switzerland	3		
Hungary	2		
Ireland	2		
Lithuania	2		
Bulgaria	1		
Czech Republic	1		
Estonia	1		
Latvia	1		
Poland	1		
Romania	1		
Spain	1		
N/A	6		
Total	104		104

Countries: 23
EU countries: 20 (of 27)
European countries: 3

* ICARS: International Centre for Antimicrobial Resistance Solutions
** One research institute also includes public health services

Pathways of AMR

This chapter details three pathways of AMR (human medicine, veterinary medicine, and the environment), and it explains its relevance and connection to the One Health approach. Antimicrobials are used to treat and prevent microbial infections of humans, animals, and plants. The main pathways through which microbial organisms can develop resistance in each of these sectors are as follows:

Human medicine—All antimicrobial use promotes AMR, of which antimicrobial misuse in human healthcare is a key modifiable driver. Misuse occurs when antimicrobials are incorrectly prescribed through either non-rational drug selection or errors in dosage or duration of therapy. Consumers (and prescribers) can lack knowledge or have adverse responses to diagnostic uncertainty and the risks of withholding antimicrobial treatment (Majumder et al., 2020). In addition, inappropriate waste management at hospitals and nursing homes can enable the spread of resistant organisms into the surrounding environment like soil and water (Hashmi, 2020).

Veterinary medicine—Antimicrobials are extensively used in animal agriculture, especially in intensively farmed animals, including aquaculture (Mennerat et al., 2010). They are employed for four different reasons (Woolhouse et al., 2015):

1. as therapeutics, when an animal is in need of treatment due to a disease or injury;
2. as metaphylactics, when a group of animals is treated, for example, due to a risk of an expected infectious disease outbreak;
3. as prophylactics to prevent a disease from occurring; and
4. as growth promotion to accelerate weight gain and finishing (banned in the EU).

Wild animals and pets, especially those in close proximity to farms, can also carry resistant microbes. Microbes are transferred between livestock and wild or pet animals through direct contact or contact with contaminated soil, manure or water (Hashmi, 2020). As is the case in human medicine, veterinarians have been found to misuse antimicrobials and in some cases have demonstrated a lack of knowledge of AMR (Smith et al., 2018).

The environment—The environment can be contaminated with resistant microorganisms and mobile genetic elements that promote AMR through a variety of pathways. Resistant microbes can be found in the soil, as there are naturally occurring antibiotics (Woolhouse et al., 2015). Contributing to this natural reservoir, resistant organisms can spread from hospitals, households, and farms to the environment through wastewater, water, manure, and soil, which then can be a pathway to other animals and humans (Collignon and McEwen, 2019; Kahn, 2017). Additionally, toxic metals can enhance AMR by causing co-resistance or cross-resistance in bacteria–industrial contamination, and the use of metals like copper as feed additives, are key examples. Resistant organisms that emerge through the use of pesticides in horticulture can contaminate the soil, water, and also food or feed products (Humboldt-Dachroeden and Mantovani, 2021; Liao et al., 2021). Accordingly, the promotion of organic agriculture, where fewer pesticides and antimicrobials are used, can aid in combating AMR.

The different pathways through which AMR can emerge clearly show that it affects all areas of One Health. As alternative therapeutics to antimicrobials are few, and resistance can develop and spread quickly, rapid responses to contain AMR are crucial (Hashmi, 2020). The complexity of AMR also demonstrates that the issue extends beyond the human–animal–environment interface, connecting and implicating a broad range of social, ethical, political, and economic issues (Degeling et al., 2015).

One Health approaches to AMR in Europe

This chapter shows European approaches to tackle AMR by highlighting activities and legislations implemented by the EU and European member states. It provides a snapshot into states' handling of AMR and their approaches to collaborate cross-sectoral.

The EU is a union of twenty-seven Member States. The institutions of the EU have different functions. For example, the European Commission (EC) is tasked with proposing legislation, whereas the European Parliament (representatives of the citizens) and the Council of the European Union (government ministers from EU countries) approve or reject legislation (Wallace et al., 2020). The EU member states are tasked to implement approved legislation. Legislation is often cross-sectoral, which can result in conflicts on national level due to different governing systems of states, for example within federal states, or through the distinct organization of agencies under ministries, which might not align with the proposed cross-sectoral EU legislation (Mathieu et al., 2021).

The EU has acknowledged the importance of approaching AMR from a One Health perspective. In 2017, Member States committed to the EU One Health Action Plan against AMR. Within this strategy, the EU pledges to enhance surveillance activities across human, animal, and environmental sectors. The aim is to promote awareness and enhance research activities relating to AMR (European Commission, 2017). The main EU AMR surveillance activity is the European Antimicrobial Resistance Surveillance Network (EARS-Net), which receives and analyses data from the EU Member States, collected and aggregated by the European Centre for Disease Control (ECDC). These data are limited to clinical antimicrobial susceptibility data and do not include veterinary-related data (ECDC, 2019). To complement human clinical data and provide information regarding resistance in animals and food sources, the ECDC and the EFSA also produce a joint report on AMR (Queenan et al., 2016). Supporting this, the EC improved the monitoring of AMR in animals (Decision 2013/652/EU) by making the reporting of the incidence of bacteria known to pose a significant risk to human health mandatory. New collaborations have also been established between the EFSA, ECDC, and the European Medicines Agency (EMA) to investigate AMR and antimicrobial use in the EU (ECDC et al., 2017). Additionally, there are several other organizations that investigate and report on different aspects of AMR, such as the European Centre for the study of Animal Health and the European Surveillance of Veterinary Antimicrobial Consumption (Queenan et al., 2016).

A key feature of a One Health approach is cross-sectoral coordination and action. The survey of experts and policy actors on One Health governance provides insights into how AMR-related tasks and responsibilities are distributed across the countries' ministries and institutions (see Figure 13.1).

Fifty-seven respondents answered for nineteen European countries regarding the potential overlap of responsibilities in ministries. Respondents representing Bulgaria, Poland, Romania, and Spain did not respond to this question. In seventeen countries, at least two or more ministries have AMR-related responsibilities. Because AMR is a major risk to human health and sustainable healthcare, the ministry commissioned with health-related issues is involved in all nineteen responding countries. The ministry commissioned for agricultural-related issues shares some responsibility in fourteen countries. In nine countries, AMR is also part of the portfolio of the ministry responsible for environment-related issues. In some countries, respondents also mentioned ministries tasked with education (Czech Republic, France, Sweden) and industry or economy (France, Norway, Sweden, Germany) that are involved in AMR-related activities. This shows that in most of the nineteen countries, AMR is an issue approached from more than

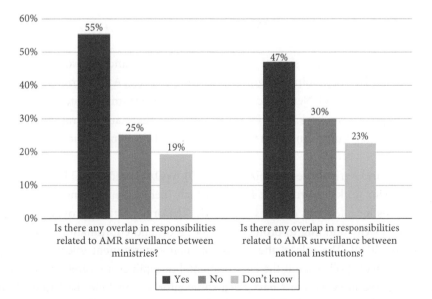

Figure 13.1 Perception of participants regarding overlap of AMR surveillance responsibilities in their countries. Institution (right) refers to national institutes or agencies that conduct AMR. surveillance.

one sectoral perspective. However, the survey only recorded a snapshot of the respondents' perspective and not of the actual activities and collaborations in the ministries. The actual work culture within the ministries might be fragmented, even though respondents recorded that AMR-related responsibilities are distributed. Within each country, it is important to understand the structures and the ways in which ministries work together. This will help to understand the specific context of the country, to curb inequalities and foster knowledge translation across sectors (Kirchhelle et al., 2020; see also Chapter 10). The survey showed that in eighteen European countries there are shared responsibilities across government agencies for AMR surveillance. For example, forty-seven respondents from eighteen countries indicated that public health, veterinary, and agriculture/food institutes are mostly tasked with AMR-related responsibilities. In seven cases (Belgium, Czech Republic, France, Germany, Hungary, Lithuania, United Kingdom), medical institutes were also involved, and in four cases (France, Germany, Switzerland, United Kingdom) the environmental institutes participated in AMR surveillance. The dedication of various agencies to AMR-related responsibilities reflects the engagement of the ministries to tackle AMR. The results also indicate that the integration of environmental agencies into AMR-related activities must be strengthened.

Approaches within Europe show that although there are initiatives and activities, a coherent approach is challenging, due to complex structures. Actors working in different sectors must compromise and collaborate to create policy change and implement One Health activities.

AMR governance—international and national opportunities

WHO initiatives

Internationally, there are several surveillance systems and networks established to combat AMR (e.g., Joint Programming Initiative on Antimicrobial Resistance (JPIAMR) and Med-Vet-Net Association). While they are important, this section focuses on approaches where the WHO is involved, as there are several initiatives and projects engaging European countries (see Chapter 11 for international One Health efforts).

The Food and Agriculture Organization (FAO), WOAH, and WHO have formed the Tripartite, who work towards One Health, which includes enhancing global surveillance systems for infectious diseases and AMR. The organizations provide tools, guidance, and capacity building to promote collaboration and coordination across sectors (FAO et al., 2019). The role of the human–animal–environment interface is emphasized in Tripartite policies, but the environmental disciplines are rarely included in its practices. In recent years, there have been some efforts to include the United Nations Environment Programme (UNEP) into the Tripartite (Tripartite Plus), but the lack of attention to the environmental dimension of One Health is still a challenge (Kirchhelle et al., 2020). The WHO is also committed in the WHO Advisory Group on Integrated

Surveillance of Antimicrobial Resistance (AGISAR), where the FAO and WOAH act as advisors. AGISAR was established in 2008 to provide guidance for establishing AMR surveillance programmes (Queenan et al., 2016), including the National Action Plans (NAPs) that WHO Member States must complete as part of the Global Action Plan on AMR (WHO, 2017).

The Global Action Plan was developed to strengthen surveillance activities on AMR and enhance the understanding and awareness of AMR as well as the use of antimicrobial agents. The objective is to reduce infections and find new treatments, diagnostics, vaccines, and other interventions (WHO, 2015). However, reporting the NAPs is challenging for many countries because of time and resource demands as well as the need for expertise from various disciplines. Further, the level of articulation of government responses around One Health principles in a country does not always lead to multisectoral collaboration in practice (Munkholm et al., 2021). Nevertheless, the NAP can be a useful tool for countries to foster their AMR surveillance activities by engaging all relevant sectors and integrating a One Health perspective. To support the development of the Global Action Plan, the WHO launched the initiative Global Antimicrobial Resistance Surveillance System (GLASS) in 2015, aiming to support national AMR surveillance and harmonize collection, analysis, and sharing of data (WHO, 2021). However, only ninety-four of 196 Member States are enrolled in GLASS, of which twenty-five out of fifty-four are from the European region. For the latest report in 2021, seventy-eight (of which twenty-three are European region) Member States reported information to GLASS (WHO, 2021). The Tripartite Plus also support the Global Leaders Group on Antimicrobial Resistance, which was established in November 2020. The group is composed of twenty-seven 'member states, civil society and the private sector' representatives, of which six are from the EU (plus two from the United Kingdom) to collaborate globally, advising and advocating for AMR, and incorporating the One Health approach (GLG, 2021).

Nationally, many European countries have established surveillance approaches and networks to combat AMR. As mentioned in relation to the GLASS, those surveillance activities are not harmonized, which challenges comparability and compatibility (Kirchhelle et al., 2020). Further, the many initiatives show that the WHO is involved and engaged but struggles to harness political awareness and interest to engage all its member states in the many initiatives.

The collaboration and coordination issue

This section outlines some of the difficulties in relation to leadership and knowledge translation that have been and can be encountered when tackling AMR with a One Health approach.

In its ideal formulation, properly resourced with appropriate measures and accountability strategies put in place, a One Health approach could be a means to establish an international multi-stakeholder engagement dedicated to fight AMR. This engagement must be mindful of all actors 'from microbes to people, to markets' as Hinchliffe et al.

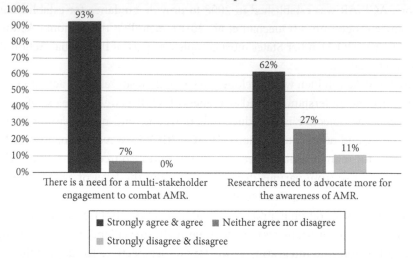

Figure 13.2 Perceptions of respondents on stakeholder engagement and advocacy for AMR.

(2018) emphasize, and a comprehensive understanding of the local context must be established, for example by interacting with local actors like farmers.

Even though a multi-stakeholder engagement is not a novel idea and multiple scholars have called for it in different forms (e.g., Katwyk et al., 2019; Kluge and Monti, 2021; Landford and Nunn, 2012; Ruckert et al., 2020; Schrijver et al., 2018), the majority of participants (ninety-three of 103 respondents) in the One Health governance survey indicated agreement or strong agreement for the need of a multi-stakeholder engagement (Figure 13.2). While 77 per cent of respondents agreed that such an engagement is realistic, some respondents pointed out challenges relating to political barriers like funding issues and conflicting political and economic interests. These concerns are recurring among scientists and policy actors (Kirchhelle, 2020). Participants' arguments for a multi-stakeholder engagement included necessity for coordinated surveillance activities, strengthening of the One Health approach, increased awareness among the public and scientists, and the need to translate knowledge from scientific findings to politicians and decision-makers.

Ideally, stakeholders and constitutive members of a multi-stakeholder engagement should come from all areas implicated in AMR (like public health, human and veterinary medicine, veterinary science, environment, food safety, agriculture, industry, etc.). Importantly, stakeholders from the political and social sciences must be engaged to ensure that the broadest set of interests are considered, promoting successful agenda setting, policy formulation and implementation. However, as seen in Switzerland (see Chapter 10), cross-sectoral collaboration has challenges, such as clearly defined boundaries and hierarchies within the sectors that lead to assumptions that cross-sectoral sharing of responsibility promotes inefficiency. This is consistent with the survey, which shows that 50 per cent of respondents see the lack of collaboration across ministries as a challenge for the implementation of the One Health approach, and 37 per cent of respondents link this challenge to inadequate governance and leadership. Coordinating interdisciplinary activities requires trust among stakeholders, synergistic and coherent activities, and tools to achieve those activities (Raymond, 2018). However, institutional traditions and internalized practices are difficult to change and leadership is needed to integrate sectors and coordinate activities (Degeling et al., 2017).

If there is political will and appropriate leadership, there is a greater chance of development and implementation of policies on AMR and One Health. Managing competing sectoral priorities and developing integrated comprehensive AMR-related policies, nationally and internationally, can provide invaluable support to tackle AMR. To promote governance and leadership, it can be helpful to employ problem brokers. Problem brokers are people who are can convey scientific information comprehensibly as they speak the language of science and politics (Rushmer et al., 2019). In this case, problem brokers can be scientists or experts from for example research institutes, EU agencies or the Tripartite organizations. They are able to frame problems, considering scientific and bureaucratic knowledge, local conditions, values, and emotions (Knaggård, 2015). Those aspects can help AMR to become tangible and real for decision- and policy-makers.

To attain legal reforms, policy changes, and promote implementation, scientists need to advocate for AMR and One Health. The One Health governance survey indicates that of 102 respondents, more than half (sixty-three respondents) agreed or strongly agreed that scientists need to advocate more for AMR (Figure 13.2). A multi-stakeholder engagement should ensure the communication of research to political actors to captivate and foster political leadership. Knowledge translation means to translate knowledge, for example scientific findings, to politicians or people working in institutes and organizations so it can be applied and used (Rushmer et al., 2019). Informing policy-makers about AMR is crucial to place the issue high on the political agenda. Further, to promote a widespread understanding of AMR, scientists must disseminate findings beyond the traditional outlets like journals, conferences, or books. A wider audience could be reached through channels like social media, news articles, blogs, citizen science projects, talks at science festivals, and more (Ross-Hellauer et al., 2020). Increased public awareness, coupled with measures that empower citizens, can foster knowledge building, behavioural changes, and increase political pressure (Hitziger et al., 2021).

The complexity of the One Health approach asks for the engagement of actors from various sectors. It highlights the importance of leaders who strengthen networks, see beyond their sectoral interests, include social as well as political actors, and facilitate knowledge translation to initiate policy change.

Performing AMR governance

This section elaborates on AMR governance, looking into existing structures like surveillance activities and AMR stewardship programmes. Important aspects for AMR
surveillance are the coherence of data and possibilities to share data. Multi-stakeholder
engagements must encourage this by providing guidance, navigating through already
existing regulations and standards, and by establishing harmonized analytical approaches and reporting (Acar and Moulin, 2013). Reinforcing initiatives like GLASS
can promote the harmonization of national AMR surveillance programmes. This will
benefit the development and reporting of the NAPs, strengthen the One Health perspective for AMR surveillance, and promote collaboration and coordination across
sectors (WHO, 2021).

On a national level, AMR stewardship programmes must be supported by governments and practitioners. Majumder et al. (2020) emphasize that AMR stewardship is
a shared responsibility across sectors and borders. It is defined as an effort to promote
appropriate antimicrobial use for humans and animals through education, reviewing
and controlling prescriptions (Majumder et al., 2020). Implementing or promoting
existing AMR stewardship programmes will aid in containing local AMR patterns
and preventing the spread of resistance to new locations. Within hospital settings,
AMR stewardship can support and monitor the handling of antimicrobials. The
same applies for veterinary practices and using therapeutic and metaphylactic antibiotics in animals (Majumder et al., 2020). In the animal sector, AMR stewardship
is needed as antimicrobials are prescribed regularly and the effects of AMR are not
always well understood by practitioners (Hardefeldt et al., 2018; Patel et al., 2020).
However, AMR stewardship must acknowledge local realities and overcome difficulties regarding the communication between farmers and veterinarians, reluctance of
farmers to use less antibiotics, or limited willingness of veterinarians to prescribe (or
sell) fewer antibiotics due to economic losses (Gerber et al., 2020). AMR is a complex issue with many drivers. Hence, AMR stewardship must be accompanied with
other approaches like the implementation of AMR policies (Aliabadi et al., 2021).
Integrating social sciences will aid in understanding the connections between actors,
their behaviours, and could identify individual or generic approaches to tackle AMR
(Hinchliffe et al., 2018).

The One Health governance survey indicated that in many European countries,
several institutes collaborate on AMR surveillance activities (e.g., public health, veterinary, agriculture/food institutes). This shows that there is an understanding of the
complexity and necessity to combine different specializations to approach AMR collectively. The existing engagements can facilitate to implement further AMR stewardship initiatives. However, the survey showed a lack of involvement of environmental
institutes. To enable comprehensive AMR stewardship and surveillance programmes,
more involvement of this sector is an essential step to broaden the scope of activities
and move towards improving the detection, prevention, and mitigation of AMR.

The challenges of translating findings and knowledge across the sectors impedes the engagement of the environmental sector as well as the harmonization of data. It emphasizes the need to engage all sectors on the human–animal–environment interface as well as other sectors such as the social sciences that take into account local to global contexts.

Actions beyond the human–animal–environment interface

This section provides an overview of other potential avenues that can be taken to tackle AMR, such as obtaining funding and resources, or the use of legal aspects on EU and international level.

Comprehensive AMR surveillance must be financed and supported, which is a major challenge. Contexts and resources of countries vary. Not only national funding is crucial, but incentives coming from the EU to support all Member States equally, tailored to their financial abilities. Although much must be invested, the returns will make such measures inexpensive in the longer term. The Organisation for Economic Co-operation and Development have developed a model to show that investment in combating AMR through policies is cost-effective (Anderson M et al., 2019). Furthermore, it can also have a positive social impact through greater workforce productivity and enhancing social capital (Queenan et al., 2016). If AMR continues to progress, however, the increased disease burden will have negative socio-economic impacts. Apart from the mortality risk, AMR can entail mental health and secondary health conditions leading to a loss in productivity and labour. Additionally, access to effective health-care will become increasingly difficult to achieve due to growing costs and inequalities, linked for example to poverty (Alvarez-Uria et al., 2016; Harbarth and Monnet, 2008).

Implementing or expanding legal frameworks or mandatory aspects can further support efforts to tackle AMR, which can easily spread across borders, and nations need to be accountable for their actions and inactions. A legal basis coupled with a One Health perspective could enforce needed measures and achieve success in tracking and preventing AMR (Hoffman et al., 2015; Ruckert et al., 2020). The EC has the tools to implement or expand legal frameworks to integrate mandatory AMR surveillance aspects. There are for example the (non-mandatory) Decision 2013/652/EU to monitor AMR in animals, and the (non-mandatory) Regulation (EU) 2021/808 to perform sampling and use analytical approaches for methods, and interpretation of results. However, mandatory aspects must be embedded in all the other areas where AMR can be found, especially in the neglected area of the environment. The EC needs to engage in discussions with stakeholders that affect AMR in environments, implementing cross-sector AMR surveillance with mandatory aspects and a One Health perspective.

Another channel to respond to AMR are the International Health regulations (IHR). The IHR are a legally binding agreement under international law between 196 states to detect, assess, report, and respond to global health threats. The international treaty provides coordinated responses to public health emergencies to minimize impact and spread of health threats. The IHR was last updated in 2005 and mentions neither One Health nor specifically includes AMR. Annex II of the IHR mentions antibiotic resistance, listing it as a potential public health impact (WHO, 2005). However, the lack of a more specific reference to AMR in the main body of the IHR hinders broader implementation. Without a clear legal commitment against AMR, this global health threat could lose relevance. Countries might dismiss the importance of AMR, fail to establish AMR surveillance, and thus lack the infrastructure to report on AMR. Integrating AMR into the IHR is complex and needs expertise from many sectors. Here, a One Health perspective can encourage the inclusion of all perspectives and actors. As the 196 Member States are legally bound to comply, this would benefit the fight against AMR, by providing a clearer picture of the prevalence and strengthening the implementation of measures to prevent AMR (Wernli et al., 2011). However, integrating AMR into the IHR is a challenge, as there is reluctance by Member States to implement legally binding agreements (Rogers Van Katwyk et al., 2020).

There are different avenues to tackle AMR. However, there is a need to catch and then harness the attention of political actors who can advance and implement resource-related and legal aspects of AMR.

Conclusion

The One Health approach is a crucial tool for AMR. It can aid and promote cross-sector collaboration and communication. Coordinating AMR activities is ambitious, as it has many pathways and various sectors need to come together. There are existing interdisciplinary initiatives within Europe and by organizations like the WHO that create networks, perform surveillance, and provide funding. However, a multi-stakeholder engagement to tackle AMR can go beyond those activities and national borders strengthening leadership, knowledge translation, setting research priorities, and advising decision- and policy-makers. Operationalizing the One Health approach will bring together experts from the human–animal–environment interface, and ideally also social and political science experts (see Chapter 9 for an illustrative example of One Health operationalization in Bangladesh). This could provide a platform for successful AMR activities based on harmonized analytical approaches that consider local to global contexts. For this, the communication of scientific knowledge to political actors must be facilitated, for example through problem brokers who can convey information from research to political actors. Additionally, scientific knowledge can be used to educate citizens about One Health and AMR. While dependent on political attention and will, the allocation of resources or initiation of legal action on EU and international level is another way to tackle AMR.

Based on the analysis of various policy initiatives and the survey on One Health governance, recommended actions to implement integrated One Health–AMR activities are to focus more attention on the environment sector. The environment is an important driver for AMR and experts can provide and integrate their knowledge of environments and ecosystems. Additionally, social and political actors must be involved to promote a better understanding of contextual factors and actors. The EU must enhance AMR surveillance, for example, by supporting multi-stakeholder engagements by providing funding and legislation for One Health activities related to AMR, and by strengthening initiatives like GLASS. This will improve the development of the NAPs and facilitate the adoption of AMR surveillance beyond the borders of the EU, leading to a more comprehensive and globally integrated overview of AMR.

References

Acar, J. F., and Moulin, G. (2013). 'Integrating Animal Health Surveillance and Food Safety: The Issue of Antimicrobial Resistance', *Revue Scientifique Et Technique (International Office of Epizootics)*, 32/ 2, 383–92. <https://doi.org/10.20506/rst.32.2.2230>. Access date: 31.01.2023.

Aliabadi, S., Anyanwu, P., Beech, E., Jauneikaite, E., Wilson, P., Hope, R., et al. (2021). 'Effect of Antibiotic Stewardship Interventions in Primary Care on Antimicrobial Resistance of Escherichia Coli Bacteraemia in England (2013–18): A Quasi-Experimental, Ecological, Data Linkage Study', *The Lancet Infectious Diseases*, 21/12, 1689–1700. <https://doi.org/10.1016/S1473-3099(21)00069-4>. Access date: 31.01.2023.

Alvarez-Uria, G., Gandra, S., and Laxminarayan, R. (2016). 'Poverty and Prevalence of Antimicrobial Resistance in Invasive Isolates', *International Journal of Infectious*, 52, 59–61. <https://doi.org/10.1016/j.ijid.2016.09.026>. Access date: 31.01.2023.

Anderson, M., Clift, C., Schulze, K., Sagan, A., Nahrgang, S., Ait Ouakrim, D., et al. (2019). 'Averting the AMR Crisis: What Are the Avenues for Policy Action for Countries in Europe?', *European Observatory on Health Systems and Policies*. Policy Brief, No. 32. <https://europepmc.org/article/med/31287637>. Access date: 31.01.2023.

Collignon, P. J., and McEwen, S. A. (2019). 'One Health—Its Importance in Helping to Better Control Antimicrobial Resistance', *Tropical Medicine and Infectious Disease*, 4/1, 22. <https://doi.org/10.3390/tropicalmed4010022>. Access date: 31.01.2023.

Degeling, C., Johnson, J., Kerridge, I., Wilson, A., Ward, M., Stewart, C., et al. (2015). 'Implementing a One Health Approach to Emerging Infectious Disease: Reflections on the Socio-Political, Ethical and Legal Dimensions', *BMC Public Health*, 15/1, 1307. <https://doi.org/10.1186/s12889-015-2617-1>. Access date: 31.01.2023.

Degeling, C., Johnson, J., Ward, M., Wilson, A., and Gilbert, G. (2017). 'A Delphi Survey and Analysis of Expert Perspectives on One Health in Australia', *EcoHealth*, 14/4, 783–92. <https://doi.org/10.1007/s10393-017-1264-7>. Access date: 31.01.2023.

ECDC. (2019). *Antimicrobial Resistance in the EU/EEA (EARS-Net)—Annual Epidemiological Report*. European Centre for Disease Prevention and Control. <https://www.ecdc.europa.eu/sites/default/files/documents/surveillance-antimicrobial-resistance-Europe-2019.pdf>. Access date: 31.01.2023.

ECDC, EFSA, and EMA. (2017). 'ECDC/EFSA/EMA Second Joint Report on the Integrated Analysis of the Consumption of Antimicrobial Agents and Occurrence of Antimicrobial Resistance in Bacteria from Humans and Food-Producing Animals', *EFSA Journal*, 15/7, 135. <https://doi.org/10.2903/j.efsa.2017.4872>. Access date: 31.01.2023.

European Commission. (2017). *A European One Health Action Plan against Antimicrobial Resistance (AMR)*. European Commission. <https://ec.europa.eu/health/sites/health/files/antimicrobial_res istance/docs/amr_2017_action-plan.pdf>. Access date: 31.01.2023.

FAO, OIE, and WHO. (2019). *Taking a Multisectoral One Health Approach: A Tripartite Guide to Addressing Zoonotic Diseases in Countries* (Geneva: Food and Agriculture Organization of the

United Nations; World Organisation for Animal Health; World Health Organization). https://apps. who.int/iris/handle/10665/325620. Access date: 31.01.2023. Geneva, Switzerland: World Health Organization.

Gerber, M., Dürr, S., and Bodmer, M. (2020). ‚Decision-Making of Swiss Farmers and the Role of the Veterinarian in Reducing Antimicrobial Use on Dairy Farms', *Frontiers in Veterinary Science*, 7, 565. <https://doi.org/10.3389/fvets.2020.00565>. Access date: 31.01.2023.

GLG. (2021). *Priorities of the Global Leaders Group on AMR for 2021–2022.* World Health Organization. <https://cdn.who.int/media/docs/default-source/antimicrobial-resistance/glg-act ion-plan-july-2021_final.pdf?sfvrsn=daa1bd02_5&download=true>. Access date: 31.01.2023.

Harbarth, S., and Monnet, D. L. (2008). 'Cultural and Socioeconomic Determinants of Antibiotic Use', in I. M. Gould and J. W. van der Meer, eds, *Antibiotic Policies: Fighting Resistance* (Boston, Massachusetts: Springer US), 29–40. <https://doi.org/10.1007/978-0-387-70841-6_3>. Access date: 31.01.2023.

Hardefeldt, L. Y., Gilkerson, J. R., Billman-Jacobe, H., Stevenson, M. A., Thursky, K., Bailey, K. E., et al. (2018). 'Barriers to and Enablers of Implementing Antimicrobial Stewardship Programs in Veterinary Practices', *Journal of Veterinary Internal Medicine*, 32/3, 1092–99. <https://doi.org/ 10.1111/jvim.15083>. Access date: 31.01.2023.

Hashmi, M. Z., ed. (2020). *Antibiotics and Antimicrobial Resistance Genes: Environmental Occurrence and Treatment Technologies* (Switzerland: Springer International Publishing). <https://doi.org/ 10.1007/978-3-030-40422-2>. Access date: 31.01.2023.

Hinchliffe, S., Butcher, A., and Rahman, M. M. (2018). 'The AMR Problem: Demanding Economies, Biological Margins, and Co-Producing Alternative Strategies', *Palgrave Communications*, 4/1, 1– 12. <http://dx.doi.org/10.1057/s41599-018-0195-4>. Access date: 31.01.2023.

Hitziger, M., Berezowski, J., Dürr, S., Falzon, L. C., Léchenne, M., Lushasi, K., et al. (2021). 'System Thinking and Citizen Participation Is Still Missing in One Health Initiatives—Lessons from Fifteen Evaluations', *Frontiers in Public Health*, 9, 653398. <https://doi.org/10.3389/fpubh.2021.653398>. Access date: 31.01.2023.

Hoffman, S. J., Caleo, G. M., Daulaire, N., Elbe, S., Matsoso, P., Mossialos, E., et al. (2015). 'Strategies for Achieving Global Collective Action on Antimicrobial Resistance', *Bulletin of the World Health Organization*, 93, 867–76. <https://doi.org/10.2471/BLT.15.153171>. Access date: 31.01.2023.

Humboldt-Dachroeden, S., and Mantovani, A. (2021). 'Assessing Environmental Factors within the One Health Approach', *Medicina*, 57/3, 240. <https://doi.org/10.3390/medicina57030240>. Access date: 31.01.2023.

Kahn, L. H. (2017). 'Antimicrobial Resistance: A One Health perspective', *Transactions of the Royal Society of Tropical Medicine and Hygiene*, 111/6, 255–60. <https://doi.org/10.1093/trstmh/trx050>. Access date: 31.01.2023.

Katwyk, S. R. V., Balasegaram, M., Boriello, P., Farrar, J., Giubilini, A., Harrison, M., et al. (2019). 'A Roadmap for Sustainably Governing the Global Antimicrobial Commons', *The Lancet*, 394/10211, 1788–9. <https://doi.org/10.1016/S0140-6736(19)32767-9>. Access date: 31.01.2023.

Kirchhelle, C. (2020). *Pyrrhic Progress: The History of Antibiotics in Anglo-American Food Production* (New Brunswick, NJ: Rutgers University Press). <http://www.ncbi.nlm.nih.gov/books/NBK554 200/>. Access date: 31.01.2023.

Kirchhelle, C., Atkinson, P., Broom, A., Chuengsatiansup, K., Ferreira, J. P., Fortané, N., et al. (2020). 'Setting the Standard: Multidisciplinary Hallmarks for Structural, Equitable and Tracked Antibiotic Policy', *BMJ Global Health*, 5/9, e003091. <https://doi.org/10.1136/bmjgh-2020-003091>. Access date: 31.01.2023.

Kluge, H. H. P., and Monti, M. (2021). *Rethinking Policy Priorities in the Light of Pandemics—A Call to Action.* Pan-European Commission. <https://www.euro.who.int/__data/assets/pdf_file/0010/495 856/Pan-European-Commission-Call-to-action-eng.pdf>. Access date: 31.01.2023.

Knaggård, Å. (2015). 'The Multiple Streams Framework and the Problem Broker', *European Journal of Political Research*, 54/3, 450–65. <https://doi.org/10.1111/1475-6765.12097>. Access date: 31.01.2023.

Landford, J., and Nunn, M. (2012). 'Good Governance in "One Health" Approaches', *Revue Scientifique Et Technique (International Office of Epizootics)*, 31/2, 561–75. doi:http://dx.doi.org/10.20506/rst.31.2.2133. Access date: 31.01.2023.

Liao, H., Li, X., Yang, Q., Bai, Y., Cui, P., Wen, C., et al. (2021). 'Herbicide Selection Promotes Antibiotic Resistance in Soil Microbiomes', *Molecular Biology and Evolution*, 38/6, 2337–50. <https://doi.org/10.1093/molbev/msab029>. Access date: 31.01.2023.

Majumder, M. A. A., Rahman, S., Cohall, D., Bharatha, A., Singh, K., Haque, M., et al. (2020). 'Antimicrobial Stewardship: Fighting Antimicrobial Resistance and Protecting Global Public Health', *Infection and Drug Resistance*, 13, 4713–38. <https://doi.org/10.2147/IDR.S290835>. Access date: 31.01.2023.

Mathieu, E., Matthys, J., Verhoest, K., and Rommel, J. (2021). 'Multilevel Regulatory Coordination: The Interplay between European Union, Federal and Regional Regulatory Agencies', *Public Policy and Administration*, 36/3, 343–60. <https://doi.org/10.1177/0952076719886736>. Access date: 31.01.2023.

Mennerat, A., Nilsen, F., Ebert, D., and Skorping, A. (2010). 'Intensive Farming: Evolutionary Implications for Parasites and Pathogens', *Evolutionary Biology*, 37/2, 59–67. <https://doi.org/10.1007/s11692-010-9089-0>. Access date: 31.01.2023.

Munkholm, L., Rubin, O., Bækkeskov, E., and Humboldt-Dachroeden, S. (2021). Attention to the Tripartite's One Health Measures in National Action Plans on Antimicrobial Resistance. *Journal of Public Health Policy*, 42/2, 236–48. <https://doi.org/10.1057/s41271-021-00277-y>. Access date: 31.01.2023.

Patel, S. J., Wellington, M., Shah, R. M., and Ferreira, M. J. (2020). 'Antibiotic Stewardship in Food-producing Animals: Challenges, Progress, and Opportunities', *Clinical Therapeutics*, 42/9, 1649–58. <https://doi.org/10.1016/j.clinthera.2020.07.004>. Access date: 31.01.2023.

Queenan, K., Häsler, B., and Rushton, J. (2016). 'A One Health Approach to Antimicrobial Resistance Surveillance: Is There a Business Case for It?', *International Journal of Antimicrobial Agents*, 48/4, 422–7. <https://doi.org/10.1016/j.ijantimicag.2016.06.014>. Access date: 31.01.2023.

Raymond, A. (2018). '"Aligning Activities": Coordination, Boundary Activities, and Agenda Setting in Interdisciplinary Research', *Science & Public Policy*, 45/5, 621–33. <https://doi.org/10.1093/SCIPOL/SCX087>. Access date: 31.01.2023.

Rogers van Katwyk, S., Giubilini, A., Kirchhelle, C., Weldon, I., Harrison, M., McLean, A., et al. (2020). 'Exploring Models for an International Legal Agreement on the Global Antimicrobial Commons: Lessons from Climate Agreements', *Health Care Analysis*, 1–22. <https://doi.org/10.1007/s10728-019-00389-3>. Access date: 31.01.2023.

Ross-Hellauer, T., Tennant, J. P., Banelytė, V., Gorogh, E., Luzi, D., Kraker, P., et al. (2020). 'Ten simple rules for innovative dissemination of research', *PLoS Computational Biology*, 16/4, e1007704. <https://doi.org/10.1371/journal.pcbi.1007704>. Access date: 31.01.2023.

Ruckert, A., Fafard, P., Hindmarch, S., Morris, A., Packer, C., Patrick, D., et al. (2020). 'Governing Antimicrobial Resistance: A Narrative Review of Global Governance Mechanisms', *Journal of Public Health Policy*, 41/4, 515–28. <https://doi.org/10.1057/s41271-020-00248-9>. Access date: 31.01.2023.

Rushmer, R., Ward, V., Nguyen, T., and Kuchenmüller, T. (2019). 'Knowledge Translation: Key Concepts, Terms and Activities', in M. Verschuuren and H. van Oers, eds, *Population Health Monitoring: Climbing the Information Pyramid* (Springer, Cham in Switzerland: Springer International Publishing), 127–50. <https://doi.org/10.1007/978-3-319-76562-4_7>. Access date: 31.01.2023.

Schrijver, R., Stijntjes, M., Rodríguez-Baño, J., Tacconelli, E., Babu Rajendran, N., and Voss, A. (2018). 'Review of Antimicrobial Resistance Surveillance Programmes in Livestock and Meat in EU with Focus on Humans', *Clinical Microbiology and Infection*, 24/6, 577–90. <https://doi.org/10.1016/j.cmi.2017.09.013>. Access date: 31.01.2023.

Smith, M., King, C., Davis, M., Dickson, A., Park, J., Smith, F., et al. (2018). 'Pet Owner and Vet Interactions: Exploring the Drivers of AMR', *Antimicrobial Resistance & Infection Control*, 7/1, 46. <https://doi.org/10.1186/s13756-018-0341-1>. Access date: 31.01.2023.

Wallace, H., Pollack, M. A., Roederer-Rynning, C., and Young, A. R. (Eds.). (2020). *Policy-Making in the European Union* (8th edn, Oxford: Oxford University Press).

Wernli, D., Haustein, T., Conly, J., Carmeli, Y., Kickbusch, I., and Harbarth, S. (2011). ‚A Call for Action: The Application of the International Health Regulations to the Global Threat of Antimicrobial Resistance', *PLoS Medicine*, 8/4, 1–6. <https://doi.org/10.1371/journal.pmed.1001 022>. Access date: 31.01.2023.

WHO. (2005). *International Health Regulations* (Geneva: World Health Organization). <https://www.who.int/publications/i/item/9789241580410>. Access date: 31.01.2023.

WHO. (2015). *Global Action Plan on Antimicrobial Resistance* (Geneva: World Health Organization). <https://apps.who.int/iris/bitstream/handle/10665/193736/9789241509763_eng.pdf?sequence=1>. Access date: 31.01.2023.

WHO. (2022). *Resource Materials for In-Country Development and Implementation of Antimicrobial Resistance National Action Plans* (Geneva: World Health Organization). <https://cdn.who.int/media/docs/default-source/antimicrobial-resistance/amr-spc-npm/nap-support-tools/amr-resource-pack-october-2022.pdf?sfvrsn=e4801d1_4 >. Access date: 31.01.2023.

WHO. (2021). *Global Antimicrobial Resistance and Use Surveillance System (GLASS) Report: 2021.* (Geneva: World Health Organization). <https://www.who.int/publications-detail-redirect/978924 0027336>. Access date: 31.01.2023.

Woolhouse, M., Ward, M., van Bunnik, B., and Farrar, J. (2015). 'Antimicrobial Resistance in Humans, Livestock and the Wider Environment', *Philosophical Transactions of the Royal Society B: Biological Sciences*, 370/1670, 20140083. <https://doi.org/10.1098/rstb.2014.0083>. Access date: 31.01.2023.

PART V
GLOBAL ADVOCACY AND AWARENESS OF AMR

14

Policy Entrepreneurship and Problem Brokering in the Global Governance of AMR

Olivier Rubin and Erik Baekkeskov

Introduction

There is little doubt that global political attention to the threat of antimicrobial resistance (AMR) has increased in recent years. Since the World Health Assembly adopted a global action plan in 2015, national governments in more than 140 countries have developed national action plans for AMR response (WHO et al., 2021). Notwithstanding this remarkable progress, several UN-sponsored reports refer to inadequate political commitment and existing global efforts that 'are currently too slow and must be accelerated' (UN Interagency Coordination Group on Antimicrobial Resistance (IACG, 2019: 6). Less than 20 per cent of the Member States, for example, have started implementation of their national action plans, although the implementation deadline given by the World Health Organization (WHO) was 2017 (WHO et al., 2021). Several scholars have called for more systematic social science research to help explain why global policies to combat AMR remain hard to implement (Anderson et al., 2019; Carlet et al., 2014; Laxminarayan et. al., 2013; Nathan and Cars, 2014; Rochford et al., 2018). The consensus is that a weak international governance regime undermines effective AMR response, and current academic debates centre on whether global governance should be strengthened through a hard law approach with binding treaties, or a soft law approach based on voluntary aims and guidelines (cf. Baekkeskov et al., 2020; Padiyara et al., 2018; Ruckert et al., 2020; Van Katwyk et al., 2020).

This chapter offers a different perspective. It applies a prominent analytical framework from political science, namely Kingdon's 1984 multiple stream approach (MSA), to shed light on the apparent puzzle that an increase in global attention and agenda-setting does not appear to have produced an equivalent increase in actual implementation of AMR policy initiatives. We argue that health experts have played a key role in successfully placing the threat of AMR on the global agenda. Indeed, during the last decade, core political institutions have acknowledged the threats from AMR, and they have signed international and national documents and agreements aimed at bolstering AMR response. However, health experts have been less successful in translating this increased attention into concrete policies and programmes, as evidenced by the inadequate implementation and funding of AMR initiatives.

Olivier Rubin and Erik Baekkeskov, *Policy Entrepreneurship and Problem Brokering in the Global Governance of AMR* In: *Steering against Superbugs*. Edited by: Olivier Rubin, Erik Baekkeskov, and Louise Munkholm, Oxford University Press. © Oxford University Press 2023. DOI: 10.1093/oso/9780192899477.003.0014

We introduce the concept of *advocacy ecology* as an important intermediating factor in translating agenda-setting into policy. A strong advocacy ecology consists of a broad range of powerful champions such as invested bureaucrats, powerful activist networks, strong industrial buy-in, continuous public engagement, social media interest, and persistent news media coverage. This advocacy ecology appears to be a necessary (but not sufficient) condition for the formation of a strong governance regime, particularly when dealing with long-term chronic crises that cannot be addressed with one set of policies at one time. Instead, continued political attention and multi-sectoral policy development that stretch for several decades are needed to address AMR.

The challenge for AMR global governance is that advocacy ecology continues to consist almost exclusively of committed medical experts that strive to drive the agenda forward in the face of strong agricultural interests, negligible public engagement, limited media coverage, and political leaders preoccupied with other challenges. We recommend concerted efforts be made to strengthen the advocacy ecology surrounding AMR. A focus on formal governance regimes (binding or non-binding), incentive structures for the pharmaceutical industry, and awareness-raising initiatives is certainly merited. We argue, however, that more attention and resources should also be devoted to broader coalition and network building with non-health stakeholders. The example of climate change policy advocacy illustrates how a multi-sectoral advocacy ecology can join effective problem brokers and policy entrepreneurs, and boost and sustain attention and action (see Chapter 15).

The chapter is structured as follows. The MSA will first be outlined and enhanced to improve the capture the global policy process of AMR. In the subsequent analytical section, the approach will be applied to provide one explanation to the puzzle that successful agenda-setting is not being translated to actual policy implementation. Finally, the chapter offers recommendations for how to strengthen the global AMR advocacy ecology.

Conceptualizing global AMR policy-making—multiple streams approach with problem brokers

How can we understand the puzzling contrast between the successful efforts to raise AMR on global and national policy agendas and then the drag in performance when it comes to actual policy implementation?- To begin to answer, this section introduces the MSA originated by John Kingdon in 1984 and applied and refined by many scholars of public policy in subsequent decades (Cairney and Jones, 2016; Sabatier and Weible, 2014). The MSA belongs to a group of evolutionary policy theories that seek to explain how and why various problems make it onto the policy agenda and the conditions under which particular policies are likely to be adopted (Yusuf et al., 2016). We describe a version MSA with the addition of new analytical concepts such as *problem brokers* and *advocacy ecology*. This 'enhanced MSA' will then be applied in the analysis section that follows this one.

MSA understands policies as outcomes from interactions between three independent but interlinked 'streams' with their own dynamics and rules (Kingdon, 2014): (i) the *problem recognition stream* where issues that require attention are identified and effective solutions outlined; (ii) the *policy/proposal stream* characterized by a 'policy primeval soup' (to use Kingdon's own expression, 2014: 16) where most policy solutions are continuously simmering but where a few manage to be turned into concrete policy ideas by invested key stakeholders; and (iii) the *political stream* that encompasses the motives and opportunities of policy-makers to advocate for a particular policy idea, which in turn depends on the national mood, pressure from interest groups, the budgetary funds available and the adaptation of politics into legal instruments. MSA introduces the key analytical concept of *policy entrepreneurs*. These are actors who attempt to couple the three streams by advocating how a policy idea could solve an important problem during politically opportune moments. Successfully coupling the three streams produces a *policy window* for advocates to enact their policy proposals. Policy entrepreneurs constantly 'lie in wait in and around government with their solution at hand, waiting for problems to float by to which they can attach their solutions, waiting for a development in the political stream they can use to their advantage' (Kingdon, 2014: 165). Policy entrepreneurs are needed to convince officials, agency bureaucrats, and the public to adopt particular solutions, and to show how particular policies will solve important problems related to AMR (see Chapter 15 for a discussion of digital policy entrepreneurs).

To apply the MSA framework to the political challenges facing AMR responses outlined earlier, we propose theoretical augmentations of the concepts of *policy window* and the *problem stream*.

First, standard MSA does not pay much attention to longevity of the policy window, characterized by the alignment of the three streams. This is likely to be because the MSA was developed to capture national policy-making processes for conventional problems where a single window of opportunity would often suffice to implement policies to address the problem. For policy-making addressing chronic crises that span generations, such as climate change and AMR, for example, prolonged or repeated windows of opportunity stretching decades are needed. These policy windows are most likely not to remain open throughout the entirety of the period but will fluctuate, opening and closing over time, providing opportunities for novel policy implementations at different points in time. We propose that the concept of *advocacy ecology* is useful in determining the temporal strength of the policy windows of opportunity. Without a healthy advocacy ecology, windows of opportunity for effective policies might wither away in the absence of visible crises, as politicians and the public turn attention to other pressing global challenges.

Second, while Kingdon in 1984 introduced the concept of *policy entrepreneurship* to explain why solutions emerge as policies, the MSA devotes less attention to the initial phase of the policy-making process where problems are first identified and framed as public and political concerns. The MSA describes that issues that are highly salient to the public, that are easily quantifiable, that have identifiable solutions, or that are

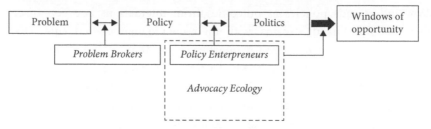

Figure 14.1   Analytical framework of the global AMR policy streams.

the product of a crisis event, all have a greater likelihood of being defined as problems deserving of attention. Solutions to these problems, in turn, can be carried forward by policy entrepreneurs. However, the role of agency in this vital first part of the process is left underexplored. Political attention not only depends on inherent characteristics of the problem itself (salient, quantifiable, and with available solutions) but also on whether invested actors are interested in carrying the problem forward into the policy process. Åsa Knaggård, therefore, sought to inject more agency into the problem stream by introducing the concept of *problem broker* (Knaggård, 2015). The role of problem brokers is to frame conditions as public problems for the consumption of policy-makers. Policy entrepreneurship primarily relates to the formulation and execution of policies by aligning the policy and politics streams. Problem brokering relates to the process of turning specific conditions into policy problems by aligning the problem and policy streams. Capturing the agency involved in problem brokering is particularly important in the case of AMR because the most active actors in the policy process, the health experts, appear to work primarily in the problem stream by linking problems with solutions and communicating these to policy-makers.

Figure 14.1 provides a graphical summary of our analytical framework based on MSA where problem brokers align the problem/policy streams and policy entrepreneurs, supported by an advocacy ecology, align the policy/politics streams to provide sustained windows of opportunity for AMR policies.

In the following, we will first analyse the successful alignment of the problem and policy streams, and subsequently, the failure to align the policy and politics streams fully.

Successful problem brokering—raising AMR on the global agenda

AMR problems have been known for decades. Famously, in his 1945 Nobel Prize acceptance speech for the discovery of penicillin, Alexander Fleming warned about the 'danger that the ignorant man may easily underdose himself and by exposing his microbes to non-lethal quantities of the drug make them resistant' (Fleming, 1945: 93). However, it took several decades before the first international coordinated response to AMR emerged. In 1998, the World Health Organization (WHO) published its resolution on antimicrobial resistance where the Member States were urged to enact responses and WHO pledged to support, assist, and sponsor key initiatives. The European Commission adopted its first AMR action plan in 2011 (based on the One Health approach) as a replacement for the 2001 community strategy on AMR. The big surge in global attention, however, came after 2013. In September 2013, WHO Strategic Technical Advisory Group on AMR recommended developing a Global Action Plan (GAP) on AMR. The recommendation was subsequently adopted in May 2014 through a World Health Assembly resolution. The WHO developed the GAP in collaboration with the Food and Agriculture Organization of the United Nations (FAO) and the World Organization for Animal Health (OIE) (collectively known as the Tripartite Organizations; see Chapters 11 and 13 for analysis of Tripartite initiatives). The GAP was endorsed in May 2015 by the WHO's 194 Member States. The Member States were urged to develop and have in place national action plans (NAPs) on AMR by 2017, modelled on the guidelines in the GAP (WHO et al., 2015). Prior to 2015, very few Member States had the equivalent of a NAP on AMR. While the 2017 deadline was not met, more than 140 Member States developed NAPs after 2015, so the push was largely successful (Munkholm and Rubin, 2020). The WHO also launched a surveillance system in 2015 aimed at standardizing AMR surveillance across countries. Again, the drive appears successful, with 105 Member States having signed up for the system (WHO, 2021).

The impact of global AMR agenda-setting and initiatives during the period around the 2015 GAP is further shown by the fact that AMR was put on the G7 agenda starting in 2015 and on the G20 agenda in 2017. In 2016, a United Nations (UN) high-level meeting on AMR resulted in a political declaration on AMR (United National General Assembly, 2016). In 2017, the UN Secretary General established the Inter-Agency Coordination Group (IACG) on AMR. The IACG published several working papers on AMR governance before finalizing and submitting its report 'No Time to Wait' to the UN General Assembly in April 2019. Key recommendations included establishing an Independent Panel on Evidence (inspired by the The Intergovernmental Panel on Climate Change (IPCC) for climate change), a multi-stakeholder partnership platform, and a Global Leadership Group on Antimicrobial Resistance. However, the report stopped short of recommending a global AMR treaty (which would carry legally binding obligations), suggesting instead 'that priority be given to adopting and implementing global standards and best practices' (IACG, 2019: 23). Following recommendations in the IACG, the UN approved the establishment of the Global Leaders Group in 2020. The Global Leaders Group is accountable to and convened by the Tripartite Organizations as a key global governance structure. It is led by current or former heads of state and includes members from Member States, civil society, and the private sector. The group primarily has an advisory and advocacy role, and it is clear from the terms of reference that the antimicrobial resistance agenda will primarily be advanced through the group's individual members 'availing their voices and expertise at the global and national level' (United Nations General Assembly, 2020).

This rise in global attention to AMR can be explained by the emergence of problem brokers that used the One Health framework to push for increased global awareness to AMR. The United Kingdom in particular appears to have been strongly involved in problem brokerage at the international stage. The WHO explicitly acknowledged the support of a small handful of countries, the Netherlands, Norway, Sweden, and the United Kingdom, for their 'support' and 'leadership' in producing the GAP (WHO, 2014ab). Over the course of the last few years, the chapter authors have spoken to multiple WHO representatives and stakeholders involved in field of AMR, and one name recurs as the principal champion of putting AMR on the international agenda. Dame Sally Davies, then Chief Medical Officer for England and Senior Medical Advisor to the UK government, in 2011 dedicated a volume of her Annual Report of the Chief Medical Office solely to the rise of AMR (Davies, 2011). She arrived at her decision to do this after discovering that AMR-related problems were repeatedly described in reports and analyses she received from many parts of the English health system, but rarely discussed as a unified and national challenge (personal communication with Dame Sally Davies, 15 December 2021). Davies has also served in several formal global policy roles related to AMR, which gave her access and voice beyond the United Kingdom.

Symptomatic of problem brokers, Davies' 2011 annual report not only pointed to the threat of AMR but made seventeen concrete recommendations to named organizations to address the threat. In 2013, she led a delegation to the World Health Assembly 'calling for international action to deal with the growing problem of fewer medicines to treat the soaring number of antibiotic-resistant infections' (UK government, 2013). Davies also approached UK Prime Minister David Cameron directly to help persuade him of the dangers of AMR (personal communication with Dame Sally Davies, 15 December 2021). Cameron publicly stated that '[i]f we fail to act, we are looking at an almost unthinkable scenario where antibiotics no longer work and we are cast back into the dark ages of medicine' (BBC, 2014). Inspired by successes in the climate change field with the UK's publication of the Stern Review in 2006, Davies also recommended to the Prime Minister that he commission a senior economist to lead an independent review on AMR (personal communication with Dame Sally Davies, 15 December 2021). The resulting two-year review, headed by the then Commercial Secretary to the UK Treasury James O'Neill, analysed the scope of the problem and proposed actions to tackle the issue internationally. With more than 2000 citations in Google Scholar, O'Neill's 2016 report remains one of the most cited publications on AMR, and the source of the much-cited statistic that AMR will cause 10 million deaths by 2050 (O'Neill, 2016: 4).

In terms of public attention (proxied by newspaper articles), 2013 again appears to be a significant turning point. Using leading US newspapers' coverage of antibiotic resistance as an indication, 197 newspaper articles on average annually mentioned antibiotic resistance or superbugs in the period 1980–2012 compared to an annual average of 508 in the period 2013–2020 (ProQuest, 2021).[1] Tying antibiotic resistance to some kind of apocalyptic scenario also appears to have increased after 2013: eighteen articles prior to

---

[1] We carried on the same analysis using only the three biggest newspapers (The Wall Street Journal, The Washington Post, and The New York Times) to account for an increase in newspapers. The result was the same with an average of fourteen articles per year in 1980 to 2012 and fifty-one from 2013 to 2020.

2013 used the term 'apocalypse' when reporting on antibiotic resistance while twenty-nine used the term from 2013 to 2020. However, it is important to recognize that these increases occur in the context of extremely low media attention. As a comparison, 3,390 articles in the period 1980–2012 and 2,960 articles in the period 2013–2020 referred to 'the apocalypse' when reporting on climate change. Similarly, 556 pandemic articles in the period 1980–2012 and 2,420 in the period 2013–2020 referred to the potential apocalyptic consequences (the latter period driven almost exclusively by the COVID-19 pandemic in 2020). This suggests that although AMR problem brokers were successful in increasing international political attention, they may not have elevated the issue on general public's agenda. This will be further substantiated and explored below.

Lacklustre policy entrepreneurship—the failure of implementation

Despite the immense success in AMR agenda-setting and problem brokerage, resulting in global initiatives, AMR policy implementation has made limited progress. The IACG concludes that the greatest challenge is not writing national action plans on AMR but implementing them and demonstrating sustained action (IACG, 2018:2). Weldon and Hoffman conclude in their review on AMR progress that 'five years later [from the 2015 GAP], progress reports suggest the implementation of AMR activities is vastly below what was initially promised' (Weldon and Hoffman, 2021: 60). Several studies have pointed to important discrepancies, between high adherence and alignment with WHO guidelines in the NAPs and low harmonization and transparency of the actual policies implemented (Munkholm et al., 2021; Munkholm and Rubin, 2020; Weldon and Hoffman, 2021). Within some countries, research suggests that subnational and individual-level actors ignore (partially or completely) national AMR directives (Thomas and Lo, 2020).

An obstacle for political entrepreneurship is AMR's character as a quintessential creeping global emergency. It possesses little of the urgency and visibility of sudden-onset health emergencies such as pandemics or bioterrorism (Baekkeskov et al., 2020). Emergencies that appear elusive to the public eye and where solutions span decades are notoriously difficult to raise and sustain on the political agenda. The scope for policy entrepreneurship suffers from the absence of highly visible focusing events because fatalities are spread out temporal and spatially. That is, there are rarely politically opportune moments for acting on AMR.

However, the political challenge in the AMR policy space is not confined to a scarcity of focusing events. There are also few powerful actors who mobilize around and work for the goals of the GAP and related strategies to mitigate AMR. We characterize this in terms of AMR's *advocacy ecology*. To appreciate the relevance of a strong advocacy ecology to sustain or create windows of opportunity over time, consider the ongoing climate change crisis. Scholars routinely compare AMR and climate change (Harring and Krockow, 2021; Rizvi and Hoffman, 2015; Rochford et al., 2018; Van Katwyk et al.,

2020) due to similarities between the crises. Both are slow-onset (or creeping) crises that flow discreetly across borders while having strong links to other transboundary crises; that is, mitigating either calls for long-term governance across many jurisdictions. However, in the context of this discussion, there are also important differences related to the advocacy ecology surrounding the issues.

International surveys suggest that the general public consistently ranks climate change among the most important global threats, even during global shocks such as the COVID-19 pandemic that put infectious diseases high on the public agenda (Fagan and Huang, 2020). Hundreds of major transnational non-governmental organizations (NGOs) advocate for curbing climate change, for instance, Greenpeace, the World Wildlife Fund (WWF), the Sierra Club, and Oxfam. More than 2,000 NGOs and civil society organizations (CSOs) are admitted each year as observers to the United Nations Framework Convention on Climate Change (UNFCCC, 2021). Greta Thunberg, one of the most prominent public figures to emerge on the global stage in the past few years, speaks for climate change mitigating policy. As many of the most prominent champions for climate change mitigation, Thunberg is no expert. Rather, she is a committed and vocal Swedish schoolgirl turned climate activist. Many political parties include climate change as a substantial part of their platform. Indeed, Green parties are among the major parties in several mature democracies. Climate change objectives figure prominently among the UN's Sustainable Development Goals (SDGs). While some industrial interests oppose climate change, many others benefit from climate policies and investments in new green energy solutions. In fact, 2018 marked the year where the worth of the green economy exceeded that of the fossil fuel industry (UNFCC, 2018). These diverse and powerful mobilized actors constitute a robust advocacy ecology, capable of sustaining attention and policy initiatives on all levels, even in periods of sluggish global international diplomatic progress. The advocacy ecology, importantly, does not ensure that the policy initiatives are adequate to counter the problem effectively (climate change being a case in point), but it does appear to produce sustained policy engagement and behavioural changes (however slow) on all levels from the local to the international.

Contrast this with the advocacy ecology surrounding AMR. No matter whether you use social media mentions, newspaper articles, or seek out relevant news coverage on search engines as metrics for public attention, attention to AMR is dwarfed by climate change. A search on Google Trends in the period 2013–2020 on the topic of climate change in the news exceeds that of antibiotic resistance by a factor of 37 (Google Trends, 2021). There are few major transnational NGOs or CSOs committed to curbing AMR as their top priority (ReAct, an international AMR network, being a notable exception). Notwithstanding the previously described acknowledgements in 2016 by the World Health Assembly and the United National General Assembly, politicians rarely mention AMR and political parties certainly do not recognize AMR as a political platform on which to win elections, much less build movements. AMR mitigation has been conspicuously absent from the SDGs. Instead, AMR debates are mostly siloed within health agencies and ministries, and policy solutions are primarily put forth by health experts using technical arguments. As a case in point, Huttner et al. (2019) find that 78 per cent of antimicrobial awareness campaigns globally were organized by public health authorities. In Khan et al.'s (2020) study of Pakistan's AMR policy implementation, all 195 identified policy actors worked in the field of either human or animal health. The consequence of this narrow advocacy ecology, consisting mostly of health experts and agencies, is limited scope for policy entrepreneurship. Mason et al.'s (2018) study on advocacy campaigns revealed that 80 per cent of the surveyed community pharmacists in London never initiated a planned antibiotic awareness campaign, stating a lack of motivation to run such campaigns. If pharmacists in one of the leading countries behind the push for greater AMR response cannot find the motivation to commit to the cause, then barriers to political or public engagement are likely to be great in contexts where there are even more issues competing for attention, resources, and time.

Recommendations

Policy issues compete for attention. Confining health community activities to AMR awareness raising falsely assumes that promulgating scientific information will alone lead to desirable health policies. *The Lancet Global Health*'s editorial has called for raising awareness of the looming antibiotic apocalypse by means of 'framing the solution as a continuum, from surveillance to infection prevention to diagnosis to treatment' (Editorial, 2017). Likewise, on a more recent occasion, a *Lancet* Global Health Viewpoint called for resetting the agenda for antibiotic resistance by building 'on relevant data, informing both policy makers and the public about the serious consequences of a lack of effective antibiotics' (Cars et al., 2021: e1023). Such perspectives perpetuate a scientific reasoning where communicating, reframing, and popularizing scientific data and information are sufficient. This limits advocacy for action on AMR to problem brokering.

Social science literature reviewed and applied in this chapter casts doubt on this assumed sufficiency. The same Viewpoint (Cars et al., 2021: e1024) argues that the 'narrative for antibiotic resistance needs drastic improvement to enable a strong civil society movement and political commitment.' Yet studies of other transboundary threats as well as health networks suggest the reverse to be the case: strong civil society movements and private actors are needed for policy entrepreneurship that strengthens the AMR narrative (Pralle, 2009; Shiffman, 2017). Indeed, numerous awareness campaigns are already undertaken regularly. Globally, a prominent example is the WHO's annual World Antibiotic Awareness Week (renamed in 2020 World Antimicrobial Awareness Week). Regionally, an example is the EU's European annual Antibiotic Awareness Day. National examples are Public Health England's Keep Antibiotics Working and the U.S. Centers for Disease Control and Prevention annual Antibiotic Awareness Week. While awareness raising matters, it needs to be supported by a robust advocacy ecology to have the desired effect on political, public, and media engagement.

To strengthen the AMR advocacy ecology, health professionals and agencies need to form stronger AMR networks by working with external partners—NGOs, CSOs, foundations, lobbyist, influencers, and donors—that are positioned and motivated to undertake the role of policy entrepreneurs. Policy entrepreneurship is part of their expertise and core activities. Such partners can frame issues to make them comprehensible to a broader target audience by relying on iconic themes and symbols, and by persistently pushing the agenda on multiple fronts. They can also be positioned to create and take advantage of political opportunities, complementing the already rich supply of AMR information with organization and mobilization of demands for political and policy action. The MSA and several other public policy theoretical frameworks identify broad coalitions of actors as crucial for policy-making and implementation (Kingdon, 2014: 53, Sabatier and Weible, 2014). For instance, interest groups are often more important for policy entrepreneurship than experts. Research on global health networks, such as the HIV/AIDS, maternal mortality, and tobacco control communities suggests that successfully portraying AMR in ways that inspire external audiences to act, and committing to forging alliances with external actors around the issue are indispensable pillars of strong networks (Shiffman et al., 2015, Shiffman, 2017). These health issues have extended their reach beyond the health community to become broader public issues with the involvement of a dedicated coalition of committed actors.

There is no reason why policy entrepreneurship on AMR should not aim to build broadly based advocacy ecology. Still, strengthening advocacy on the global and national level does not constitute a short-term panacea for improving AMR response policies and programmes. As other chapters in this book make apparent, mitigating AMR is multifaceted and complex, but without a stronger advocacy ecology, it will be difficult consistently to exert the pressure and attention necessary to implement effective AMR policies, in many jurisdictions, at all levels of organization, and for the long haul.

Conclusion

AMR figures prominently on the international agenda, but concrete commitment in the form of funding and policy implementation is lagging behind. We account for this pattern of agenda-setting success but implementation failure by applying an enhanced version of the MSA. In global AMR agenda-setting, health experts can be recognized as problem brokers who succeeded in linking the problem and policy stream, particularly from about 2013. But health experts and agencies have often lacked the reach of policy entrepreneurs, who link policy with politics streams. In particular, climate change policy advocacy suggests how policy entrepreneurship in a creeping and global crisis such as AMR calls for a far more robust movement than expert agencies and scientific specialists alone can provide. A broad-based advocacy ecology, where health specialists partner with NGOs, political parties, and numerous other interests, stands a greater chance of repeatedly raising and sustaining AMR in agenda-setting, through policy-making, and into policy implementation.

The world is awash with global threats and just causes for costly global and national interventions. Issues compete for attention. Only a select few global threats manage to lead to concrete policy initiatives. The main political challenge for effective AMR response is not popularizing scientific knowledge but rather overcoming a deficit in mobilizing sufficient numbers and kinds of powerful actors to push forward policy and its implementation. Promulgating scientific information is vital for understanding the problem and how to solve it, but knowledge alone will not automatically translate into desirable health policies and programs, however widely it is shared across the world. For effective AMR policy, powerful networks and coalitions are essential. Hence, our focus here on robust advocacy ecologies. In other related transboundary challenges, for example that of climate change, the role of policy entrepreneurship is shared among many actors. The IPCC publishes important scientific reports aimed at problem brokering but the main messages are then carried forward by a broad coalition of the (social) media, numerous NGOs and CSOs, invested private stakeholders, and political parties. To strengthen the fight against AMR, we suggest refocusing some of the efforts and funding from awareness raising to network and coalition building. In other words, strengthening and broadening the advocacy ecology. This would create fertile grounds for stronger and persistent policy entrepreneurship to improve AMR responses globally.

References

Anderson, M., Schulze, K., Cassini, A., Plachouras, D., and Mossialos, E. (2019). 'A Governance Framework for Development and Assessment of National Action Plans on Antimicrobial Resistance', *The Lancet Infectious Diseases*, 19/11, e371–e384.

Baekkeskov, E., Rubin, O., Munkholm, L., and Zaman, W. (2020). 'Antimicrobial Resistance as a Global Health Crisis', *Oxford Research Encyclopedia of Politics*. Retrieved 27 January 2023, from https://oxfordre.com/politics/view/10.1093/acrefore/9780190228637.001.0001/acrefore-9780190228637-e-1626

BBC. (2014). 'Antibiotic resistance: Cameron warns of medical "dark ages"', 2 July 2014, <https://www.bbc.com/news/health-28098838> accessed 27 August 2021.

Cairney, P., and Jones, M. D. (2016). 'Kingdon's Multiple Streams Approach: What Is the Empirical Impact of this Universal Theory?', *Policy Studies Journal*, 44/1, 37–58.

Carlet, J., Pulcini, C., and Piddock, L. J. V. (2014). 'Antibiotic Resistance: A Geopolitical Issue', *Clinical Microbiology and Infection*, 20, 949–53.

Cars, O., Chandy, S. J., Mpundu, M., Peralta, A. Q., Zorzet, A., and So, A. D. (2021). 'Resetting the Agenda for Antibiotic Resistance through a Health Systems Perspective', *The Lancet Global Health*, 9/7, e1022–e1027.

Davies, S., ed. (2011). *Annual Report of the Chief Medical Officer, Volume Two, Infections and the Rise of Antimicrobial Resistance*. <https://assets.publishing.service.gov.uk/government/uploads/system/uploads/attachment_data/file/138331/CMO_Annual_Report_Volume_2_2011.pdf> accessed 27 August 2021.

Editorial. (2017). 'Fighting Antimicrobial Resistance on All Fronts', *The Lancet Global Health*, 5/12, e1161.

Fagan, M., and Huang, C. (2020). 'Many Globally Are as Concerned about Climate Change as About the Spread of Infectious Diseases', Pew Research Center, 26 October 2020. <https://www.pewresea

rch.org/fact-tank/2020/10/16/many-globally-are-as-concerned-about-climate-change-as-about-the-spread-of-infectious-diseases> accessed 27 August 2021.

Fleming, A. (1945). Nobel Lecture 'Penicillin', <https://www.nobelprize.org/prizes/medicine/1945/fleming/lecture/> accessed 27 August 2021.

Google Trends. (2021). News database. <https://trends.google.com/trends/explore?date=2013-01-01%202020-12-31&gprop=news&q=%2Fm%2F0v5b,%2Fm%2F0d063v> accessed 27 August 2021.

Harring, N., and Krockow, E. M. (2021). 'The Social Dilemmas of Climate Change and Antibiotic Resistance: An Analytic Comparison and Discussion of Policy Implications', *Humanities and Social Sciences Communications*, 8/1, 1–9.

Huttner, B., Saam, M., Moja, L., Mah, K., Sprenger, M., Harbarth, S., and Magrini, N. (2019). 'How to Improve Antibiotic Awareness Campaigns: Findings of a WHO Global Survey', *BMJ Global Health*, 4/3, e001239.

IACG. (2018). *Antimicrobial Resistance: National Action Plans.* <https://www.who.int/antimicrobial-resistance/interagency-coordination-group/IACG_AMR_National_Action_Plans_110618.pdf> accessed 27 August 2021.

IACG. (2019). No Time to Wait: Securing the Future from Drug-Resistant Infections. Report to the Secretary-General of the United Nations. <https://cdn.who.int/media/docs/default-source/documents/no-time-to-wait-securing-the-future-from-drug-resistant-infections-en.pdf?sfvrsn=5b424d7_6&download=true accessed 27 January 2023.

Khan, M. S., Durrance-Bagale, A., Mateus, A., Sultana, Z., Hasan, R., and Hanefeld, J. (2020). 'What Are the Barriers to Implementing National Antimicrobial Resistance Action Plans? A Novel Mixed-Methods Policy Analysis in Pakistan', *Health Policy and Planning*, 35/8, 973–82.

Kingdon, J. W. (2014). *Agendas, Alternatives, and Public Policies* (2nd edn, Essex: Pearson Education Ltd).

Knaggård, Å. (2015). 'The Multiple Streams Framework and the Problem Broker', *European Journal of Political Research*, 54/3, 450–65.

Laxminarayan, R., Duse, A., Wattal, C., Zaidi, A. K., Wertheim, H. F., Sumpradit, N., et al. (2013). 'Antibiotic Resistance—The Need for Global Solutions', *The Lancet Infectious Diseases*, 13/12, 1057–98.

Mason, T., Trochez, C., Thomas, R., Babar, M., Hesso, I., and Kayyali, R. (2018). 'Knowledge and Awareness of the General Public and Perception of Pharmacists about Antibiotic Resistance', *BMC Public Health*, 18/1, 1–10.

Munkholm, L., and Rubin, O. (2020). 'The Global Governance of Antimicrobial Resistance: A Cross-Country Study of Alignment between the Global Action Plan and National Action Plans', *Globalization and Health*, 16/1, 1–11.

Munkholm, L., Rubin, O., Bækkeskov, E., and Humboldt-Dachroeden, S. (2021). 'Attention to the Tripartite's One Health Measures in National Action Plans on Antimicrobial Resistance', *Journal of Public Health Policy*, 42, 236–48.

Nathan, C., and Cars, O. (2014). 'Antibiotic Resistance—Problems, Progress, and Prospects', *New England Journal of Medicine*, 371/19, 1761–3.

Padiyara, P., Inoue, H., and Sprenger, M. (2018). 'Global Governance Mechanisms to Address Antimicrobial Resistance', *Infectious Diseases: Research and Treatment*, 11, 1–4.

O'Neil, J. (2016). *Tackling Drug-resistant Infections Globally—Final Report and Recommendations.* <https://amr-review.org/sites/default/files/160525_Final%20paper_with%20cover.pdf> accessed 27 August 2021.

Pralle, S. B. (2009). 'Agenda-setting and Climate Change', *Environmental Politics*, 18/5, 781–99.

ProQuest. (2021). US Newsstream Database. <https://www-proquest-com.ep.fjernadgang.kb.dk/usnews/fromDatabasesLayer?accountid=13607> accessed 27 August 2021.

Rizvi, Z., and Hoffman, S. J. (2015). 'Effective Global Action on Antibiotic Resistance Requires Careful Consideration of Convening Forums', *Journal of Law, Medicine & Ethics*, 43/S3, 74–8.

Rochford, C., Sridhar, D., Woods, N., Saleh, Z., Hartenstein, L., Ahlawat, H., et al. (2018). 'Global Governance of Antimicrobial Resistance', *The Lancet*, 391/10134, 1976–8.

Ruckert, A., Fafard, P., Hindmarch, S., Morris, A., Packer, C., Patrick, D., et al. (2020). 'Governing Antimicrobial Resistance: A Narrative Review of Global Governance Mechanisms', *Journal of Public Health Policy*, 41, 515–28.

Sabatier, P., and Weible, C. (eds.). 2014. *Theories of the Policy Process* (3rd edn, Boulder, CO: Westview Press).

Shiffman, J. (2017). 'Four Challenges that Global Health Networks Face', *International Journal of Health Policy and Management*, 6/4, 183–89.

Shiffman, J., Quissell, K., Schmitz, H. P., Pelletier, D. L., Smith, S. L., Berlan, D., et al. (2015). 'A Framework on the Emergence and Effectiveness of Global Health Networks', *Health Policy and Planning*, 31(suppl_1), i3–i16.

Thomas, N., and Lo, C. Y. P. (2020). 'The Macrosecuritization of Antimicrobial Resistance in China', *Journal of Global Security Studies*, 5/2, 361–78.

UK Government. (2013). 'UK calls for international action on antimicrobial resistance', <https://www.gov.uk/government/news/uk-calls-for-international-action-on-antimicrobial-resistance> accessed 27 August 2021.

UNFCC. (2018). *Green Economy Overtaking Fossil Fuel Industry—FTSE Russel Report*. <https://unfccc.int/news/green-economy-overtaking-fossil-fuel-industry-ftse-russel-report> accessed 27 August 2021.

UNFCCC. (2021). Overview of non-party stakeholders. <https://unfccc.int/process-and-meetings/parties-non-party-stakeholders/non-party-stakeholders/overview> accessed 27 August 2021.

United Nations General Assembly. (2016). Political Declaration of the high-level meeting of the General Assembly on antimicrobial resistance. <https://digitallibrary.un.org/record/842813> accessed 27 August 2021.

United Nations General Assembly. (2020). Final Terms of Reference for the Global Leaders Group on Antimicrobial Resistance. <https://cdn.who.int/media/docs/default-source/antimicrobial-resistance/global-leaders-group-on-amr-terms-of-reference.pdf?sfvrsn=9402309d_16> accessed 27 August 2021.

Van Katwyk, S. R., Giubilini, A., Kirchhelle, C., Weldon, I., Harrison, M., McLean, et al. (2020). 'Exploring Models for an International Legal Agreement on the Global Antimicrobial Commons: Lessons from Climate Agreements', *Health Care Analysis*, 1–22. <https://doi.org/10.1007/s10728-019-00389-3>.

Weldon, I., and Hoffman, S. J. (2021). 'Bridging the Commitment-Compliance Gap in Global Health Politics: Lessons from International Relations for the Global Action Plan on Antimicrobial Resistance', *Global Public Health*, 16/1, 60–74.

WHO, FAO, and OIE. (2015). *Global Action Plan on Antimicrobial Resistance*. (Geneva: World Health Organization). <https://www.who.int/publications/i/item/9789241509763> accessed 27 August 2021.

WHO, FAO, and OIE. (2021). *Monitoring Global Progress on Antimicrobial Resistance: Tripartite AMR Country Self-Assessment Survey* (TrACSS) 2019–2020. Global analysis report. <https://www.who.int/publications/i/item/monitoring-global-progress-on-antimicrobial-resistance-tripartite-amr-country-self-assessment-survey-(tracss)-2019-2020> accessed 27 August 2021.

WHO. (2021). Global Antimicrobial Resistance and Use Surveillance System (GLASS). <https://www.who.int/initiatives/glass> accessed 27 August 2021.

WHO. (2014a). Strategic and Technical Advisory Group on Antimicrobial Resistance (STAG-AMR) Report of Second Meeting, 14–16 April 2014 (Geneva: WHO). <https://apps.who.int/iris/handle/10665/128675?locale-attribute=zh&>.

WHO. (2014b). 'Report of the 64th Session of the WHO Regional Committee for Europe', Copenhagen, Denmark, 15–18 September 2014. https://apps.who.int/iris/bitstream/handle/10665/337451/64rp00e-Rep-140754.pdf?sequence=1&isAllowed=y, 1-101

Yusuf, J. E. W., Neill, K., St John, B., Ash, I. K., and Mahar, K. (2016). 'The Sea Is Rising . . . But Not onto the Policy Agenda: A Multiple Streams Approach to Understanding Sea Level Rise Policies', *Environment and Planning C: Government and Policy*, 34/2, 228–43.

15

Global Attention to Antimicrobial Resistance and Climate Change in the Era of Social Media

Ahmad Wesal Zaman

Introduction

Two years of real-time data collection through a streaming Application Programming Interface (API), shows that 71,000 tweets have engaged in discussing the topic of anti-microbial resistance (AMR) and during the same time, more than 3.5 million tweets have engaged in the climate change debate. While the two complex global problems share many similarities, the difference in Twitter engagement between the two is captivating, particularly as to why such a difference exists. AMR and climate change are both transboundary crises. They are both future threats but with consequences that are already being felt. They both suffer from the tragedy of common and are collective problems that pose social dilemmas, where the benefits from the actions that cause these collective and transboundary problems are mostly local, but the negative consequences of these actions are felt at global and collective levels (Baekkeskov et al., 2020; Harring and Krockow, 2021; Lazarus, 2009; Levin et al., 2012). The use of fossil fuels, for instance, is beneficial for easy travel or for profit at local level, but the increase in CO_2 levels causes climate change, which could potentially threaten our existence. Similarly, the use of antibiotics could be considered beneficial for purposes of quick treatment or rapid animal growth, but the consequences of increasing antibacterial resistance could potentially make the treatment of simple infections such as a knife cut almost impossible and this could harm us at the collective level. AMR already kills more than 1.2 million people globally every year, and the pace shows no sign of slowing down (Laxminarayan, 2022). By 2050, another 10 million people are expected to die of AMR complications resulting in billions of dollars in losses to the global economy (Harring and Krockow, 2021; O'Neill, 2016). Similarly, climate change is already causing many catastrophes, such as rising sea levels, natural disasters, and more. Scientists warn that a temperature increase above 1.5 degrees Celsius will cause more extensive droughts, floods, and many other natural disasters, and if serious action is not taken the global temperatures could rise above 2 degrees Celsius with catastrophic consequences (IPCC, 2021).

Furthermore, scholars argue that AMR is one of the leading slow-burning and complex global health crisis of our time (Engström, 2021; Prestinaci et al., 2015; see also

Ahmad Wesal Zaman, *Global Attention to Antimicrobial Resistance and Climate Change in the Era of Social Media* In: *Steering against Superbugs*. Edited by: Olivier Rubin, Erik Baekkeskov, and Louise Munkholm, Oxford University Press. © Oxford University Press 2023.
DOI: 10.1093/oso/9780192899477.003.0015

Chapter 4). Both the nature of the problem, as a problem with many faces and dimensions, and perception of public and political domains about AMR, as a problem in the future, establish it as a slow-burning and complex crisis (Boin et al., 2021; Gil-Gil et al., 2019). Climate change is also considered a complex crisis, especially when it comes to economic and behavioural activities that lead to an increase in the creation and circulation of greenhouse gases and the many conflicting value systems that come into play in finding solutions to the problem (Baekkeskov et al., 2020; Lazarus, 2009; Levin et al., 2012).

While both problems share these similarities, AMR still lacks similar global attention. Intrigued by this difference in Twitter engagement of the two global crises that share many similarities, this chapter thoroughly analyses the collected tweets to explain the difference in global attention directed towards AMR and climate change. Although AMR is a global health problem and climate change an environmental one, comparing them provides valuable knowledge and lessons learned from climate change to AMR, as seen in other studies (e.g., Rogers Van Katwyk et al., 2020). Climate change studies often focus on the challenges facing and the inadequacy of climate change policies, however what is often neglected is how successful climate change has been in terms of the agenda-setting processes. The study of this success can provide invaluable lessons for AMR advocates and policy-makers. To study how and why climate change has received more attention than AMR, this chapter investigates social media attention paid to both climate change and AMR.

In an era where information travels fast, global disasters strike continually, and problems and issues for both public and political organizations change rapidly, keeping one issue at the forefront of public and political attention is an arduous task, at both national and global levels. This is particularly because public and political attention spans are short and organizational attention spans are challenged by multiple issues, all demanding solutions (Downs, 2016; Jones and Baumgartner, 2005). Limited attention spans and competing issues crowding for public, political, and scientific attention mean that attention to any given issue will fade over time (Downs, 2016; Jones and Baumgartner, 2004; Zhu, 192). The dilemma therefore is that if attention to problems eventually ends then how do complex and slow-burning global problems like climate change and AMR, both of which have the potential to last for generations and which potentially require being on the public and political agenda for decades, maintain global attention? Furthermore, attention to a problem is a prerequisite of global governance; without public, political, or expert attention directed at a problem, a solution runs the risk of not being found because the resources allocated to that issue will tend not to be sufficient to design, let alone implement, that solution (see Chapter 14 for further discussion).

While attracting attention to any global problem is a challenge at the best of times, doing so during slow-onset crises or slow-burning and complex global crises is much more complex than during rapid-onset crises (Boins et al., 2021; Downs, 2016). Attracting attention to a rapid-onset crisis, such as COVID-19, is more or less straightforward since the crisis can be felt, seen, and understood by both public and policy-makers, in this instance because of the rise in number of infections and the consequent loss of lives. However, the nature of slow-onset and complex global crises often makes it difficult for the public and policy-makers to comprehend the risks associated with these as the consequent losses from them are not clearly observed and understood. Therefore, in these cases, justification of resource allocation is not easy for policy-makers and hence poses a governance challenge.

The tripartite dimensions of social media attention

To explain global attention through Twitter engagement, the chapter looks at three dimensions, which I have labelled as the tripartite dimensions of social media attention. I have studied these dimensions by combining social media studies; looking at agenda setting, organizational communication, collective action literature; and observations from the collected Twitter data. This chapter theoretically argues that these three dimensions can explain differences in social media attention towards AMR and climate change. These three dimensions are *the origins of tweeter attention*, *the nature of tweets*, and *the nature of communities*. The definitions of these three dimensions are developed through an iterative process—going back and forth between theories and observations. While the concepts have some basis in multiple disciplines, the definitions applied here are unique to this chapter.

The origins of tweeter attention

The *origins of tweeter attention* refers to the sources that produce the tweets and sources that attract most attention. An individual or an organization can contribute to Twitter attention on a topic by either tweeting about an issue or being mentioned by other users in relation to that issue. Whether it is an organization or an individual as the origins of tweeter attention is telling in a sense that it shows the level of attention amongst different actors, the purpose of engagement, and sheds light on the role that individuals and organizations play on Twitter in brining attention to an issue.

Organizational origins of tweeter attention: this refers to tweets that are produced by organizations and, in this case, mainly international organizations (IOs) such as the United Nations Framework Convention on Climate Change (UNFCCC), the World Health Organization (WHO), the Intergovernmental Panel on Climate Change (IPCC), etc. According to theories of collective action and organizational communications, networking and communication are extremely important for an organization's relationship building and goal attainment (Kapucu, 2005; Wang and Guan, 2020). Relationship building and organizational communication play an important role in creating positive public relations outcomes. The relationship[building and organizational communication is intended at achieving common goals and outcomes (Kapucu, 2005; Wang and Guan, 2020). Organizations use Twitter communication not only as a tool to disseminate information to the public but also to establish connections with other organizations (Wang and Guan, 2020). Many studies focus on how and why IOs use media and social media, whether it is to advocate for a cause or to propagate a certain image of themselves (Jones, 2017; Lang, 2010; Lehman, 2007). This chapter looks at how IOs' use of social media brings attention to a global problem like that of AMR and climate change. To do so, the chapter looks at the reactions that an organization's tweets create and looks at how these kinds of tweets increase debates about a given problems amongst Twitter users. Through an iterative process, I argue that an organization's tweets do not always generate attention to an issue, and there is need for a much more complex engagement from other actors to generate attention towards a specific issue and to keep the wheel of attention rolling. More than the organizational-generated tweets, individual tweets with *digital entrepreneurial features* are more effective in generating attention.

Digital individual entrepreneurs

Individuals tweeting as ordinary people in a creative and provoking manner can generate attention on Twitter. I call this *digital individual entrepreneurship*. This phenomenon has been previously studied under many different titles in different fields and from multiple perspectives such as policy-making studies, agenda setting studies, and social media studies. I developed the concept of *digital individual entrepreneurship* taking inspirations from the concept of policy entrepreneurship. The concept of policy entrepreneurship has emerged from a combination of concepts from established theories of policy-making such as those developed by Baumgartner and Jones (1993), Kingdon (1995), and Sabatier et al. (2014) (see also Chapter 14). Policy entrepreneurs share similar characteristics to business entreprenurs. They are individuals who are willing to allocate their resources to a cause where their actions 'require creativity, energy and political skill' (Mintrom and Norman, 2009: 650). It is important to realize that policy entrepreneurs cannot be credited with all changes made to a specific policy, but Mintrom and Norman (2009) argue that at times when the likelihood of change in several policy areas was low, policy entreprenuers have shown to be decisive in bringing about change. Although this chpater is not concerned with policy change; the point I wish to make is that policy entrepreneurs play an important role in bringing about policy change or attracting attention to an issue. For individuals to be considered policy entrepreneurs in policy-making studies, it is important that they display four elements of entrepreneurship—namely, social acuity, defining problems, building teams, and leading by example. When they define problem, their aim is to highlight failures of current policy settings and to draw attention of actors outside the immediate scope of the problem (Minitrom and Norman, 2009). Inspired by this, I argue that for individuals to be considred *digital individual enrepreneurs*, it is important to show creativity in a provocative manner on Twitter. Minitrom and Norman (2009) argue that the strenghth of policy entrepeneurs comes from their ability to build networks, not just from their ideas, and this is also true in the case of *digital individual entrepreneurs.* They also lead by example by taking action in a way that inspires others or at least builds momentum for change (Minitrom and Norman, 2009). *Digital indiviual advocacy entrepreneurs* share similar charactersitics with policy enterpreneurs; however, combining these characteristics with a simplified presentation of their ideas on social media with theatrical and dramatical visualizations that intensifies polarized debates, makes them successful in a social media setting. While tradition policy entrepreneurs are concerned with the formation and maintainance of networks in the real world, the digital ones are concerned with both the social media enviroment and the world beyond it (Mintrom and Norman 2009; Sabatier et al., 2014).

Nature of tweets and nature of communities on Twitter

The nature of tweets refers to the manner in which Twitter users communicate their message. I argue that tweets that are clearly emotional in tone have the ability to generate more attention than tweets that are presented as emotionless or highly scientific. Tweets from organizations and individuals can both be effective in generating attention if they show some emotion. These emotions can be in the form of anger, sadness, or worry. While conducting the analysis, I found that the nature of tweets is more effective at generating attention, especially if they are from *digital individual entrepreneurs.* While emotional tweets can generate more attention than emotionless and scientific tweets, it is important that for this attention to maintain momentum, it is necessary that the communities that engage with these issues engage in the topic in a polarized manner. Tweets with emotions attract attention, and in addition to attracting attention, they generate debate and form *affective digital publics.* I define the *digital affective publics* as groups who show passion for a topic and they express that passion through tweets for a purpose. This purpose is mainly to convince others in their Twitter community to join their cause or to engage in disagreements with opposing groups, sometimes simply to express their frustration. Such communication often forms polarizing debates and these debates increase participation in the communities. To increase participation in and generate attention towards a problem on social media, controversy and polarization of debates from opposing groups of users is vital. In other words, what generates attention to a matter is not just the collective agreement over a problem but also a disagreement and polarization (Lee et al., 2014).

The affective public (public that demonstrates affection and passion towards an issue and take action to bring about change) intends to bring about change and to do so, it produces statements and strategies that are based either on opinion or on scientific knowledge (Papacharissi, 2016; Roelvink, 2010). The more the public express their political opinion the more the political debate intensifies, connecting those that share the same opinion and dividing those with the opposing point of view. In other words, increased political expressions increases debate and consequently could result into increasing polarization. Either way, it keeps debate alive between different groups

(Papacharissi, 2016; Roelvink, 2010). 'Affective publics are powered by affective statements of opinion, fact, or a blend of both, which in turn produce ambient, always on feeds further connecting and pluralizing expression' (Papacharissi, 2016: 316). These publics have a performative, theatrical, or aesthetic approach to politics, where these approaches, either in form of visualizations, presentation of ideas, or opinion and dramatic statements, will pluralize the debate (Roelvink, 2010: 85).

Methods

To study the difference in global attention directed towards AMR and climate change, I have looked at Twitter's use as a social media platform. It is one of the most widely used social media platforms frequented by politicians, individuals, organizations, and other actors. Geographically, those who engage with Twitter are dispersed around the globe. The platform is most famous for studies relating to engagement of citizens with politicians (Harder et al., 2017; Tromble, 2018: 226; williams et al., 2015).

This chapter relies on sequential explanatory strategies mainly considered suitable for mixed methods that combine qualitative and quantitative methods (Creswell, 2014). Data were collected from Twitter using a streaming API (application programming interface) called T-CAT (Twitter Capturing and Analysis Toolset). The hashtags (#climatechange #globalwarming) were used to carry out data-mining on climate change, and the hashtags (#antimicrobialresistance #antibioticresistance) were used for data queries on AMR. The API collected any tweets using these phrases as either a hashtag or a keyword, and it would also capture retweets and replies to those tweets that used these hashtags.

One of the disadvantages of using APIs is because they function as *the black box* (Driscoll and Walker, 2014). The API software has some programming limitations that are not possible to account for comprehensively in this chapter. This is because API may have some specific programming code that limits the collection of certain types of data which is not possible to identify. Secondly, API does not collect all tweets as there is a limit on how many tweets it can collect at a given time. This limit is not fully transparent because it depends on a protocol agreed by Twitter and the software developer (Driscoll and Walker, 2014). These two limitations did not hinder our current research; there were sufficient tweets available to conduct the analysis.

After the data were collected, Gephi was used for network analysis in carrying out a number of analyses relevant for this study—namely, clustering coefficient or modularity tests and network centrality tests. These analyses provided an understanding of the density of the network, the type of communities, and identified the most important nodes in the networks.

Qualitative analysis was carried out on tweets that had received most attention and on individuals who were identified as the most important nodes to study these communities and individuals in more depth.

Analysis

Individuals, emotions, and provocations

From November 2019 to August 2021, 71,552 tweets from 34,727 users have engaged in the AMR debate. In comparison to this, over 3.5 million tweets (3,553,948 tweets) from over 1 million users (1,039,421 users) have engaged in the climate change debate. This shows that there is a massive difference in Twitter interaction and engagement between AMR and climate change, with climate change receiving higher attention on Twitter than has AMR over those two years. The average overall tweets per source is 126.84 on AMR and 594.95 on climate change, showing that climate change Twitter users are almost five times more active on Twitter than users discussing AMR. There is overall higher engagement and a higher active individual engagement per user on climate change than on AMR.

Additionally, the network analysis was set to identify top 500 users in the data and after *clustering coefficient or modularity test* on approximately 1.5 million tweets, thirty-seven different communities were identified within the topic of climate change. Using similar parameters on Gephi that were applied to analysing activity surrounding climate change, analysis was carried out on 28,000 tweets obtained from T-CAT concerning AMR and ultimately, only thirteen communities were identified. The climate change network is also denser (has more nodes and ties) than the AMR: the density score for AMR is 0.007, and for climate change it is 0.015, implying that the climate change network is more than twice as dense than the AMR network.

The two largest modularity classes or communities of climate change Twitter users are mostly individuals, and the third largest community is largely made up of organizations. Even though there is interaction between the three communities, most of the interactions occur in the first two communities, amongst individuals. On the contrary, the largest community on AMR is mainly made up of organizations and almost no community was identified to be formed by ordinary individuals who would interact with one another like those identified as belonging to the climate change communities. While looking at nodes on AMR, every individual in the network is either a natural scientist, medical doctor, or someone who is, in one way or another, related to an organization or company that works with AMR-related matters.

The most influential nodes in the two networks identified as the WHO in the AMR network, which is the most mentioned node (with 4,808 mentions). Greta Thunberg (with 18,073 mentions) is the most mentioned node within the climate change network. The most mentioned user for AMR is an organization and for climate change it is an individual.

Greta Thunberg is the most mentioned node within the climate change network. Thunberg, a teenage Swedish environmental activist and founder of the 'Fridays for Future' movement, joined Twitter in 2018 and since then attracted over 4.1 million followers. Her most famous Twitter interaction was with US former President Donald Trump, which created what is referred to as a Twitter storm. After Thunberg was named

Time Magazine's Person of the year in 2019, Trump tweeted: 'So ridiculous. Greta must work on her anger management problem, then go to a good old-fashioned movie with a friend! Chill, Greta, chill!' Right after this tweet, Greta Thunberg changed her Twitter biography to 'A teenager working on her anger management problem, currently chilling and watching a good old-fashioned movie with a friend.'

This interaction followed a number of tweets back and forth between Thunberg and Trump and resulted in millions of Twitter interactions in the form of tweets, retweets, and likes. The matter went beyond social media and became an issue that was discussed in the traditional media such as *The New York Times* and on several TV programmes in the United States and around the globe, including CNN and the BBC. Both individuals also attended the Climate Action Summit in September, where the United States did not make a statement. Thunberg gave an emotional speech, saying:

> You have stolen my dreams and my childhood with your empty words. And yet I'm one of the lucky ones. People are suffering. People are dying. Entire ecosystems are collapsing. We are in the beginning of a mass extinction, and all you can talk about is money and fairy tales of eternal economic growth. How dare you! (Thunberg, 2019)

After the 2019 incident with Trump, tweets directed at Thunberg have come from both her supporters and those who oppose her. Hashtags such as #climatcriminal, #climatesaviors, and #tiredearth are common amongst her supporters, while hashtags like #climatehoax and #climatebrawl are common amongst her opponents. More than 100,000 tweets and retweets of her tweets and Trump's tweets are a mix of both supporters and opponents of them both.

Even though Thunberg was named *Time Magazine*'s Person of the year, what created a tweeter storm was the fact that Trump attacked her on Twitter. The interaction between Trump and Thunberg also dragged millions of their followers in the debate. This resulted in increased attention not just on the two individuals but also on the topic of climate change. The fact that Thunberg changed her Twitter biography in response to the attack by Trump can be considered both creative and politically skilful. Likewise, Trump's attack on Thunberg also attracted a lot of attention. Therefore, both Trump and Thunberg can be considered *digital individual entrepreneurs*.

Scott Morrison, Australia's Prime Minister at the time of the data collection for this chapter, with the twitter ID (@ScottMorrisonMP), was the second-highest most mentioned user in the climate change network above. He was mentioned 14,255 times using the #climatechange and #globalwarming. Morrison faced a backlash after his comments that 'this is not the time to talk about climate change' in 2019 during terrible bushfires that ravaged his country. He argued that there was no direct link between Australia's greenhouse gas emissions and the unprecedented bushfires in Australia (Karp, 2019). His comments were not well received by many on social media, and the backlash was in the order of hundreds and thousands of tweets by many ordinary users, mainly people who were affected by the bushfires, as well as celebrities took to Twitter to condemn his words. For instance, a related tweet on 3 January 2020 by US singer Bette Midler got over 130,000 reactions within hours of being posted.[1]

A week after the Twitter backlash, Morrison's senior ministers discussed how to reposition climate policies in a cabinet meeting (Martin, 2020). Although no solid policy for climate change was proposed immediately following the backlash, the Twitter backlash, combined with bushfire disaster, helped to bring the issue to the attention of the Australian public and the Australia's cabinet. Morrison also criticized Thunberg's stance and stated it caused 'needless anxiety' to Australian children (Murphy, 2019). Every tweet Morrison made about climate change was accompanied by reactions from both his supporters and his opponents,[2] as was Bette Midler's tweet mentioned earlier.

AMR tweets are different from climate change: they are mostly from organizations. The majority of top users on Twitter who engage with the hashtags #antimicrobialresistance and #antibioticresistance are international organizations. WHO is the highest mentioned user with 13,540 mentions. The US Centers for Disease Control and Prevention (CDC), with the Twitter ID @cdcgov, scores the second highest mentions (2,065) in the AMR network. The only two individuals that are in the top ten highest mentioned tweeters in the AMR network are Tedros Ahdanom Ghebreyesus, with the twitter ID @DrTedros, who is the director general of the WHO and Ángel Rod-Villodres, with the twitter ID @1797angel, who is a microbiologist. Ghebreyesus is mentioned 2,000 times and RodVillodres 1,300. Regarding their tweets about AMR, none has generated more than 100 reactions.

Scientific and emotionless representation from individuals and organizations

Even the most prominent advocate of AMR who fits the criteria of a policy entrepreneur, Professor Dame Sally Davies, with the twitter ID @UKAMREnvoy, has not generated significant reaction to her tweets. While looking at the AMR network and Twitter users, there are almost no individuals outside the immediate scope of the problem who are able to establish a large network. Most of the users within the AMR network are either organizations or individuals working with AMR.

AMR users on Twitter engage in scientific debates to persuade people and policymakers of the dire consequences of AMR. Even though the profile of several of the individuals who engage in the debate do fit the criteria of being policy entrepreneurs, in none of their tweets do they generate polarized debate or make statements that would trigger an ideological or dramatic response. In other words, AMR policy entrepreneurs have not been able to build networks on Twitter beyond the immediate of scope of the AMR problem. Since only those within the medical community or those within the

---

[1] <https://twitter.com/bettemidler/status/1212897346423599105>. Accessed: 20/02/2020.
[2] One example of a Morrison tweet on CC can be found here: <https://mobile.twitter.com/ScottMorrisonMP/status/1193419641705492480>. Accessed: 20/02/2020.

natural sciences, who are either working with AMR or are directly affiliated with an AMR-connected project, engage in social media debates on AMR.

However, what is interesting here is that while there is less interaction amongst the network itself within AMR than that found within the climate change community, the Twitter activity of policy entrepreneurs of AMR largely targets the WHO. Even though policy entrepreneurs of AMR have not been successful in terms of building their network beyond the immediate scope of the problem, they have been successful at communicating directly with the WHO. However, during the interviews with WHO's social media team in their regional offices, interviewees stated that they mostly focus on information dissemination and outward communication to the public rather than receiving information on social media. However, the only times they focus on information received is when they look at the performance on Twitter of a particular post to get a general view about the WHO's reputation and clarify health messages to the public (Interviewee 1 and Interviewee 2). Both interviewees insisted that they pay attention to information that comes from well-known individuals, especially if it is controversial.

Interviewee 1 stated:

If a well-known individual … puts out information that is maybe against what we would advise, or attack us or … something like that, then we will definitely be … tracking it to see what is going on and what kind of rumours [are] circulating. We might not necessarily reply to it on social media, but we will definitely be checking it internally.

Interviewee 2 stated:

We mostly use social media for information dissemination, but in case there are false information or roamers that is putting WHO's reputation at risk, and especially if it is coming [from] a popular figure [on] social media, then we do take that into consideration and look at ways to approach it.

Both interviewees from WHO confirm that they use social media for information dissemination and communication to partner organizations. However, the only time that they pay attention to the received information is when it is from a well-known individual and if there is some sort of controversy. It can also be observed in the interviews that performance on Twitter matters to the WHO: if a tweet gets a large number of likes and retweets they pay attention to that and monitor it.

Interestingly, no independent advocate or person who is not affiliated to any of the organizations that deal with AMR or who is not an expert in microbiology or medicine was identified in the network. This indicates that the discussion of AMR on Twitter has not gone beyond experts and public is not yet engaged with the topic. The AMR debate is highly technical and limited to experts and practitioners of AMR from different disciplines rather than ordinary people having moral, ideological, and political discussions that are observable in the climate change debate.

While looking at the top 200 hashtags of AMR, none has been able to spark any controversial debate, which include the ordinary public or affective publics. The only time the use of hashtags #antimicrobialresistance, #antibioticresistance, or #amr have increased has been during the WHO's awareness week on AMR. Even looking at the tweets in that period, no major controversy or polarization can be identified. The only minor polarized discussion on the issue of AMR is between the human and animal industries that use antibiotics. One thousand random generated tweets from the 28,000 total show that the issue regarding antibiotic use on animals is the only major controversy on Twitter with regards to AMR. The following tweets are examples of this.

@FAO: Healthy animals do not need antibiotics or other antimicrobials. #AntimicrobialResistance #WAAW2019 <https://t.co/hNUKGEzAn0>.

This tweet has created fifty-five retweets and 106 likes on Twitter. This is still a very high number compared to other posts about FAO concerning AMR. No discussion stemmed from this tweet, no spark of debate was caused by it.

Another tweet shows that the food industry, one that relies a great deal on animal farming, occasionally interacts with the topic, but in terms of volume of tweets and reactions to an initial tweet about the topic, that is still minimal and has not caused any major increase in the network engagement.

RT @ConsumerReports: When food animals like cattle are given antibiotics they don't need, it contributes to #AntibioticResistance that threatens public health. How does your favorite fast-food chain fare on our latest #chainreaction scorecard? #USAAW2019 <https://t.co/MaHJbovpNN>.

This tweet created a very brief discussion between Twitter users, where two users have criticized the @ConsumerReports claims, but they both have not received any reply, retweet, or like from other users. On the contrary, when one looks at climate change, a high number of tweets that engage two polarized groups, as witnessed in the tweet above by Thunberg, receives thousands of likes, retweets, and replies, generating debate and hence increasing the number of participants in the network and in the debate on climate change.

Conclusion

AMR as one of the leading global health crises of our time but has received lower social media attention than the leading environmental crisis of our time—namely, climate change. AMR's Twitter engagements have been limited to scientific and emotionless communications from experts and organizations. Users who discuss AMR on Twitter do not show similar characteristics to those of climate change users. First, there are not as many individuals discussing AMR compared to those discussing climate change.

Secondly, there are few emotional, aesthetic, provocative, and polarized tweets and groups that discuss AMR. In contrast, the climate change's Twitter engagements are full of emotion and polarized engagement with provocative language and actions. The climate change debate has moved beyond experts and expert organizations: the largest communities in the network analysis are formed of many individuals who are not necessarily connected to any expert group or organization. Such a community of users does not exist in the Twitter debate on AMR. Hardly any individual who is not an expert or strongly involved in AMR can be noticed in the AMR network analysis.

The AMR digital individual entrepreneurs' communication is limited to expert-oriented individuals and groups who have not been able to bring AMR to the attention of public outside the immediate scope of the AMR problem on Twitter (for a related point about AMR's reach in policy-making, see Chapter 14). The very scientific nature of both the digital entrepreneurs' communication to the public and to organizations has prevented any dramatic and aesthetic presentation of the AMR problem, which could have resulted in any ideological and controversial debate that would have been able to increase Twitter engagement by common users. This has not just prevented AMR from receiving more public attention on social media but has also failed to catch the attention of WHO's social media team. The team monitors Twitter and other social media outlets on a daily basis and staff pay attention to the information received on social media only if something posted on Twitter performs well or if there is a controversy regarding WHO advice.

AMR networks can be identified as issue-driven publics who are clear of any affective action that would cause any ideological debate. This has resulted in smaller communities, since communication amongst the nodes is very low, but communication directed at organizations like WHO and CDC is still high.

On the contrary, climate change's digital entrepreneurs have been successful in using dramatic and aesthetic means to present the climate change problem and therefore they have been successful in raising attention to the problem. Individuals like Thunberg and Trump, who have been at opposite poles of the debate, have contributed immensely to the increase of the climate change debate on social media. The digital policy entrepreneurs of climate change have been able to build polarized networks which reach beyond the immediate scope of the problem.

Ideological interactions amongst the believers and deniers of climate change have formed larger communities who interact on Twitter. The heterogeneity of the communities in terms of ideology have contributed to the increase in attention paid to climate change on Twitter.

Policy recommendations

There is a need for transformation of the language of communication, from designated individuals and organizations working with AMR in social media, from a scientifically oriented language to common language that touches people's emotions. The scientific language and emotionless presentation of the problem has hindered public engagement because for the public to engage affectively in the debate about the problem of AMR there needs to be a level of emotional attachment and room to express public opinion, which would then lead to effective advocacy. Such communication can be achieved through simplified and symbolic communication strategies that would attract public and political attention without compromising scientific facts.

References

Baekkeskov, E., Rubin, O., Mumkholm, L., and Zaman, A. W. (2020). 'Antimicrobial Resistance as a Global Health Crisis Antimicrobial Resistance as a Global Health Crisis Dimensions of Antimicrobial Resistance', in E. Stern, ed., *Oxford Research Encyclopedia of Politics: Oxford Encyclopedia of Crisis Analysis* (Oxford Research Encyclopedias: Oxford University Press), 2050/ October, 1–26. doi:10.1093/acrefore/9780190228637.013.1626.

Baumgartner, F. R., and Jones, B. B. (1993). *Agendas and Instability in American Politics, Choice Reviews Online.* doi:10.5860/choice.31-0574. *Journal of Politic*, 1164–6.

Boin, A., Ekengren, M., and Rhinard, M. (2021). *Understanding the Creeping Crisis, Understanding the Creeping Crisis* (Cham, Switzerland: Palgrave Macmillan). doi:10.1007/978-3-030-70692-0.

Creswell, J. W. (2014). *Research Design: Qualitative, Quantitative, and Mixed Methods Approaches* (Thousand Oaks, CA: Sage). doi:10.1017/CBO9781107413324.004.

Downs, A. (2016). 'Up and Down with Ecology: The "Issue-Attention Cycle"', in Kristen Eichorn and Don Stacks, eds, *Agenda Setting: Readings on Media, Public Opinion, and Policymaking* (Chapter 8. New York: Routledge), 165–174. doi:10.4324/9781315538389.

Driscoll, K., and Walker, S. (2014). 'Working within a Black Box: Transparency in the Collection and Production of Big Twitter Data', *International Journal of Communication*, 8/1, 1746–64.

Engström, A. (2021). 'Antimicrobial Resistance as a Creeping Crisis', in A. Boin, M. Ekengren, and M. Rhinard, eds, *Understanding the Creeping Crisis* (Palgrave Macmillan, Cham), 19–36. doi:10.1007/978-3-030-70692-0_2.

Gil-Gil, T., Laborda, P., Sanz-García, F., Hernando-Amado, S., Blanco, P., and Martínez, J. L. (2019). 'Antimicrobial Resistance: A Multifaceted Problem with Multipronged Solutions', *MicrobiologyOpen*, 8/11, e945. doi:10.1002/mbo3.945.

Harder, R. A., Sevenans, J., and Van Aelst, P. (2017). 'Intermedia Agenda Setting in the Social Media Age: How Traditional Players Dominate the News Agenda in Election Times', *International Journal of Press/Politics*, 22/3, 275–93. doi:10.1177/1940161217704969.

Harring, N., and Krockow, E. M. (2021). 'The Social Dilemmas of Climate Change and Antibiotic Resistance: An Analytic Comparison and Discussion of Policy Implications', *Humanities and Social Sciences Communications*, 8/1, 1–9. doi:10.1057/s41599-021-00800-2.

IPCC (2021). 'Climate Change 2021', *The Physical Science Basis. Contribution of Working Group 1 to Sixth Assessment Report of the Intergovernmental Panel on Climate Change* (Cambridge, United Kingdom: Cambridge University Press).

Jones, B. (2017). 'Looking Good: Mediatisation and International NGOs', *European Journal of Development Research*, 29/1. doi:10.1057/ejdr.2015.87.

Jones, B. D., and Baumgartner, F. R. (2004). 'Representation and Agenda Setting', *Policy Studies Journal*, 32/1, 1–24. doi:10.1111/j.0190-292X.2004.00050.x.

Jones, B. D., and Baumgartner, F. R. (2005). *The Politics of Attention: How Government Prioritizes Problems* (Chicago, IL: University of Chicago Press).

Kapucu, N. (2005). 'Interorganizational Coordination in Dynamic Context: Networks in Emergency Response Management', *Connections*, 26/2.

Karp, P. (2019). 'Scott Morrison says no evidence links Australia's carbon emissions to bushfires', *The Guardian*.

Kingdon, J. (1995). *Agendas, Alternatives and Public Policies* (2nd edn, HarperCollins Publishers, New York).

Lang, S. (2010). *NGOs, Civil Society, and the Public Sphere* (Cambridge: Cambridge University Press). doi:10.1017/CBO9781139177146.

Laxminarayan, R. (2022). 'The Overlooked Pandemic of Antimicrobial Resistance', *The Lancet*. doi.org/10.1016/S0140-6736(22)00087-3.

Lazarus, R. J. (2009). 'Super wicked problems and climate change: Restraining the present to liberate the future', *Cornell Law Review*.

Lee, J. K. et al. (2014). 'Social Media, Network Heterogeneity, and Opinion Polarization', *Journal of Communication*, 64/4, 702–22. doi:10.1111/jcom.12077.

Lehman, G. (2007). 'The Accountability of NGOs in Civil Society and its Public Spheres', *Critical Perspectives on Accounting*, 18(6), 645–69. doi:10.1016/j.cpa.2006.04.002.

Levin, K., Cashore, B., Bernstein, S., Graeme, A. (2012). 'Overcoming the Tragedy of Super Wicked Problems: Constraining Our Future Selves to Ameliorate Global Climate Change', *Policy Sciences*. doi:10.1007/s11077-012-9151-0.

Martin, S. (2020). 'Scott Morrison's senior ministers discuss how to reposition climate policies', <https://www.theguardian.com/australia-news/2020/jan/22/scott-morrisons-senior-ministers-discuss-how-to-reposition-climate-policies>. *The Guardian*, United Kingdom, Accessed: 20/02/2020.

Mintrom, M., and Norman, P. 2009). 'Policy Entrepreneurship and Policy Change', *Policy Studies Journal*, 37/4, 649–67. doi:10.1111/j.1541-0072.2009.00329.x.

Mintrom, M., and Norman, P. (2009). 'Policy Entrepreneurship and Policy Change', *Policy Studies Journal*, 649–67. doi:10.1111/j.1541-0072.2009.00329.x.

Murphy, K. (2019). 'Morrison responds to Greta Thunberg by warning children against "needless" climate anxiety', *The Guardian*, 25 September. <https://www.theguardian.com/australia-news/2019/sep/25/morrison-responds-to-greta-thunberg-speech-by-warning-children-against-needless-climate-anxiety>. Accessed: 21/02/2020.

O'Neill, J. (2016). *Tackling Drug-Resistant Infections Globally: Final Report and Recommendations: The Review on Antimicrobial Resistance, 2016*. <https://amr-review.org/sites/default/files/160525_Finalpaper_with cover.pdf>.

Papacharissi, Z. (2016). 'Affective Publics and Structures of Storytelling: Sentiment, Events and Mediality', *Information Communication and Society*, 19/3, 307–24. doi:10.1080/1369118X.2015.1109697.

Prestinaci, F., Pezzotti, P., and Pantosti, A. (2015). 'Antimicrobial Resistance: A Global Multifaceted Phenomenon', *Pathogens and Global Health*. doi:10.1179/2047773215Y.0000000030.

Roelvink, G. (2010). 'Collective Action and the Politics of Affect', *Emotion, Space and Society*. doi:10.1016/j.emospa.2009.10.004.

Rogers Van Katwyk, S., Giubilini, A., Kirchhelle, C., Weldon, I., Harrison, I., McLean, A., et al. (2020). 'Exploring Models for an International Legal Agreement on the Global Antimicrobial Commons: Lessons from Climate Agreements', *Health Care Analysis*, 31, 25–46. doi:10.1007/s10728-019-00389-3.

Sabatier, P., and Weible, M. C. (2014). *Theories of the Policy Process* (New York, Routeledge). doi:10.1081/E-EPAP2-120041405.

Thunberg, G. (2019). 'Greta Thunberg's Speech at the U.N. Climate Action Summit: NPR', *National Public Radio*. Date of broadcast: September 23, 2019, Link: <https://www.npr.org/2019/09/23/763452863/transcript-greta-thunbergs-speech-at-the-u-n-climate-action-summit>, Accessed: 24/02/2020.

Tromble, R. (2018). 'The Great Leveler? Comparing Citizen-Politician Twitter Engagement across Three Western Democracies', *European Political Science*, 17, 223–9. doi:10.1057/s41304-016-0022-6.

Wang, Y. and Guan, L. (2020). 'Mapping the Structures of International Communication Organizations' Networks and Cross-Sector Relationships on Social Media and Exploring Their Antecedents', *Public Relations Review*, 46/4. doi:10.1016/j.pubrev.2020.101951.

Williams, H. T. P., McMurray, J. R., Kurz, T., and Lambert, F. H. (2015). 'Network Analysis Reveals Open Forums and Echo Chambers in Social Media Discussions of Climate Change', *Global Environmental Change*. doi:10.1016/j.gloenvcha.2015.03.006.

Zhu, J. H. (1992). 'Issue Competition and Attention Distraction: A Zero-Sum Theory of Agenda-Setting', *Journalism & Mass Communication Quarterly*, 69/4, 825–36. doi:10.1177/107769909206900403.

16

The Policy Context for Responses to Antimicrobial Resistance in India

Arjun Rajkhowa, Karin Thursky, and Kabir Rajkhowa

Introduction

In this chapter, we describe the policy and governance context for AMR mitigation in India and highlight areas for future exploration. In order to contextualize the policy framework for AMR control in India, it is important to recognize the role of the United Nations (UN), and the World Health Organization (WHO) specifically, in prioritizing and driving political momentum on the issue internationally. The WHO is recognized globally as a mediator of international efforts to tackle the AMR problem and as the primary locus of biopolitical conceptualization of the primacy of the problem (WHO, 2001, 2015a, 2015b). Addressing concerns about inappropriate antimicrobial use is one of the key planks of the WHO's global strategy for the containment of AMR, published in 2001 (WHO, 2001). This strategy, and the action plan that followed in 2015, identify key elements of the response to AMR, which are as follows: comprehensive and co-ordinated national strategies for AMR, laboratory capacity for surveillance of AMR, access to safe and effective antimicrobial drugs, control of the misuse of antimicrobial drugs, awareness of the threat of AMR and the importance of appropriate antimicrobial use in the community, and effective infection prevention and control (IPC) (WHO, 2015a). This framework, endorsed by WHO Member States, serves as the blueprint for most national action plans on AMR control, including in India (GoI, 2017b). As described later, this blueprint enables conceptualization and endorsement of ambitious aspirations which, had a strictly pragmatic and grounded approach been adopted in the Indian context, may not have been articulated as policy. Globally, the context for AMR mitigation across different WHO regions remains complex, with varying levels of achievement of target goals in crucial areas such as microbiology infrastructure, infection surveillance, access to quality medicines, antimicrobial stewardship (AMS) (i.e., efforts aimed at promoting the judicious use of antimicrobials), public awareness and education about antibiotic use and AMR, and IPC (UN, 2018; WHO, 2015b). From a health system perspective, the absence of infrastructure for microbiological testing, infection control, prescribing guidelines development and uptake, and AMS can limit the value of AMR mitigation commitments (WHO, 2015b). The absence of such infrastructure can be linked to systemic healthcare governance and delivery challenges, solutions

Arjun Rajkhowa, Karin Thursky, and Kabir Rajkhowa, *The Policy Context for Responses to Antimicrobial Resistance in India* In: *Steering against Superbugs*. Edited by: Olivier Rubin, Erik Baekkeskov, and Louise Munkholm, Oxford University Press.
© Oxford University Press 2023. DOI: 10.1093/oso/9780192899477.003.0016

for which often require significant political guidance and investment (Collignon et al., 2015). The problem of antimicrobial misuse has socio-political dimensions. It can be linked to the governance arrangements that underpin healthcare delivery and the complexities of approaches to regulating healthcare and medication access and delivery (Collignon et al., 2018). These complexities take on particular significance in the context of low- and middle-income countries like India (Laxminarayan and Chaudhury, 2016; see also Chapters 7, 9, 17, and 18).

The strategic framing of the AMR problem in various international and national declarations arguably evinces a unique form of politically endorsed consensus-making in the policy domain globally. Clare Chandler provides a useful discourse analysis of global political articulations of (and policy responses to) AMR (Chandler, 2019). Chandler writes, '[s]ensitive to the controversy around the science of climate change, those engaged with AMR advocacy have been careful to develop a "political narrative" that comprises consistent messaging and a coherent voice within a science-policy complex'. This emphasis on consensus-based political mobilization of discourses focalizing the crisis and promoting the need for effective mitigation actions, and coherence of advocacy, is reflected in the large (and growing) corpus of international agreements, consensus statements, and national action plans on the issue (Rochford et al., 2018). The UN—particularly the tripartite formation of the WHO, World Organization for Animal Health, and Food and Agriculture Organization—has been central to mobilizing and securing in-principle agreements from UN members about the need for AMR mitigation (UN, 2016). This political consensus has been mirrored by corresponding articulations of commitments to combatting AMR from industry groups (AMR Industry Alliance, 2016; Wellcome Trust, 2017). Following the work of Andrew Lakoff (Lakoff, 2015), Chandler charts the emergence of 'sentinel' and 'actuarial' frames in global biopolitical discourses about AMR; the 'sentinel' frame emphasizes 'vigilant attention and speculative intervention for a surprise and potentially catastrophic' emergence of AMR, whereas the 'actuarial' frame 'justifies action through the statistical calculation of risk' relating to AMR (Chandler, 2019; see also Chapter 4). These frames guide biopolitical discourses about AMR and shape both governmental and scholarly articulations of the problem. The 'actuarial' frame—promoting surveillance of both AMR and the quantity and quality of antimicrobial use—has been used to generate politically endorsed AMR mitigation policy and facilitate significant outputs in countries such as Australia (ACSQHC, 2019; NCAS and ACSQHC, 2020) and Japan (Tsutsui and Suzuki, 2018), where nationally coordinated surveillance efforts have been framed in policy as generating bodies of actionable knowledge, although, invariably, gaps remain.

In the next section, we chart the chronology of policy-making on AMR mitigation in India, highlighting the role of expert-led strategic communications in prompting government formulation and endorsement of a national action plan and declaration modelled on WHO-led international frameworks. This is followed by an analysis of implementation gaps and policy translation challenges in the country and a discussion of the role of research-led initiatives in sustaining infrastructure development and quality improvement action in the apparent absence of system-wide facilitation of interventions envisaged in policy. We argue that the imperative to conform to consensus-based international policy frameworks has led to endorsement of aspirational goals in policy; however, this has ostensibly not been accompanied by a recognition of the importance of adapting policy to local contexts and translating policy.

The policy context for AMR mitigation in India

India's relevance to global AMR mitigation efforts derives from both the significant burden of the AMR problem in India as well as the magnitude of antimicrobial consumption in the country; moreover, in terms of the dichotomy between purportedly 'excessive' medication consumption and still-inadequate healthcare access, it typifies many of the challenges that developing countries face (Laxminarayan and Chaudhury, 2016; see also Chapter 7). India has been specifically described in the biomedical literature as a key hub of the global AMR challenge (Kumar et al., 2013). Clinicians and researchers report a high burden of drug-resistant infections (CDDEP, 2017; Datta et al., 2012; Gandra et al., 2016). Health analysts surmise that a 'convergence of factors such as poor public health infrastructure, rising incomes, a high burden of disease, and cheap, unregulated sales of antibiotics has created ideal conditions for a rapid rise in resistant infections in India' (Laxminarayan and Chaudhury, 2016). In 2013, the ramifications of the AMR crisis and the urgent steps that were required for its control were articulated comprehensively in the Chennai Declaration, a document generated by infectious diseases and other medical experts through an inter-disciplinary symposium in 2012 (Ghafur et al., 2013). This document, which preceded the first government policy documents on AMR by four years, may be described as a salient catalyst for AMR policy action in India, and it is framed by the expert authors as an appeal to the Indian government to partner with medical societies and interested clinicians to establish a national roadmap for AMR mitigation. The authors write, '[t]he Indian medical community is seriously concerned about the high resistance rate in our country and would like to partner with Indian authorities in tackling the issue and joining the global fight against antimicrobial resistance' (Ghafur et al., 2013) The declaration frames the appeal to government as one that is underpinned by significant concern among clinicians about the deleterious impact of AMR on clinical outcomes and the discrepancy between growing international efforts to consolidate AMR mitigation strategies and an absence of cohesive action and government support for mitigation action in India. The Chennai Declaration explicitly articulates clinicians' requirements for pragmatic and programmatic action, including ministerial and regulatory policy-making on rationalization of antimicrobial use at the federal level, ministerial support for infection control and AMS infrastructure (including implementation policies and funding for resources) at the state level, the incorporation of mandatory infection control and AMS criteria into the hospital accreditation framework by the National Accreditation Board for Hospitals and Healthcare Providers, and systemic changes in programmes for clinical and research workforce training by the Medical Council of India and Indian

Council of Medical Research respectively. In its explicit enumeration of proposed actions to be undertaken by specific agencies, and its clarity of role assignment, it is a unique publication in India. The Chennai Declaration also looks beyond medical-infrastructural issues to demand societal interventions such as educational campaigns focused on raising awareness of the dangers and challenges associated with antimicrobial misuse through the news media and other educational avenues. The publication of the Chennai Declaration may be described as a key milestone in India's journey towards AMR mitigation, setting the scene for later policy interventions such as the Indian national action plan on AMR. Formulated as an explicitly political declaration, the Chennai Declaration is a work of strategic communication that emphatically articulates clinicians' and medical experts' investment in policy-making on antimicrobial consumption in India and their interest in catalysing interventionist political action driven by clinical and societal needs. It exemplifies expert-led awareness-raising and mobilization of political recognition of a pressing health issue. Arguably, its most important feature is its pragmatism and realistic emphasis on 'implementable' (rather than ideal) strategies for AMR mitigation (Ghafur et al., 2013). It eschews the aspiration to create ideal conditions for interventions: '[A]sking for a complete and strict antibiotic policy in a country where there is currently no functioning antibiotic policy at all may not be an intelligent or immediately viable option without the political will to make such a drastic change' (Ghafur et al., 2013). It posits the need for solutions that can be introduced and progressed despite current resource and other limitations. In this respect, it echoes international clinical consensus statements on AMR mitigation, which emphasize pragmatic, implementable strategies (Cox et al., 2017).

In April 2017, the Indian federal government published the *National Action Plan on Antimicrobial Resistance (2017–2021)* (NAP-AMR) (GoI, 2017b). Explicitly based on the WHO's framework, the NAP-AMR sets up six overarching strategic objectives in priority areas: (i) improve awareness of AMR and appropriate antimicrobial use through communications for the general public, and education and training for professionals; (ii) strengthen knowledge and evidence on AMR through surveillance and laboratory capacity-building; (iii) improve IPC in healthcare, community, and agricultural settings; (iv) support initiatives to improve antimicrobial use through regulations, and AMS initiatives in human and animal healthcare and agricultural settings; (v) promote investments in research and development initiatives; and (vi) strengthen India's capabilities and leadership in AMR mitigation through national, state, and international collaborations.

The first objective encompasses both general public education and professional education and training. The second objective entails strengthening laboratory capacity across human and animal health, and food and environment sectors, and specifically establishing and strengthening AMR surveillance capacity. The third and fourth objectives (covering IPC and AMS) are ambitiously articulated as encompassing human and animal health, community, and environmental settings. Aspirational goals of establishing coordination mechanisms, enforceable regulatory frameworks (and practice guidelines), surveillance programmes, and functional infection control and AMS programmes for healthcare settings are mentioned in the plan. These would fall primarily within the remit of the states. The fifth and sixth objectives relate to federal political functions such as supporting health funding for research and development, and facilitating coordination among national, state, and international stakeholders.

In 2017, in order to strategically communicate political will to intervene in the AMR health crisis, the federal government separately published a manifesto alongside the technical NAP-AMR. The Delhi Declaration, published in April 2017, reiterates the priority areas enumerated in the NAP-AMR but, importantly, also articulates and confirms political commitments to the implementation of the NAP-AMR (GoI, 2017a). It commits the government to developing and implementing national and state action plans on AMR; implementing these plans with a focus on strengthening surveillance of AMR and regulation of antimicrobial use; mobilizing and maintaining funding for implementation strategies in the healthcare sector; initiating and sustaining educational and public awareness-raising efforts focused on infection control and quality use of medicines, including through existing programmes such as the 'Swachh Bharat Abhiyan' (Clean India Mission); and adopting a 'mission' approach to addressing AMR. It commits to mitigation efforts across human and animal health (taking a 'One Health' approach; see Chapters 11, 12, and 13), and formalizes political commitment at the federal level to all-round AMR control. In this respect, it is a much more explicitly political document that conveys promises of political (rather than technical or agency-based) commitment to mitigation actions. While the NAP-AMR enumerates priority areas and aspirational goals for each of these areas, the Delhi Declaration serves to affirm government support for the implementation of the NAP-AMR. This political strategy of separately endorsing policy and confirming political will to implement policy is intended to signal prioritization of the issue on the part of the federal government. The document appears to echo the Chennai Declaration (2013) deliberately, and, in this respect, the Delhi Declaration arguably represents government affirmation of the expert-led demands for interventions that were first systematically articulated in the Chennai Declaration and the concretization of mitigation goals as policy. Despite the explicit political support, however, there appear to be several barriers to policy translation.

The NAP-AMR classifies goals into short-, medium- and long-term goals, and, where possible, lists institutions and ministries as being responsible for particular objectives. The federal government-funded National Centre for Disease Control (NCDC) and Indian Council of Medical Research (ICMR) are given responsibility for several objectives, particularly in priority areas 2 to 6. Interestingly, the NAP-AMR names a National Authority for Containment of Antibiotic Resistance (a new statutory body specifically for AMR), and describes it as being accountable for a significant proportion of the education and professional training (and key regulatory and coordination-related) functions envisaged in the plan. At the time of writing, this body had ostensibly not yet been established. Instead, the grey literature indicates that the NCDC's National

Program on AMR Containment has become the broader rubric under which progress on AMR mitigation is being monitored.

While the NAP-AMR mainly names federal institutions and ministries as being accountable for different objectives of the plan, it is intended primarily as a template for state action plans, as public hospitals in India are state-run. Information on state-level implementation of the NAP-AMR is scarce. The absence of publicly accessible information on assessment or evaluation of NAP-AMR implementation progress indicates that, at the federal level to begin with, there has been insufficient attention paid to communicating progress on AMR policy implementation on the ground. There is insufficient information in the public domain on whether the coordination mechanisms and institutional collaborations that were envisaged in the NAP-AMR have actually been established. This speaks to the challenge of health policy implementation lags in India (Ramani and Mavalankar, 2006).

In July 2018, over a year after the NAP-AMR was published, the federal government also published a document to guide the development of state action plans on AMR (GoI, 2018). This document recommends that the states undertake a stakeholder-mapping exercise, formulate a state action plan, and establish governance mechanisms such as a multi-sectoral steering committee and a technical working group. Its defining feature is that it provides a template for states to undertake stakeholder mapping (listing potential key groups across state health department affiliates and state medical colleges) and a basic terms of reference template for advisory groups. It also proposes key targets or outputs for each of the priorities of the NAP-AMR (which, it suggests, should be replicated in the state action plans). Only two state-based policy documents were publicly accessible at the time of writing. The Kerala (October 2018) and Madhya Pradesh (July 2019) state action plans demonstrate conformity with this guidance, specifying individual government departments, and healthcare and educational institutions that should take responsibility for the different activities specified in the priority areas, and key preliminary achievements and outputs that may be expected from these parties within a time frame of one to three years (GoK, 2018; GoMP, 2019). However, for many of the priorities, non-institution-specific clinical specialties or groups (e.g., microbiology and infection control specialties) are listed as the responsible party without further information on formalized structures of operation, and who they would report to or how they would coordinate their actions. This framing indicates a lack of strategic prioritizing of operational support and accountability mechanisms.

Most states have ostensibly not formulated state action plans, and those that have done so have not publicly evaluated them or reported progress on their implementation. An expert's observations on the development phase of the Kerala state government- and NCDC-coordinated Kerala state action plan, which was anticipated to be 'the guiding lamp for the whole country', indicate that insufficient planning and tensions over the involvement of non-governmental organizations stymied both the formulation and publication of the plan and its implementation (Ghafur, 2018). Kerala's state action plan, the first in the country, was, however, successfully launched in October 2018. On the other hand, across most of the country, the preliminary goals of formulating state action plans, mapping stakeholders, and establishing steering and technical advisory groups have ostensibly not been achieved. Gaps in the political stewardship of policy-making have allegedly contributed to this. For example, it was observed that over half of states did not participate in a federally led consultation in 2017 on state-level implementation actions, and that, while the NCDC was a co-organizer, most of the responsibility for coordinating this inter-governmental consultation was left to the WHO, an external advisory body, which lacked ministerial authority to mandate state participation (Ghafur, 2018). Expert commentary on the political dynamics underpinning coordination of initiatives following the launch of the NAP-AMR indicates that, overall, accountability for strategic communication and management of strategies remains diffuse and uncertain, leading to a fragmented response (Ghafur, 2018).

Seen collectively, this policy-related context for AMR control in India signals political and medical-professional recognition of the need to publicly commit to AMR mitigation goals, primarily (though not exclusively) to maintain parity with international efforts in this domain (Chandra et al., 2020; Dixit et al., 2019). However, NAP formulation is an essential but preliminary mitigation strategy, and there is a need to assess whether politically and professionally endorsed declarations have been strategically communicated to stakeholders, particularly those at the state level, and translated into practice in India (Chandra et al., 2020). Since the publication of the Chennai Declaration in 2013 and the NAP-AMR and Delhi Declaration in 2017, many of the proposed implementation strategies relating to devolution of accountability for various containment and quality improvement mechanisms to state governments and related institutions apparently remain unrealized. Particularly, in the health policy formulation domain, many (if not most) aspirational goals remain unfulfilled, as few states have enacted state action plans or initiated the complex processes that the NAP-AMR explicitly states are necessary for AMR control at the state level.

Despite these and other political and technical challenges, pockets of the Indian healthcare system continue to demonstrate progressive adoption of some mitigation strategies mentioned in policy documents (Bhattacharya et al., 2019). For example, reports indicate that, by late 2019, in the state of Kerala, seen as a state leader in healthcare improvement more generally, infection control protocols and AMS initiatives had been established in pockets of the tertiary care sector, and an AMR surveillance network comprising both public and private laboratories had also been established, despite a reported lack of dedicated state funding for these initiatives (Maya, 2019). While the challenges of the development phase might have stymied progress in this particular state, the accumulation of practical initiatives ultimately facilitated attainment of some key goals.

Importantly, nationally, it is evident that several critical health management initiatives relevant to AMR control preceded the publication of the NAP-AMR. The inclusion of selected antibiotics in Schedule H1 by the Central Drugs Standard Control Organisation (CDSCO) in 2014 served as a milestone in national antimicrobial use-related policy in India (Hazra, 2014). In 2014, the list included thirty-five critically important antibiotics (more frequently used in acute, rather than community, settings) such as some third- and fourth-generation cephalosporins, carbapenems, antituberculosis drugs and fluoroquinolones, but excluded others such as some aminoglycosides, cephalosporins, and macrolides (Hazra, 2014). The regulation stipulated more stringent record-keeping (of patient, prescriber, and prescription details, for a period of three years) for these prescription-only medications and specified penalties (such as license cancellation) for breaches by pharmacy owners. There have been reports of occasional regulatory enforcement and punitive actions against pharmacies found guilty of non-compliance (Laxminarayan and Chaudhury, 2016). Hailed as an appropriate intervention for the problem of over-the-counter consumption, this reform portends more stringent self-regulation by pharmacy operators, and the likely improvement of compliance with Schedule H (which includes other antimicrobials not included in H1) provisions. (Schedule H drugs cannot be sold without a prescription but do not require as stringent record-keeping as H1 drugs do). However, medical experts surmise that because the practice of non-prescription antimicrobial procurement has remained entrenched for so long (Salunkhe et al., 2013), regulatory changes need to be augmented with educational campaigns and awareness-raising efforts among both the general public and healthcare workforce. Experts note that many antibiotics that are more frequently used in the community remain off the Schedule H1 list, and, therefore, it may be difficult to monitor non-prescription sales of these antibiotics (Ghafur, 2018). As such, the primary effect of the introduction of Schedule H1 may have been to create greater awareness of the need for regulatory oversight among stakeholders (Hazra, 2014). The Red Line Campaign, for example, has led to the modification of medication packaging by pharmaceutical manufacturers, with a red line on antimicrobial drugs' packets drawing pharmacy workers' and consumers' attention to their regulated nature (Travasso, 2016). The extent to which awareness of initiatives to curtail non-prescription antimicrobial use has increased and prompted concomitant AMS efforts among the relevant professional groups and in the community is not yet well-understood.

The literature indicates that national bodies initiated pathogen surveillance prior to the publication of the NAP-AMR (Walia, Madhumathi, et al., 2019). Nationally endorsed guidelines (i.e., guidelines endorsed by a regulatory body for national use) for antimicrobial prescribing in India were first published by the NCDC in 2016 (National Centre for Disease Control, 2016), which were followed by additional treatment guidelines from the ICMR in 2017 (updated in 2019) (Indian Council of Medical Research, 2017). The ICMR published a framework for improving antimicrobial prescribing practices in acute care settings (which, importantly, enjoins the development of resources such as formularies and guidelines) (Walia, Ohri, et al., 2019) and established a research network to support the coordination of AMR surveillance activities (Walia, Madhumathi, et al., 2019). The ICMR used its pathogen surveillance data to frame its treatment guidelines (Indian Council of Medical Research, 2017). These guidelines complement its hospital infection control (Indian Council of Medical Research, 2016) and AMS (Indian Council of Medical Research, 2018) guidelines. The NCDC has also established an AMR surveillance network (Chandra et al., 2020). The two networks now comprise thirty and twenty tertiary hospitals respectively (Walia and Gangakhedkar, 2021). These initiatives by leading public institutions are important to the enablement of AMR mitigation. There is a need for more information on the up-take of available policies and guidelines across healthcare settings. Reportedly, IPC and AMS initiatives remain scattered and restricted to small pockets of the acute care set-ting, and are largely institution-driven (without external monitoring or coordination) (Bhattacharya et al., 2019).

Conclusion and discussion

While international medical and technical experts (and inter-governmental organiza-tions) repeatedly emphasize the importance of political leadership on control of AMR, in India, despite the publication of policy documents strategically communicating both stakeholder and government commitment to AMR mitigation, there appears to be insufficient acknowledgement of the significance of ongoing political leadership for AMR mitigation, and for the devolution of accountability for mitigation actions to the state level, where most of healthcare is controlled, despite the existence of an federally endorsed policy framework recommending this (Ghafur, 2018). Both the biomedical literature and policy documents signal the primacy of nascent institutional networks in taking the lead on facilitating AMR mitigation and AMS across tertiary human health sectors. This institution- and research-driven approach relies on specialist expertise in developing capacity among selected stakeholders and in facilitating sufficient up-take of capabilities and guidelines through professional and research communications targeting those stakeholders. This approach may be generally contrasted with health department-led approaches that reflect greater governmental stewardship of efforts to horizontally spread new initiatives (e.g., surveillance) and quality and safety require-ments (e.g., IPC and AMS). While government-coordinated mechanisms were en-visaged in the Indian federal NAP-AMR, the current evidence indicates that the onus on research institutions to carry out AMR surveillance and to promote AMS among selected stakeholders (and thus assume most of the burden of AMR mitigation) re-mains in place (Chandra et al., 2021; Walia and Gangakhedkar, 2021). The need for a transition from research-led to government-led or health department-led facilitation of AMR mitigation and AMS has been averred in media commentary by a former head of the ICMR (Ganguly, 2021). Expert commentary on the emergence of new govern-ment funding for infectious diseases management-related infrastructure and initiatives in the context of the COVID-19 pandemic, and the specific challenges the pandemic posed, indicates that there is potential for investment of resources (including labora-tory and human resources) and greater awareness and uptake of mitigation initiatives among (primarily acute care) stakeholders on the ground (Walia and Gangakhedkar, 2021), which could potentially facilitate more systematic adoption of AMR policy aims.

The strategic framing of the government's intention to conform with international commitments and efforts—the drive to develop a 'political narrative' on the AMR problem through declarations that confirm the support of the 'science-policy complex'—has resulted in the actualization of a publicly accessible 'sentinel' policy frame for AMR mitigation in India (Chandler, 2019); however, it may be argued, the transition to an 'actuarial' approach to framing the problem or implementing policy has not yet been realized or publicly communicated. The policy literature, biomedical literature, and grey literature indicate that the 'sentinel' framing has achieved the aim of demonstrating consensus at the federal level on the need for recognition of the problem and in-principle commitment to a template for the enablement of mitigation efforts. However, this has not been accompanied by dissemination of accessible information on the outcomes of initiatives and efforts towards policy translation. This arguably signals the potential difficulty of facilitating goals envisaged in a policy framework that was modelled on an ambitious international blueprint. Moreover, it is apparent that the endorsement of multisectoral regulatory aims in the NAP-AMR—across human and animal health domains and agriculture—has not necessarily led to multisectoral initiatives and achievements. Achievements highlighted in the literature, mainly concerning infrastructure development through research networks, pertain to the acute care setting (Walia and Gangakhedkar, 2021). Other priority areas, including agriculture, are ostensibly not currently the subject of systematic effort. Also important are issues not explicitly addressed in the grey literature but identified as critical to AMR mitigation; these include the contribution of pharmaceutical manufacturing and discharge of antibiotic-containing effluents to the environmental burden of AMR (see Chapter 17), and of the production and illicit sale of sub-standard and 'spurious' antibiotic medications (among other sub-standard medications) to the AMR problem in human health. These industry-related problems ostensibly have not been explicitly addressed in research-led initiatives and remain diffuse and neglected areas of concern (Ganguly, 2021).

Given the pre-NAP-AMR initiation of some key policies and programmes, an issue for future AMR-related health policy and governance research relates to whether the NAP-AMR has provided an effective and cohesive framework for the ongoing operationalization and communication of policies and strategies. Future research on the policy and governance context for AMR mitigation and control in India can examine whether, and to what extent, the existing governance framework for AMR mitigation has facilitated programme cohesion and stakeholder awareness, and what stakeholders' perspectives on existing challenges and barriers to effective health policy translation may be. There is a need for greater understanding of the gaps that characterize the translation of international policy frameworks and modalities in India and the region more broadly. The centrality of the WHO in supporting AMR mitigation in India, and comprehensive reliance on the WHO framework as a 'template that can aid in systematising AMR containment in India... [to] make it comparable to global efforts' should be seen as beneficial, and a facilitator of multinational research collaboration and engagement (GoI and WHO, 2016). At the same time, there is a need for greater reflection on the gaps between political commitments to international frameworks and the concretization of domestic and local efforts. In a closely related context, these gaps have been characterized as the result of 'local political and economic dynamics [that] may be more salient to policy actors influencing implementation of AMR national action plans than solutions presented in global guidelines that rely on implementation of hard regulations' (Khan et al., 2020). The 'disconnect' in countries like India between international frameworks endorsed by national governments and the realities of the 'local contexts where implementation takes place' (Khan et al., 2020) should be critically analysed (see also Chapters 7, 9, 10, and 12).

In exploring the salience of local contexts, attention may be paid to sub-national political arrangements and factors (e.g., centre–state relations); strategic communication of health policy aims and perceptions regarding the implementability of desired activities; and facilitators and barriers of translating international frameworks (beyond AMR) and related political discourses and works of strategic communication (including declarations and political pronouncements) into domestic policy. Opportunities and challenges relating to the role of federalism in shaping healthcare policy in India have been previously highlighted as a key topic area (Peters et al., 2003). These opportunities and challenges undoubtedly have a role to play in shaping AMR policy too, and there is a need for critical analysis of how the existing structural features of government and modes of communication affect the way policies are conceptualized, communicated, and implemented. The contemporary Indian healthcare landscape remains governed by a relatively static governmental framework that was established under conditions different to those that exist today, and recommendations about the 'splitting' of healthcare policy have been anchored in demands for greater recognition of 'inter- and intra-state differences in contexts and processes' and the need for state-level 'innovation and local accountability' (Peters et al., 2003). The process of consolidating local accountability can be accompanied by a simultaneous 'lumping of policy issues' at the federal level, with an emphasis on coordination of systemic efforts and the 'development of systems for quality assurance and regulation of the private sector' (Peters et al., 2003). The desirability and attainability of this differential approach can be gauged through qualitative research with federal and state policy-makers.

In the domain of stakeholder awareness, analysis of medical professionals' perspectives on AMR mitigation rhetoric indicates that there is significant uncertainty about the feasibility and implementability of quality improvement actions, and a general sense of resignation (besides apprehension) about the AMR problem at a local level (Broom and Doron, 2020). This analysis suggests that externalization of the AMR threat (as a problem that lies 'elsewhere', even though it is proximate and immediate) is a common trope in stakeholders' discourses (Broom and Doron, 2020). Analysing what responsible institutional experts can do to improve their understanding of the contextual barriers and facilitators experienced by intended stakeholders such as acute care professionals, and how the latter can better engage with strategically developed messages to promote a sense of ownership of mitigation efforts, is likely to be essential. Many policy-makers posit that understanding behavioural and social-contextual factors should constitute a crucial (if not fundamental) element of the overarching response to the problem of antimicrobial misuse, and that reinforcing accountability for individual contributions to antimicrobial misuse should be a key mitigation activity (Ashiru-Oredope and Hopkins, 2015; Price et al., 2018). An exploration of whether 'individualization' of the problem of AMR—the diffuse attribution of responsibility for the problem to individuals (in various settings) who may contribute to suboptimal use or misuse of antimicrobials, and who, consequently, may become cognizant of their putative agency to curtail any individual contributions to the problem (Chandler, 2019)—may have a role in augmenting stakeholder awareness in India could be explored through qualitative research with different stakeholder groups.

This chapter briefly describes the policy and governance context for AMR mitigation in India. It highlights facets of extant policy frameworks for the problem and goals for mitigation actions, contextualized with observations on reported implementation challenges. This chapter forms a point of departure for further inquiry into policy-making and communication on AMR mitigation in India. Particularly, inquiries into how, and to what extent, existing policy and emerging stakeholder awareness, and sectoral barriers and facilitators, have influenced policy translation and communication of strategies in health departments, healthcare settings, professional bodies, and agricultural and environmental settings, may be pursued. Such inquiries may take the form of qualitative research with stakeholders and experts, and may inform strategies to bolster policy translation and communication.

References

ACSQHC. (2019). *AURA 2019: Third Australian Report on Antimicrobial Use and Resistance in Human Health*. <https://www.safetyandquality.gov.au/our-work/antimicrobial-resistance/antimicrobial-use-and-resistance-australia-surveillance-system/aura-2019>. Accessed 01.03.2023.

AMR Industry Alliance. (2016). *Declaration by the Pharmaceutical, Biotechnology and Diagnostics Industries on Combating Antimicrobial Resistance*. AMR Industry Alliance. <https://www.amrindustryalliance.org/wp-content/uploads/2017/12/AMR-Industry-Declaration.pdf>. Accessed 01.03.2023.

Ashiru-Oredope, D., and Hopkins, S. (2015). 'Antimicrobial Resistance: Moving from Professional Engagement to Public Action'. *Journal of Antimicrobial Chemotherapy*, 70/11, 2927–30.

Bhattacharya, S., Joy, V. M., Goel, G., Nath, S. R., Santosh, S., George, K., et al. (2019). 'Antimicrobial Stewardship Programme—From Policies to Practices: A Survey of Antimicrobial Stewardship Programme Practices from 25 Centres in India'. *Journal of The Academy of Clinical Microbiologists*, 21/1, 4.

Broom, A., and Doron, A. (2020). 'Antimicrobial Resistance, Politics, and Practice in India'. *Qualitative Health Research*, 30/11, 1684–96.

CDDEP. (2017). *Resistance Map*. Center for Disease Dynamics Economics and Policy. <https://resistancemap.cddep.org> accessed 29 October 2021.

Chandler, C. I. (2019). 'Current Accounts of Antimicrobial Resistance: Stabilisation, Individualisation and Antibiotics as Infrastructure'. *Palgrave Communications*, 5/1, 1–13.

Chandra, P., Mk, U., Ke, V., Mukhopadhyay, C., U, D. A., and V, R. (2021). Antimicrobial Resistance and the Post Antibiotic Era: Better Late Than Never Effort. *Expert Opinion on Drug Safety*, 20/11, 1375–90.

Chandra, S., Prithvi, P., Srija, K., Jauhari, S., and Grover, A. (2020). 'Antimicrobial Resistance: Call for Rational Antibiotics Practice in India'. *Journal of Family Medicine and Primary Care*, 9(5), 2192.

Collignon, P., Athukorala, P.-C., Senanayake, S., and Khan, F. (2015). 'Antimicrobial Resistance: The Major Contribution of Poor Governance and Corruption to This Growing Problem'. *PLoS One*, 10/3, e0116746.

Collignon, P., Beggs, J. J., Walsh, T. R., Gandra, S., and Laxminarayan, R. (2018, 2018/09/01/). 'Anthropological and Socioeconomic Factors Contributing to Global Antimicrobial Resistance: A Univariate and Multivariable Analysis'. *The Lancet Planetary Health*, 2/9, e398–e405. <https://doi.org/https://doi.org/10.1016/S2542-5196(18)30186-4>.

Cox, J. A., Vlieghe, E., Mendelson, M., Wertheim, H., Ndegwa, L., Villegas, M. V., et al. (2017). 'Antibiotic Stewardship in Low- and Middle-income countries: the Same but Different?', *Clinical Microbiology and Infection*, 23/11, 812-818.

Datta, S., Wattal, C., Goel, N., Oberoi, J. K., Raveendran, R., and Prasad, K. (2012). 'A Ten Year Analysis of Multi-drug Resistant Blood Stream Infections caused by Escherichia coli & Klebsiella pneumoniae in a Tertiary Care Hospital'. *The Indian Journal of Medical Research*, 135/6, 907.

Dixit, A., Kumar, N., Kumar, S., and Trigun, V. (2019). 'Antimicrobial Resistance: Progress in the Decade since Emergence of New Delhi Metallo-β-lactamase in India'. *Indian Journal of Community Medicine*, 44/1, 4.

Gandra, S., Mojica, N., Klein, E. Y., Ashok, A., Nerurkar, V., Kumari, M., et al. (2016). 'Trends in Antibiotic Resistance among Major Bacterial Pathogens Isolated from Blood Cultures Tested at a Large Private Laboratory Network in India, 2008–2014'. *International Journal of Infectious Diseases*, 50, 75–82. <https://doi.org/https://doi.org/10.1016/j.ijid.2016.08.002>.

Ganguly, N. K. (2021, 4 March). 'Antimicrobial resistance is a serious threat to public health in India'. *The Wire*. <https://science.thewire.in/health/antimicrobial-resistance-is-a-serious-threat-to-public-health-in-india/>. Accessed 01.03.2023.

Ghafur, A. (2018). 'State-Level AMR Action Plans in India: Progress at a Snail's Pace!', in J. Carlet and G. Upham, eds, *AMR Control 2018* (Global Health Dynamics), 22 25.

Ghafur, A., Mathai, D., Muruganathan, A., Jayalal, J., Kant, R., Chaudhary, D., et al. (2013). 'The Chennai Declaration: A Roadmap to Tackle the Challenge of Antimicrobial Resistance'. *Indian Journal of Cancer*, 50/1, 71.

GoI. (2017a). *Delhi Declaration on Antimicrobial Resistance—An Inter-ministerial Consensus* (New Delhi: Government of India).

GoI. (2017b). *National Action Plan on Antimicrobial Resistance (2017–2021)*. (New Delhi: Government of India).

GoI. (2018). *Guidance for Developing State Action Plans for Containment of Antimicrobial Resistance* (New Delhi: Government of India).

GoI and WHO. (2016). *Antimicrobial Resistance and its Containment in India*. <https://www.who.int/docs/default-source/searo/india/antimicrobial-resistance/amr-containment.pdf?sfvrsn=2d7c49a2_2>. Accessed 01.03.2023.

GoK. (2018). *Kerala Antimicrobial Resistance Strategic Action Plan*. Government of Kerala.

GoMP. (2019). *Madhya Pradesh State Action Plan for Containment of Antimicrobial Resistance*. Government of Madhya Pradesh.

Hazra, A. (2014). 'Schedule H1: Hope or Hype?', *Indian Journal of Pharmacology*, 46/4, 361.

Indian Council of Medical Research. (2016). *Hospital Infection Control Guidelines* (New Delhi: Indian Council of Medical Research). <https://main.icmr.nic.in/sites/default/files/guidelines/Hospital_Infection_control_guidelines.pdf>. Accessed 01.03.2023.

Indian Council of Medical Research. (2017). *Treatment Guidelines for Antimicrobial Use in Common Syndromes* (New Delhi: Indian Council of Medical Research). <http://iamrsn.icmr.org.in/images/pdf/STG270217.pdf>.

Indian Council of Medical Research. (2018). *Antimicrobial Stewardship Program Guidelines*. (New Delhi: Indian Council of Medical Research). <http://iamrsn.icmr.org.in/images/pdf/AMSP_Guidelines_final.pdf>.

Khan, M. S., Durrance-Bagale, A., Mateus, A., Sultana, Z., Hasan, R., and Hanefeld, J. (2020). 'What Are the Barriers to Implementing National Antimicrobial Resistance Action Plans? A Novel Mixed-Methods Policy Analysis in Pakistan'. *Health Policy and Planning*, 35/8, 973–82. <https://doi.org/10.1093/heapol/czaa065>.

Kumar, S. G., Adithan, C., Harish, B., Sujatha, S., Roy, G., and Malini, A. (2013). 'Antimicrobial Resistance in India: A Review'. *Journal of Natural Science, Biology, and Medicine*, 4/2, 286.

Lakoff, A. (2015). 'Real-time Biopolitics: The Actuary and the Sentinel in Global Public health'. *Economy and Society*, 44/1, 40–59.

Laxminarayan, R., and Chaudhury, R. R. (2016). 'Antibiotic Resistance in India: Drivers and Opportunities for Action'. *PLoS Medicine*, 13/3, e1001974.

Maya, C. (2019, 27 October). 'Antimicrobial resistance action plan losing steam'. *Hindu*. <https://www.thehindu.com/news/national/kerala/antimicrobial-resistance-action-plan-losing-steam/article29810532.ece>.

National Centre for Disease Control. (2016). *National Treatment Guidelines for Antimicrobial Use in Infectious Diseases–Version 1.0* (New Delhi: Government of India).

NCAS and ACSQHC. (2020). *Antimicrobial Prescribing Practice in Australian Hospitals: Results of the 2018 Hospital National Antimicrobial Prescribing Survey*. (Canberra: Australian Commission for Safety and Quality in Health Care) <https://www.safetyandquality.gov.au/our-work/antimicrobial-resistance/antimicrobial-use-and-resistance-australia-surveillance-system-aura/hospital-antimicrobial-use/appropriateness-antimicrobial-use-australian-hospitals-naps>. Accessed 01.03.2023.

Peters, D. H., Rao, K. S., and Fryatt, R. (2003). 'Lumping and Splitting: The Health Policy Agenda in India'. *Health Policy and Planning*, 18/3, 249–60.

Price, L., Gozdzielewska, L., Young, M., Smith, F., MacDonald, J., McParland, J., et al. (2018). 'Effectiveness of Interventions to Improve the Public's Antimicrobial Resistance Awareness and Behaviours Associated with Prudent Use of Antimicrobials: A Systematic Review'. *Journal of Antimicrobial Chemotherapy*, 73/6, 1464–78.

Ramani, K., and Mavalankar, D. (2006). 'Health System in India: Opportunities and Challenges for Improvements'. *Journal of Health Organization and Management*, 20/6, 560–72.

Rochford, C., Sridhar, D., Woods, N., Saleh, Z., Hartenstein, L., Ahlawat, H., et al. (2018). 'Global Governance of Antimicrobial Resistance'. *The Lancet*, 391/10134, 1976–8.

Salunkhe, S., Pandit, V., Dawane, J., Sarda, K., and More, C. (2013). 'Study of over the Counter Sale of Antimicrobials in Pharmacy Outlets in Pune, India: A Cross Sectional Study'. *International Journal of Pharmacology and Biological Science*, 4/2, 616–22.

Travasso, C. (2016). 'India Draws a Red Line under Antibiotic Misuse'. *British Medical Journal*. <https://www.bmj.com/content/352/bmj.i1202> accessed 28 October 2021.

Tsutsui, A., and Suzuki, S. (2018). 'Japan Nosocomial Infections Surveillance (JANIS): A Model of Sustainable National Antimicrobial Resistance Surveillance Based on Hospital Diagnostic Microbiology Laboratories'. *BMC Health Services Research*, 18/1, 799.

UN. (2016). *Political Declaration of the High-Level Meeting of the General Assembly on Antimicrobial Resistance* (New York, NY: United Nations). <https://digitallibrary.un.org/record/842813?ln=en>.

UN. (2018). *Monitoring Global Progress on Addressing Antimicrobial Resistance: Analysis Report of the Second Round of Results of AMR Country Self-Assessment Survey*. <https://apps.who.int/iris/bitstream/handle/10665/273128/9789241514422-eng.pdf?ua=1>.

Walia, K., and Gangakhedkar, R. R. (2021). 'Infectious Disease Blocks in District Hospitals to Augment India's Resolve to Contain Antimicrobial Resistance'. *Indian Journal of Medical Research*, 153/4, 416.

Walia, K., Madhumathi, J., Veeraraghavan, B., Chakrabarti, A., Kapil, A., Ray, P., et al. (2019). 'Establishing Antimicrobial Resistance Surveillance & Research Network in India: Journey So Far'. *The Indian Journal of Medical Research*, 149/2, 164.

Walia, K., Ohri, V., Madhumathi, J., and Ramasubramanian, V. (2019). 'Policy Document on Antimicrobial Stewardship Practices in India'. *The Indian Journal of Medical Research*, 149/2, 180.

Wellcome Trust. (2017). *Sustaining Global Action on Antimicrobial Resistance* (London: Wellcome Trust and United Nations Foundation) <https://wellcome.ac.uk/sites/default/files/sustaining-global-action-on-antimicrobial-resistance.pdf> accessed 1 September 2021.

WHO. (2001). *WHO Global Strategy for Containment of Antimicrobial Resistance* (Geneva: World Health Organization).

WHO. (2015a). *Global Action Plan on Antimicrobial Resistance* (Geneva: World Health Organization). <http://apps.who.int/iris/bitstream/10665/193736/1/9789241509763_eng.pdf?ua=1>.

WHO. (2015b). *Worldwide Country Situation Analysis: Response to Antimicrobial Resistance* (Geneva: World Health Organization). <https://apps.who.int/iris/handle/10665/163468>. Accessed 01.03.2023.

PART VI
REGULATORY RESPONSES TO AMR

17

A Case for the Global Governance of AMR by Regulating the Pharmaceutical Supply Chain

Ipshita Chaturvedi and Natasha Kavalakkat

Introduction

While there are several reasons for the global rise in antimicrobial resistance (AMR), studies have shown that improper drug manufacturing methods in countries like India and China are a significant cause (Fouz et al., 2020). The pharmaceutical industry comprises (i) active pharmaceutical ingredients (APIs) manufacturing units that manufacture the raw material or an intermediate for the antibiotic and (ii) formulations or finished pharmaceutical product (FPP) manufacturing units that combine the active ingredient to produce a final pharmaceutical product (Nahar, 2020). Over the past three decades, India and China have emerged as the leading sources of APIs for the pharmaceutical sector (Arnum, 2013; Gandra et al., 2017). The increase in antibiotic manufacturing capacity has caused a consequent rise in the industry's pharmaceutical effluent. The effluents generated from both types of antibiotic manufacturing units (APIs and FPPs) contain antibiotic residues. Since effluents from pharmaceutical manufacturing sites contain concentrated amounts of APIs and intermediates, these sites act as hotspots for environmental contamination and the spread of AMR (Kotwani et al., 2021). Scientifically, Topp et al. (2018) have shown that the highest concentrations of antibiotics and the highest abundances of antibiotic-resistant genes detected in the environment have been found in sites polluted by direct discharges from the manufacturing of antibiotics. That is why it is incumbent that when discussing AMR, drug manufacturing must be key point. Even though agricultural and human sources are big contributors to AMR, industrial point sources for antibiotics are considerably fewer, making them an easier problem to solve.

According to Navadhi (2019), by 2023, the global pharmaceutical industry is expected to be worth US$ 1.57 trillion. With a projected 24.07 per cent market share, the Asia-Pacific region would continue to be the second largest in the world. Many low- and middle-income countries in this region invest in the pharmaceutical industry due to its high contribution to their per capita gross domestic product (GDP). However, in the efforts to industrialize, these countries do not have the finance and technology, or the luxury, to regulate polluting industries (Metcalf et al., 2017). Additionally, such countries also tend to host 'shadow economies' for drug production where even if

Ipshita Chaturvedi and Natasha Kavalakkat, *A Case for the Global Governance of AMR by Regulating the Pharmaceutical Supply Chain*
In: *Steering against Superbugs*. Edited by: Olivier Rubin, Erik Baekkeskov, and Louise Munkholm, Oxford University Press.
© Oxford University Press 2023. DOI: 10.1093/oso/9780192899477.003.0017

governments attempt to curb pollution, firms engage in corruptive practices and avoid environmental regulations (Biswas et al., 2012) to keep the costs low by offsetting them against wastewater treatment and public health. In line with the 'pollution haven' hypothesis, ineffective regulations and/or poor enforcement in these low- to middle-income countries is what makes them attractive to polluting industries that shift their bases out of heavily regulated high-income countries (Ederington et al., 2005; Tang, 2015).

Taking the example of India, the India Brand Equity Foundation (n.d.) has reported that the annual turnover of the pharmaceutical industry in India was estimated at around US$ 42 billion during 2020–2021 and is likely to grow threefold in the next decade. Further, in that period, India's drugs and pharmaceuticals exports stood at US$ 24.44 billion. One of the biggest beneficiaries of foreign direct investment, between 2000 and 2020, India received US$ 16.5 billion from foreign sources, giving credence to the pollution haven hypothesis above. With the focus on the financial incentive that drug manufacturing provides, there is no plan of regulating or abating drug manufacturing in India. According to the Indian government's Make in India initiative,[1] India plans to continue being known as the 'Pharmacy of the World' (Make in India, n.d.). Drug exports from India reach more than 200 countries globally, making it the fourth largest by volume and tenth largest in value. The Patancheru–Bollaram industrial belt in the Indian state of Telangana is one of the biggest pharmaceutical manufacturing hubs in India.

In 2007, Swedish professor Joakim Larsson, a leading scientist in this area, published the first in a series of papers that showed the link between high pharmaceutical emissions from drug manufacturers in the Patancheru–Bollaram region and the alarming increase in AMR. The findings of Professor Larsson's studies (discussed below) were followed up and corroborated by various other scientists.

To identify and address AMR arising from pharmaceutical manufacturing:

1. antibiotic discharges and sewage treatment processes have to be scientifically managed;
2. the re-use of wastewater, which is an economic necessity in countries like India, needs to be incentivized; and
3. monitoring systems testing antibiotics in water have to be developed.

Various causes including the lack of the finance and technology as well as issues around water pricing are impediments to address the problem from an economic perspective.

While regulatory mechanisms are in place on paper, they are ineffective in practice. There are various government bodies and functionaries involved in water and wastewater planning at all levels—national, state, and local municipalities. Some

---

[1] The Make in India initiative is a major national programme launched by the Government of India in September 2014 to enhance domestic production capacity, strengthen the manufacturing sector, and attract foreign investment.

municipalities handle all sewage-related issues directly, while others outsource different parts of the system, such as maintenance or design, building and operation. A study undertaken as late as in 2018 found that many municipalities were without strategic plans for the wastewater sector (Never and Stepping, 2018).

Metcalf et al. (2017) suggested that the reduction of water pollution from industries is dependent on both developing and enforcing regulations on wastewater quality. However, in countries such as India with poor implementation of laws, it is proposed that the enforcement of regulations is a distant idea. For example, despite a judicial order requiring the government to clean up water bodies and a national action plan on AMR (discussed below), there appears to be no difference on the ground—either in terms of wastewater treatment plants or reduction in effluent pollution. As a result, we are obliged to think beyond national laws and explore how the global supply chain may be regulated through a demand for cleaner drugs from those buying from Indian manufacturers (see Chapter 18 for a further discussion of procurement schemes as solution).

An example from India: The drug production industry in the Patancheru region and the failure of domestic systems to handle the pollution crisis

The industrial estates of Telangana, a state in the south of India (formerly part of Andhra Pradesh, until its separation in 2014), are a mega industrial hub hosting a sizeable proportion of India's pharmaceutical manufacturing and processing companies. The capital city of Telangana is Hyderabad, a major city, which emerged as the 'bulk drug capital of India', singlehandedly accounting for nearly a fifth of India's pharmaceutical exports (Indian Brand Equity Foundation, n.d.). At its outskirts, lies the Patancheru–Bollaram cluster—the subject of the study by Larsson mentioned above. This drug manufacturing hub has been identified by the Central Pollution Control Board of India (2010) as one of the most polluted areas in India. An early study by Shivkumar et al. (1997) found that the industrial estates in Patancheru and Bollaram together generated a cumulative 8 million litres of effluents which were being discharged without treatment into surrounding land, irrigation fields, and surface water bodies each day, gravely threatening human health and the environment. The accounts of the surrounding 60,000 acres covering around twenty-three water bodies and twenty-three inhabited villages have been nothing short of horrifying–murky waters, nauseating vapours, infertile and barren land, dying trees and cattle, and innumerable human diseases (Nordea, 2016; Pulla, 2017).

To remedy this, several citizens and non-governmental organizations (NGOs) took to the courts seeking the help of judiciary. The environmental litigation surrounding the Patancheru–Bollaram cluster has been the biggest and most significant on pollution from drug manufacturing in India. It has a prolonged and chequered history, spanning over twenty-five years and involving thirteen applications filed between 1989 and

2016 by 216 litigants including affected residents, environmental activists, and NGOs, before the Supreme Court, the High Court of Andhra Pradesh and the National Green Tribunal (NGT) of India.[2] While various interim orders and directions were issued by the courts in relation to the earlier applications, the situation in the Patancheru–Bollaram cluster kept worsening and the applications kept increasing. It was in this background that the thirteen applications were joined and heard altogether by the NGT (Southern Zone, Chennai), and a 350-page judgment delivered on 24 October 2017.

According to regulations, toxic waste including antibiotics from drug manufacturing, in Patancheru is first required to be treated at source by the industries, then transported in tankers to two common effluent treatment plants—Patancheru Enviro Tech Ltd (PETL) at Patancheru and Progressive Effluent Treatment Plant Ltd (PETPL) at Bollaram—for further treatment. The treated effluent is then transported through an 18-kilometre (km) pipeline to the sewage treatment plant (STP) in a suburb called Amberpet, where it mixes with domestic sewage as well as discharge from another plant containing pharmaceutical waste. On treatment, the blend is released into the Musi River, which is part of a larger river basin.

However, the NGT in its judgment noted that the regulations were not complied with. Some of the NGT's observations are as follows:

- Certain recalcitrant pharmaceutical manufacturers, against the directions of the courts and in violation of the law, had been sending untreated waste to the common plants. Since legal implementation is low, such breaches of law regularly go unnoticed.
- Shortly after their operations began, PETL and PETPL had come under public scrutiny for inadequate infrastructure. As per a news report by *Times of India* (2009, February), the prominent environmental activist and a litigant in the case, K. Purushottam Reddy, was quoted stating that the PETL did not have the technology to treat the hazardous waste and was an attempt to deflect public attention from the real dangers of environmental pollution from drug manufacturing.
- The 18-km pipeline carrying pharmaceutical effluents from PETL to the STP had been sanctioned by the Supreme Court after relying on an Environmental Impact Assessment (EIA). However, halfway during the construction of the pipeline, the EIA was found to be inadequate, but construction of the faulty pipeline could not be stopped mainly because of investment.

---

[2] Before the establishment of the NGT in 2010, the earlier applications were filed before either the Supreme Court or the Andhra Pradesh High Court as civil writ petitions. In Indian law, a writ is a formal order by a competent court directing a state organ to protect fundamental rights prescribed by the Constitution of India. Since all the applications dealt with issues closely related to the pollution caused by industries in the Patancheru-Bollaram cluster, those in the Supreme Court were transferred to the the Andhra Pradesh High Court to be jointly heard. On 12 February 2013, the Andhra Pradesh High Court transferred all these applications to the NGT (Southern Zone, Chennai). Since then, the NGT alone has handled the litigation in this matter. Given the complicated judicial history across the thirteen applications, this litigation is generally referred to simply as the 'Patancheru case'. However, it may be cited as *Kasala Malla Reddy & Ors. v State of Andhra Pradesh & Ors.*, National Green Tribunal (Southern Zone, Chennai), Application Nos 69–72, 82, 86–91 of 2013, and 190 & 192 of 2016 (24 October 2017).

It was in this background of an abject breakdown of regulation and legal implementation, that the NGT passed its voluminous judgment issuing directions to various government bodies. Whilst the judgment addressed various aspects of the pollution in the area, this chapter concentrates only on those which addressed AMR.

The link between AMR and the pharmaceutical sector

Larsson et al. (2007) had found that the concentrations in the effluent from a treatment plant receiving wastewater from about ninety manufacturing units were, for some pharmaceuticals, greater than those found in the blood of patients taking antibiotic medicines. The concentration of ciprofloxacin, which is a broad-spectrum antibiotic, was as high as 31 milligrams (mg) per litre, which is approximately 1 million times greater than the levels that are regularly found in treated municipal sewage effluents elsewhere in the world. The estimated total release of ciprofloxacin for one day was 44 kilograms, which is equivalent to Sweden's entire consumption over five days, or, expressed in another manner, sufficient to treat everyone in a city with 44,000 inhabitants.

In a follow-up study, Fick et al. (2009) further reported the presence of norfloxacin, cetrizine, terbinafine, citalopram, and enoxacin in water samples taken from Patancheru. More recently, Lubbert et al. (2017) reported antibiotic residues from twenty-eight environmental sampling sites in the sewers in the area. Further, tests of groundwater and surface water used for drinking and recreation revealed 100 per cent rate of *E. coli*, resistant to third-generation cephalosporin. Gothwal and Shashidhar (2017) compared samples from various points in the city, finding that the concentration of antibiotics steadily rose downstream and were highest at the inlet to the STP, indicating that neither individual treatment nor the PETL was effective in ridding the waters of antibiotics.

Apart from the manufacturing itself, a key finding by Fick et al. (2009) from testing samples of water from the PETL, was that the plant used 'activated sludge' containing approximately 20 per cent raw human faeces. The study notes that close contact between pathogens from faecal matter, resistant bacteria, and antibiotic pathogens facilitates the transfer of resistance to pathogens, resulting in increasing AMR and the incidence of 'superbugs'. Therefore, the treated effluent from PETL on introduction to domestic waste in the STP exacerbates the problem. Larsson et al. (2014) also surmises that bacteria in these environments are able to share or exchange genetic material which can also occur between different bacterial species and can spread through other mediums.

The NGT's addressing of the AMR issue

The Patancheru case is much older than many of these findings showing the link between drug manufacturing and AMR. Accordingly, this link was introduced much later in the litigation. When the evidence was presented to the NGT, the tribunal briefly recorded the findings of Professor Larsson's studies and flagged the arguments as an issue in need of deliberation but did not treat it as a key concern. This is important to note because there is a gap between scientific evidence and establishing legal causation that AMR is caused because of improper drug manufacturing. The NGT acknowledged that AMR was a problem but did not attribute drug manufacturing as the cause of it.

At the very least, the studies conducted by the former scientists suggested two things:

- that neither industries nor the PETL are effective in eliminating antibiotics from the water, since almost all samples including those at the inlet of the STP showed concentrations of antibiotics and drug-resistant pathogens, and
- that the mechanism of mixing pharmaceutical waste with domestic waste exacerbates AMR.

The NGT's judgment attempted no deliberation or analysis on the implications of these aspects, and simply rested at a decision that the causal link between drug-resistant pathogens in the water samples and pharmaceutical effluent is not conclusive. In this breath, the tribunal merely called on the government's duty to 'rule out' AMR and directed the state government to constitute an expert committee to conduct an epidemiological and genetic study and survey in the region and address whether the activities of the pharmaceutical industries have led to AMR and, if so, enlist the health consequences and suggest remedial measures.

Two years on, the expert committee appointed pursuant to the NGT's directions themselves heavily relied on the same studies that were presented before the NGT. The committee confirmed that drug-resistant bacteria were indeed present in the waterbodies in the Patancheru–Bollaram belt, calling AMR an 'imminent public health disaster, waiting to happen' (Kapur, 2019). All ninety bacterial strains isolated from fifty-four water samples were found to be resistant to at least four and at maximum thirteen of the antibiotics they were tested against. However, the report itself is underanalysed and presents no suggestions apart from regular water quality monitoring.

The case is currently dormant and there is no change on ground.

Domestic regulation of AMR in countries with economic incentives for clean drug manufacturing (or the lack thereof)

A report by Nordea Asset Management (2016) that shone light on the Patancheru case bringing it to global spotlight stated that '[i]t is felt that the Government intends to continue to pursue a pro-industry line regardless of human, social or environmental costs, and will turn a blind eye to the manipulation or overriding of regulatory legislation by industry, in the service of profit-driven production'.

Countries like India are a long way from being able to address the problems of pharmaceutical waste, let alone the nuanced implications and causal links to AMR. The NGT's own expert committee observed that the high costs associated with regular monitoring of antimicrobial levels in pharmaceutical wastewater makes it a low-priority objective for India, and potentially 'AMR-rich' municipal wastewater is finally discharged into the nearby water bodies (Kapur, 2019).

The National Action Plan on Antimicrobial Resistance (NAP) by the Ministry of Health and Family Welfare of India (2017) comprehensively outlines the priorities and implementation strategies for curbing AMR in India (see Chapter 16 for a further analysis of the Indian NAP). The NAP covers all five major objectives of the WHO's 2015 Global Action Plan (GAP) on AMR, adding an additional objective to strengthen India's AMR leadership. While the NAP predominantly deals with AMR from sources other than the pharmaceutical manufacturing process, it does call on authorities to establish the surveillance of antimicrobial residues in pharmaceutical waste and develop standards for antibiotic residues in industrial effluents.

Following from the NAP, in January 2020, the Indian Ministry of Environment, Forests and Climate Change, published a draft on environmental standards for the pharmaceutical manufacturing industry, limiting the concentration of 121 antibiotics in bulk drug manufacturing effluents. This draft was welcomed and praised by both environmental activists and health experts. However, no less than seven months later, the newly notified draft rules titled 'Environment (Protection) Second Amendment Rules, 2021' no longer mention antibiotic pollution and has omitted all the previously prescribed limits.

This makes it apparent that when it comes to the teeth of AMR regulation—case law and precedents as well as the law itself, India does not acknowledge AMR in a way drug manufacturing may be regulated. It is therefore safe to conclude that domestic systems, at least in India, cannot be strongly relied on for tackling the growing AMR issue.

Industry and international initiatives on AMR: Effective or merely ornamental?

In the lack of legal responses to addressing AMR from pharmaceutical pollution, can the industry regulate itself? Are there any differences in industry standards in developing countries and developed ones?

In India, when confronted with the findings that the pharmaceutical industry is responsible for AMR, the executive director of the Bulk Drug Manufacturers Association of India (BDMAI) responded that these were 'doubtful', suggesting that it was suspicious that most studies were from foreign countries, and would have to be locally verified (Pulla, 2017). The BDMAI had gone to the extent of publishing a contradicting report that showed no difference in the numbers of drug-resistance bacteria near the industrial units. Industry associations of international pharmaceutical companies, however, tell a different story.

Industry initiatives in addressing AMR from pharmaceuticals

1. The AMR Industry Alliance

In January 2016, over 100 biotech, diagnostic, generic, and research-based pharmaceutical companies signed the Davos Declaration welcoming global action and political focus on AMR, forming the AMR Industry Alliance. In an industry roadmap published by the AMR Industry Alliance (2016), the pharmaceutical industry recognized their responsibility in the battle against AMR and undertook to review their manufacturing and supply chains to assess good practices in controlling releases of antibiotics into the environment under a common framework. As per the latest progress report by AMR Industry Alliance (2020), 56 per cent of products made at member-owned sites are expected to be made in accordance with discharge targets within the next three years and 88 per cent within the next seven years, whereas 24 per cent of products made at supplier sites are expected to be made in accordance with discharge targets within three years and a further 70 per cent of products made at supplier sites are expected to be made in accordance with these targets within four to seven years.

2. The Pharmaceutical Supply Chain Initiative

The Pharmaceutical Supply Chain Initiative (PSCI) is a not-for-profit association of pharmaceutical and healthcare companies to collectively define, establish and promote responsible supply chain practices and environmental sustainability. The PSCI regularly issues Principles for Responsible Supply Chain Management to provide a framework for self-regulation by members. PSCI's membership includes major pharmaceutical and healthcare companies from across the globe. Many of the suppliers to the major companies are based in Patancheru and have been named in the Nordea report mentioned above.

The principles in PSCI (2019) require suppliers to operate in an environmentally responsible and efficient manner to minimize adverse impacts on the environment. This includes the management, control and treatment of API before their release into the environment. They also call for sustainable sourcing and traceability within the supply chain. An implementation guide by PSCI (2015) lays down guidelines including periodic compliance audits, allocation of necessary finances for waste management, whistleblower mechanisms, systems to report violations or exceptions, and internal accountability.

However, because voluntary frameworks are non-binding and cannot be challenged or enforced, it is difficult to use the PSCI and the AMR Industry Alliance to solicit change on the ground in India. A review by Tamimi and Sebastianelli (2017) of environmental, social and governance scores on disclosures by the biggest 500 companies showed that the lowest levels of disclosures pertained to environmental safeguards. Releasing effluents directly in waterbodies is an environmental risk. Because of the nature of the risk and existing data which puts environmental disclosures last, there is a gap between AMR-related declarations by industry and the actual setting up of/investment in wastewater systems where AMR pollution occurs.

Exploring international frameworks for addressing AMR

1. World Health Organization
The WHO (2016) guide on good trade and distribution practices for pharmaceutical starting materials has established key pharmaceutical good manufacturing practices (GMP) requirements. They start at the beginning with quality management, providing a clearly documented procedure for approving suppliers of pharmaceutical starting materials and services. They go on to regulate all involved processes including possession, repacking, relabelling, distribution, or storage of APIs or API intermediates. It attempts to attribute responsibility to all parties involved in the manufacture and supply chain to ensure the quality and safety of the materials and products, as well as proper and safe storage of waste materials awaiting disposal. While the principle of GMP could be applied to the 18-km pipeline carrying toxic materials in Patancheru, the lack of whistleblowing provisions and a reticence from Indian manufacturers make the GMP Guidelines difficult to enforce extra-judicially in India. Additionally, the guidelines do not separately address AMR as one of the issues from drug manufacturing.

2. The EU REACH
The EU REACH regulation[3] aims to protect human health and the environment from risks from chemicals (European Chemicals Agency, n.d). REACH applies to all EU companies that deal in chemical substances. Therefore, although the REACH does not specifically address the pharmaceutical industry in India, it covers pharmaceutical companies that manufacture and market within the EU. Notably, the REACH cannot be enforced on companies outside the EU, even if they export to the EU.

In principle, pharmaceutical importers based in the EU have mandatory obligations under REACH to identify and manage the risks and register products and processes. Importers are required to provide relevant information on their supply chains in safety data sheet and exposure scenarios, and obtain compliance proof from their suppliers. While this assists in promoting transparency in the supply chain and disclosing suppliers, the REACH focuses on the risk for human health and environment posed by the chemical substance itself. It does not address the impact of environmentally

---

[3] REACH stands for Registration, Evaluation, Authorization, and Restriction of Chemicals.

unsustainable manufacturing process that do not affect the EU. Therefore, the REACH too falls short in regulating AMR contamination outside of the EU.

While industry and international attempts at reducing AMR from manufacturing are noteworthy, there is no accountability or liability (because of the nature of these frameworks), and there is no manner of determining whether there is compliance on the ground. The AMR Industry Alliance itself includes many companies that have manufacturing units in Patancheru whose effluents were part of the studies mentioned above and named in the Nordea report (2016). Yet, they continue to be part of the alliance.

A report by the European Parliamenthas shown that voluntary, self-regulation is not enough (Zamfir, 2020). This report relies on various studies to highlight that most companies do not voluntarily undertake human rights and environment due diligence (Faracik, 2017). In March 2021, the European Parliament backed a legislative initiative paving the way for a new EU directive on Corporate Due Diligence and Corporate Accountability. As part of this initiative, lawmakers called for the urgent adoption of an EU-wide regulation that will require companies to identify, address, and remedy the environmental, social, and governance (ESG) risks in their supply chains. A new law is expected to follow in the coming months, whilst Germany already has come up with a new law that will apply to pharmaceutical companies as well.

Regulating the supply chain: A possible solution?

Having found that domestic systems are ineffective and unreliable, and industry and international initiatives are inadequate, the authors propose a supply chain-focused regulatory framework to address the problem. Such a framework has been in progress in several parts of the world. These laws attempt to regulate the entire supply chain in order to mitigate environmental and social risks involved in the manufacture and global trade of goods. Examples of these initiatives in Europe are the EU Conflict Minerals Regulation, the EU Timber Trade Regulation, the CSR Directive and its planned adaptations, the EU Taxonomy Regulation, the EU Guidance on Due Diligence for EU businesses to address the risk of forced labour in their operations and supply chains and, as mentioned above, the planned EU Directive for a European Supply Chain Act. In national levels, there have been regulatory attempts in supply chain regulation such as the UK Modern Slavery Act, the French *Loi de Vigilance*, and the Dutch Child Labour Due Diligence Act.

While these legislations mostly address human rights violations along supply chains, Germany has announced a new law addressing both human rights as well as environmental violations in supply chains. The *Lieferketten-Gesetz*, commonly known as the German Supply Chain Law, comes into force from 2023 and imposes due diligence obligations on companies covering both direct and indirect suppliers. The law is foreseen to govern manufacturing practices in countries other than Germany—such as factories manufacturing pharmaceuticals in India. To this end, big pharmaceutical MNCs will be required to identify and eliminate risk anywhere in the supply chain. What makes this new law cutting-edge is the whistleblower provision. Companies are obligated to introduce or extend whistleblower systems so that citizens and NGOs are able to report violations (particularly in manufacturing sites).[4]

This law shines light on a new possible pathway to securing environmental justice for the river basin and communities in Patancheru from Germany.

1. The supply chain approach could force German buyers to go beyond standard disclosures because of the fear of penalties in Germany for sourcing drugs with adverse environmental impacts. If there is a pressure from buyers, Indian drug manufacturers might have to invest in functioning wastewater systems. Because domestic regulation is ineffective, drug manufacturers were getting away with releasing effluents in the environment. By including environmental risk, the German Supply Chain Act could potentially change the situation on the ground.

2. Pharmaceutical companies in Germany now have a legal obligation to ensure that all levels of their supply chain are 'clean'. The whistleblower provisions allow anyone to report environmental damage. This makes it relatively easier for citizens and NGOs to report manufacturers that are not adequately treating their waste. If the board of a pharmaceutical company has knowledge of such an environmental damage, they have to demonstrate mitigation of the problem as per the law. This will encourage buyers in Europe to impose stricter rules on their suppliers from India.

3. The threat of the loss of their buyers from Germany and other European countries could work towards enforcing compliance on industries in India and other manufacturing countries following a top-down approach.

Regulatory requirements for manufacturing sites and emission control worldwide vary from being non-existent to the application of high standards. Where they exist, environmental permits are provided and controlled by individual countries or states, again with vast differences in requirements and enforcement. A supply chain approach harmonizes the differences in requirements to a certain extent. The production and supply chain for antibiotics often involves several steps and actors in different parts of the world, providing challenges for the end producer, and to an even larger extent the consumer, to gain insight into and influence over the degree of environmental pollution control in the early, most critical steps of production of APIs (Topp et al., 2018). It is important to note that activists and litigators who are trying to address this issue are not anti-industry. The requirement is that manufacturing units install working wastewater treatment systems so that effluents are not discharged in the environment. The actors working in different parts of the water-wastewater chain, policy-makers as well as the

---

[4] The law is in German and an English translation is not available yet. However, for details, please see <https://www.dentons.com/en/insights/articles/2021/august/5/setting-your-2022-compliance-goals-supply-chain>. Accessed 23 October 2021.

consumers of water, have a certain mindset, management capacities, skills and personal preferences which either perpetuate or help to disrupt existing wastewater systems. India is generally geared towards conventional, centralized wastewater systems, largely disregarding energy efficiency and re-use options (Never and Stepping, 2018) which is an added hindrance to incentivizing wastewater treatment.

Conclusion

Domestic systems have thus far not been able to resolve the abatement of polluting pharmaceutical industries discharging APIs directly into the environment. This is a combination of a variety of factors—the lack of clear regulations, problems with law enforcement, ineffectiveness of local litigation as evidenced by the Patancheru case, and a lack of economic incentives, particularly around wastewater re-use. Furthermore, existing voluntary industry frameworks and endeavours by international organizations have also stopped short in treating the issue on the ground primarily because of difficulties in the enforcement of the measures as well reluctance by the industry to correct itself to keep prices of medicines down. In this backdrop, the AMR problem due to drug manufacturing is only on the rise. Another pharmaceutical manufacturing area— the Baddi industrial hub in North India has emerged as the next Patancheru with evidence of AMR because of improper drug manufacturing (Bisht, 2021).

In that light, it is suggested that applying a supply chain-based regulatory framework which binds manufacturers and retailers to the lifecycle of a pharmaceutical product could be an effective solution to treat effluents adequately in the path towards AMR mitigation.

References

AMR Industry Alliance. (2016). *Industry Roadmap for Progress on Combating Antimicrobial Resistance.* <https://www.amrindustryalliance.org/wp-content/uploads/2017/12/AMR-Industry-Declaration.pdf>.

AMR Industry Alliance. (n.d.). *AMR Industry Alliance Members.* <https://www.amrindustryalliance.org/report-members/>. Accessed 27 October 2021.

Arnum, P. (2013). 'The Weaknesses and Strengths of the Global API Market', *Pharmaceutical Technology Sourcing and Management*, 9/3. <https://www.pharmtech.com/view/weaknesses-and-strengths-global-api-market>.

Bisht, G. (2021, 24 May). 'Antibiotic pollution in Sirsa river flowing through Baddi pharma hub', *Hindustan Times*. <https://www.hindustantimes.com/cities/chandigarh-news/antibiotic-pollution-in-sirsa-river-flowing-through-baddi-pharma-hub-101621851789448.html>.

Biswas, A., Farzanegan, M., and Thum, M. (2012). 'Pollution, Shadow Economy and Corruption: Theory and Evidence', *Ecological Economics*, 75, 114–25.

Central Pollution Control Board. (2010). *Final Action Plan for Improvement of Environmental Parameters in Critically Polluted Areas of 'Patancheru-Bollaram Cluster' Andhra Pradesh.* <https://cpcb.nic.in/displaypdf.php?id=UGF0YW5jaGVydS1Cb2xsYXJhbS5wZGY>.

Ederington, J., Levinson, A., and Minier, J. (2005). 'Footloose and Pollution-free', *Review of Economics and Statistics*, 87, 92–9.

European Chemicals Agency. (n.d.). 'About the REACH Regulation'. <https://echa.europa.eu/docume nts/10162/22372335/reach_clp_tips_reach_regulation_en.pdf/e095595e-b986-4af3-aeb7-e670f 26e1f0c>.

Faracik, B. (2017). Implementation of the UN Guiding Principles on Business and Human Rights. European Parliament. <https://www.europarl.europa.eu/RegData/etudes/STUD/2017/578031/ EXPO_STU(2017)578031_EN.pdf>

Fick, J. et al. (2009). 'Contamination of Surface, Ground, and Drinking Water from Pharmaceutical Production', *Environmental Toxicology and Chemistry*, 28(12), 2522–7.

Fouz, N. et al. (2020). 'The Contribution of Wastewater to the Transmission of Antimicrobial Resistance in the Environment: Implications of Mass Gathering Settings', *Tropical Medicine and Infectious Disease*, 5/1, 33. <https://doi.org/10.3390/tropicalmed5010033>.

Gandra, S. et al. (2017). 'Scoping Report on Antimicrobial Resistance in India', *Center for Disease Dynamics, Economics & Policy*. <https://cddep.org/wp-content/uploads/2017/11/AMR-INDIA-SCOPING-REPORT.pdf>.

Gothwal, R., and Shashidhar, T. (2017). 'Occurrence of High Levels of Fluoroquinolones in Aquatic Environment Due to Effluent Discharges from Bulk Drug Manufacturers', *Journal of Hazardous, Toxic, and Radioactive Waste*, 21/3. <https://doi.org/10.1061/(ASCE)HZ.2153-5515.0000346>.

India Brand Equity Foundation. (n.d.). *Snapshot: About Telangana State*. <https://www.ibef.org/sta tes/telangana.aspx> accessed 27 October 2021.

India Brand Equity Foundation. (n.d.). *Snapshot: Indian Pharmaceuticals Report*. <https://www.ibef. org/industry/pharmaceutical-india.aspx> accessed 27 October 2021.

Kapur, S. (2019). *Guidelines for Monitoring of River Hygiene. Central Pollution Control Board*. <https:// cpcb.nic.in/wqm/Draft_Guidelines_Monitoring_of_River_Hygiene.pdf>.

Kotwani, A., Joshi, J., and Kaloni, D. (2021). 'Pharmaceutical Effluent: A Critical Link in the Interconnected Ecosystem Promoting Antimicrobial Resistance', *Environmental Science Pollution Research*, 28, 32111–2124.

Larsson, D. (2014). 'Pollution from Drug Manufacturing: Review and Perspectives', *Philosophical Transactions of the Royal Society of London, B: Biological Sciences*, 369. <https://doi.org/10.1098/ rstb.2013.0571>.

Larsson, D., de Pedro, C., and Paxeus, N. (2007). 'Effluent from Drug Manufactures Contains Extremely High Levels of Pharmaceuticals', *Journal for Hazardous Material*, 148, 751–5. <doi:http:// dx.doi.org/10.1016/j.jhazmat.2007.07.008>.

Lübbert, C., Baars, C., Dayakar, A., Lippmann, N., Rodloff, A. C., Kinzig, M., and Sörgel, F. (2017). 'Environmental Pollution with Antimicrobial Agents from Bulk Drug Manufacturing Industries in Hyderabad, South India, is Associated with Dissemination of Extended-spectrum Beta-lactamase and Carbapenemase-producing Pathogens', *Infection*, 45/4, 479–91.

Make in India. (n.d.). *Sector Highlights: Pharmaceuticals*. <https://www.makeinindia.com/sector-hig hlights-pharmaceuticals> accessed 27 October 2021.

Ministry of Health and Family Welfare of India. (2017). *National Action Plan on Antimicrobial Resistance (NAP-AMR) 2017–2021*. <https://cdn.who.int/media/docs/default-source/antimicrob ial-resistance/amr-spc-npm/nap-library/national-action-plan-on-amr-(india).pdf?sfvrsn=9f3 96e90_1&download=true>.

Nahar, S. (2020). *Understanding How the Indian Pharmaceutical Industry Works—Part 2*. <https:// www.alphainvesco.com/blog/understanding-how-the-indian-pharmaceutical-industry-works-part-2/>.

Navadhi Market Research. (2019). *Global Pharmaceuticals Industry Analysis and Trends 2023*. (Publication ID: NAV0319001)

Never, B., and Stepping, K. (2018). 'Comparing Urban Wastewater Systems in India and Brazil: Options for Energy Efficiency and Wastewater Reuse', *Water Policy*, 20/6, 1129–44.

Nordea Asset Management. (2016). *Impact of Pharmaceutical Pollution on Communities and Environment in India*. <https://www.nordea.com/en/doc/impacts-of-pharmaceutical-pollution-on-communities-and-environment-in-india.pdf>.

Pharmaceutical Supply Chain Initiative. (2015). Pharmaceutical Industry Principles for Responsible Supply Chain Management. <https://pscinitiative.org/resource?resource=2>.

Pharmaceutical Supply Chain Initiative. (2019). *The PSCI Principles for Responsible Supply Chain Management*. <https://pscinitiative.org/resource?resource=1>.

Pulla, P. (2017, 18 November). 'The superbugs of Hyderabad', *The Hindu*. <https://www.thehindu.com/opinion/op-ed/the-superbugs-of-hyderabad/article20536685.ece>.

Schefold, C., and Haas, G. (2021). *The new German Supply Chain Act – also a challenge for foreign operations in Germany*. Dentons. <https://www.dentons.com/en/insights/articles/2021/august/5/setting-your-2022-compliance-goals-supply-chain>.

Shivkumar, K., Pande, A., and Biksham, G. (1997). 'Toxic Trace Element Pollution in Ground Waters around Patancheru and Bollaram Industrial areas, Andhra Pradesh, India: A Graphical Approach', *Environmental Monitoring and Assessment*, 24/1, 57–80.

Tamimi, N., and Sebastianelli, R. (2017). 'Transparency among S&P 500 Companies: An Analysis of ESG Disclosure Scores', *Management Decision*, 55/8, 1660–80.

Tang, J. (2015). 'Testing the Pollution Haven Effect: Does the Type of FDI Matter?', *Environmental and Resource Economics*, 60/4. <https://doi.org/10.1007/s10640-014-9779-7>.

Times of India. (2009, 3 February). 'Pantancheru effluent treatment plant a fraud', *Times of India*. <https://timesofindia.indiatimes.com/city/hyderabad/pantancheru-effluent-treatment-plant-a-fraud/articleshow/4067197.cms>.

Topp, E. et al. (2018). 'Antimicrobial Resistance and the Environment: Assessment of Advances, Gaps and Recommendations for Agriculture, Aquaculture and Pharmaceutical Manufacturing', *FEMS Microbiology Ecology*, 94/3, 3.

World Health Organization. (2015). *Global Action Plan on Antimicrobial Resistance*. World Health Organization. <https://www.amcra.be/swfiles/files/WHO%20actieplan_90.pdf>

Zamfir, I. (2020). Towards a Mandatory EU System of Due Diligence for Supply Chains. European Parliament. <https://www.europarl.europa.eu/RegData/etudes/BRIE/2020/659299/EPRS_BRI(2020)659299_EN.pdf>.

18

Sustainable Procurement of Pharmaceuticals

A Tool to Combat Global Antimicrobial Resistance

Katerina Mitkidis

Introduction

The progress in treatment of infections has been astonishing. The production of life-saving treatments though ironically also accelerates the spread of antimicrobial resistance (AMR), as manufacturing effluents carry active pharmaceutical ingredients (APIs) in high concentration into the environment where antimicrobial-resistant bacteria are then formed. This can compromise our future ability to treat diseases nowadays considered minor (Marschang, 2017). The World Health Organization (WHO) lists AMR among the ten most severe threats to humans in the immediate future (WHO, 2020). Nowadays, AMR causes around 33,000 deaths in the European Union (EU) per year (Cassini et al., 2019) and this number is estimated to rise exponentially to almost 400,000 by 2050 (European Commission, 2017a). The detrimental effect of AMR can be lowered by effective governance and regulation. As law, which is jurisdictionally limited, provides insufficient help in governing transnational supply chains, governance by contract presents a possible part of the solution. 'Governance by contract' is understood here as the use of the contract and procurement process in general where discreet transactions impact interests beyond those of the contractual parties (Grundmann et al., 2015).[1]

This chapter first presents the need for governance by contract in the AMR context. Then, taking the EU law as its starting point, it reviews recent EU initiatives that seek to use public procurement processes to combat AMR. The EU has been one of the frontrunners both in pharmaceutical consumption as well as addressing the pharmaceuticals in the environment (PiE) problem. The EU thus presents a good example to study here as it has a high potential of influencing actions outside its borders through its market power and regulatory authority. After reviewing the legal and policy framework, the chapter presents lessons from private responsible procurement before turning to the possibility of mutual learning between public and private sustainable procurement practices. The chapter concludes with reviewing policy implications for the use of contractual governance to contain AMR.

---

[1] The use of procurement processes thus encompasses here what is known as 'contractual governance'.

Katerina Mitkidis, *Sustainable Procurement of Pharmaceuticals* In: *Steering against Superbugs*. Edited by:
Olivier Rubin, Erik Baekkeskov, and Louise Munkholm, Oxford University Press. © Oxford University Press 2023.
DOI: 10.1093/oso/9780192899477.003.0018

The need for governance by contract in the AMR context

AMR is mostly discussed as a by-product of antibiotics' consumption (Polianciuc et al., 2020). Indeed, approximately 40–90 per cent of administered active pharmaceutical ingredients (APIs) is excreted in an active form and eventually reaches the environment (Polianciuc et al., 2020: 231). APIs enter the environment through other routes too, namely in connection to manufacturing and as end-of-life waste (AMR Industry Alliance, 2019; Mitkidis et al., 2018). It is the manufacturing effluents that are responsible for releases of APIs in the highest concentrations (Larsson, 2014|: 2), thus posing the highest immediate danger to the natural environment (Larsson et al., 2007), yet the scope of the AMR-related threats of pharmaceutical manufacturing effluents has been recognized only slowly. One of the reasons is that manufacturing takes mainly place in developing countries (see Chapter 2), where monitoring of environmentally detrimental effluents has not been in focus. China and India are of particular concern, as China produces 80–90 per cent of antibiotic APIs and India is the world leader in producing finished antibiotics (SumOfUs, 2015; see also Chapter 17).

While we have known about the problem for a long time now, the regulation of pharmaceutical manufacturing remains at the outskirts of AMR action. This might seem natural, as prescribing, implementing, and monitoring of stricter environmental standards within manufacturing processes require extraterritorial regulation, and cooperation among stakeholders in complex and transnational supply chains. Extraterritorial regulation, that is the regulation adopted in one jurisdiction with the aim to influence the behaviour of subjects in another, is needed as the level of environmental protection differs and is often weaker in developing countries. Therefore, jurisdictions with stricter standards, such as the EU, strive to extend their standards to countries where they source from (European Commission, 2019: 8). Cooperation for environmental protection through transnational supply chains is then difficult due to varying cultural, social, and legal norms. When it comes to the access to treatment, the tragedy of the commons is intense, thus making the pharmaceutical industry particularly difficult to regulate. Access to treatment by an individual in need is of utmost importance and, in fact, became a norm in the developed part of the World (Stevens and Huys, 2017). But access should not tilt to overuse and thus unnecessary pollution, as it has largely happened in the developed parts of the world (European Centre for Disease Prevention and Control, 2021).

Overcoming the complexities of extraterritorial regulation combined with the necessary coordination of transnational supply chains crossing countries with varying environmental regulation and the level of access to medicines is difficult, but it is not unsurmountable (Schaaf, 2020). In this chapter, I propose that the coordination of and mutual reinforcement among public and private procurement present an unused possibility for availing contractual governance to fight global AMR. Procurement is a tool that is recognized within policies on AMR but it has seldom been researched, despite governance by contract being extensively researched in the context of transnational supply chains' sustainability in general.

Missing drivers for sustainable procurement in the pharmaceutical industry

Procurement processes have been widely used to drive the sustainability agenda both in the private and public spheres (Andrecka and Mitkidis, 2017). This chapter focuses on their use to control pharmaceutical industrial discharges, leaving aside other sustainability areas.

Responding to the lack of hard internationally applicable laws in respect to environmental protection and/or the lack of enforcement of the existing ones, private parties resorted to the use of governance by contract to fill this regulatory vacuum. The inclusion of sustainability criteria into business contracts has become a widespread practice (EcoVadis and Affectio Mutandi, 2018: 13). The idea is that by regulating their suppliers' environmental performance through procurement processes and chains of contracts, companies can avoid negative publicity on unethical behaviours in their supply chains and to build their reputation as environmentally responsible entities. Ultimately, these efforts would turn into long-term business and financial benefits as well as contribute to the global sustainability. This win-win situation has been coined as the business case of corporate social responsibility (Kurucz et al., 2008).

The fear of negative publicity and following loss of consumers meant that close-to-consumer markets have been most keen on adopting sustainability into their business strategy and throughout their supply chains (Haddock-Fraser and Fraser, 2008). While pharmaceutical companies produce and sell products used and consumed by consumers, they are not a typical close-to-consumer industry, such as for example the food industry. The reason is that when it comes to prescription-only medicines it is not the consumer but a healthcare professional who decides, which treatment the consumer buys. Moreover, even in respect to over-the-counter medicines, although consumers who take environmental protection into consideration when buying other products, such as food or cosmetics, rarely question environmental responsibility of the processes through which their medicine is manufactured (Schaaf, 2020). Instead, it is the therapeutic effect that drives the buying decisions. There is thus a missing incentive for pharmaceutical companies to engage with their supply chains' environmental sustainability. This has also led pharmaceutical companies to focus instead on sustainability issues directly impacting their reputation, such as bribery and access to medicines questions (see e.g., Lee and Kohler, 2010; Leisinger, 2005). The gap of missing incentives can be filled by the demands of the public buyers, buying for hospitals and other healthcare providers. If public buyers require pharmaceutical companies to adhere to high environmental standards during manufacturing, pharmaceutical companies may intensify already existing influence over their suppliers in this respect. I posit that in this way public and private procurement can reinforce each other's efforts to protect the environment and fight global AMR.

Regulation of sustainable public procurement in the EU

In 2014, the Public Procurement Directive (Directive 2014/24/EU) introduced new options for sustainable procurement in the EU. Most importantly, it made clear that sustainability considerations in public procurement are supported (Andhov et al., 2020: 5; Directive 2014/24/EU, recital 91)[2] and can be implemented in all stages of the procurement process: pre-tender stage, competitive tender, contract's execution, and contract implementation (Andrecka and Mitkidis, 2017: 69). The first two stages—pre-tender and tender phases—have progressed significantly further in encompassing sustainability criteria.

Even though the Public Procurement Directive provides the space for sustainable public procurement, the use of sustainability criteria in practice remains limited. As of 2017, most public procurement contracts were still awarded based on the lowest price criteria (in 55 per cent of procurement procedures the lowest price was applied as the award criterion) (European Commission, 2017b: 5). This is also true when it comes to medicines, where public healthcare providers are under the pressure to lower costs (Medicines for Europe, 2021: 4; VIVE et al., 2018: 19).

One reason is that most of the sustainability-related provisions in the Public Procurement Directive are of facilitative rather than mandatory nature. Yet, there is one provision that mandates public authorities to reflect on sustainability performance of economic operators (Andrecka and Mitkidis, 2017: 71). Namely, Article 69(3) requires the contracting public authorities to 'reject the tender, where they have established that the tender is abnormally low because it does not comply with applicable obligations referred to in Article 18(2)'. These include obligations imposed by applicable environmental law, for example concerning wastewater treatment in manufacturing facilities.

While the Public Procurement Directive theoretically allows for sustainability to be considered in public procurement, it contains one aspect raising doubts about the legality of the use of sustainability criteria within the procurement processes: the requirement of the 'link to the subject-matter' of the contract (L2SM) (Directive 2014/24/EU, Articles 42, 43, 67(3), and 70). This requirement was developed through case law of the Court of Justice of the EU (Case C-513/99; Case C-368/) in order to prevent public authorities to demand on procurement participants general sustainability requirements, such as the existence of a corporate environmental policy, without a clear connection to the procured goods or services (Semple, 2015). While the L2SM requirement aims to inhibit the use of sustainability criteria for the purpose of hidden unequal

---

[2] See Directive 2014/24/EU, recital 91: The Public Procurement Directive 'clarifies how the contracting authorities can contribute to the protection of the environment and the promotion of sustainable development while ensuring that they can obtain the best value for money for their contracts'.

treatment and discrimination, the exact meaning of the requirement is poorly defined. This may discourage public authorities from engaging with sustainability (Andhov et al., 2020: 38). For example, it might be difficult (although not always impossible) to argue that the requirement of having a high-quality wastewater treatment facility at the manufacturer's site in a developing country is linked to the subject matter, for instance a specific antibiotic, of a sourcing agreement with a hospital in a developed country.

The European One Health Action Plan against AMR of 2017 called for addressing better the role of the environment in AMR (European Commission, 2017c). The Committee on Antimicrobial Resistance of the European Health Parliament, a movement that provides input to the European Commission regarding health issues in Europe, and others then suggested that a broader use of green public procurement could create a competitive environment among pharmaceutical manufacturers leading towards eco-innovation in drug manufacturing (Committee on Antimicrobial Resistance, 2018: 10; Guiu Segura et al., 2019). The leading idea in the suggestion of the Committee on Antimicrobial Resistance was that in case of two medicines with an equivalent therapeutic effect, a preference should be given to the one that is more environmentally friendly. What this meant though was not specified. Especially, the economic aspects were not addressed; how should public procurers proceed if one antibiotic is more environmentally friendly, but more expensive? At other occasion, the European Health Parliament also suggested that 'EU Member States should expand the use of green public procurement of antibiotics to promote a "race to the top" in terms of sustainability' (Committee on Antimicrobial Resistance, 2018: para 8). The long-awaited EU Strategic Approach to PiE then restated the importance of promoting greener manufacturing through public procurement policy (European Commission, 2019: 8–9). The EU has reinforced its position towards this issue also in the latest Pharmaceutical Strategy for Europe, where public procurement is considered a flagship initiative for developing novel antimicrobials (European Commission, 2020: 5). During negotiating and preparation of the strategy, a group of organizations signed a joint position paper demanding, among others, that the EU 'promote[s] and improve[s] green public procurement policies to increase demand for more sustainable production of medicines and the development of pharmaceuticals that are less harmful for the environment' (JPPPSE, 2020: 9). One of the signatories of the joint position paper was a non-profit network (Health Care Without Harm (HCWH)) that earlier called on the EU to step up the fight against AMR by leveraging its purchasing power to address pharmaceutical pollution from pharmaceutical manufacturing (HCWH, 2019: 6–7).

In summary, while the EU can be considered a frontrunner in the area of sustainable public procurement regulation, its use remains limited. The untapped potential of sustainable public procurement has then been called upon in recent years to help solve the growing global AMR threat.

Sustainable procurement in the private sector

Procurement practices, including supply chain contracts, have been extensively used by private actors for about two decades now to drive environmental sustainability agenda throughout transnational supply chains (see e.g., Affolder, 2018; Cafaggi, 2016; EcoVadis and Affectio Mutandi, 2018: 19). Best practice has developed, encompassing inclusion of sustainability criteria in suppliers' selection, contract negotiation, the text of contract, and contract execution. Yet, the last two are mostly used to cover the sustainability topics. The Pharmaceutical Supply Chain Initiative (PSCI) is an example of an industrial collaboration engaging with sustainable procurement. The PSCI Principles for Responsible Supply Chain Management (PSCI Principles, 2019), which are included in supply chain contracts by the Initiative's members, cover manufacturing discharges of pharmaceuticals into the environment. They require that '[a]ny waste, wastewater or emissions with the potential to adversely impact human or environmental health shall be appropriately managed, controlled and treated prior to release into the environment' (PSCI Principles, 2019: 7).

While the practice of engaging pharmaceutical suppliers with production-related environmental issues exists in the private sphere, several challenges remain. Those include vagueness in stipulating suppliers' obligations, insufficient enforcement of environmental provisions in supply chain contracts, a lack of motivation for deeper engagement of both buyers and suppliers with sustainability issues, and, not least, an absence of the AMR agenda from supply chain policy instruments.

Imprecise language when communicating sustainability requirements to suppliers throughout procurement documents (including contracts, codes of conduct, and corporate and procurement policies) has long been criticized (Mitkidis, 2015: chapters 7.2.4 and 8.2). Taking the PSCI Principles as an example, on the one hand, they do not provide concrete implementation guidelines for suppliers, who sincerely want to comply with the requirement. For example, how is the potential adverse effect of APIs' release to be established? Are only intentional discharges covered and what does it mean 'appropriately' in this context? Should any adverse effect be avoided or is a hazard of AMR also considered? On the other hand, the PSCI Principles allow for flexible compliance of suppliers that do not intend to follow the requirements' spirit (Deva, 2006: 129). And yet, there is also a range of reasons for keeping the requirements flexible (Peterkova, 2014), an important one being the main purpose of the requirement: do we want to motivate a change in suppliers' processes or enforce concrete actions?

Insufficient enforcement is then the Achilles heel for governance by contract when it comes to sustainability. The private sector operates within what can be called a four-step monitoring and enforcement process (Mitkidis, 2015: 233). The steps are often used in a progressive manner—first, suppliers conduct a self-assessment. If the self-assessment or an internal audit raises a red flag, then external audit is conducted. If a breach is identified during the audit, the parties work on a corrective action plan and only when the breach is not remedied within the stipulated framework, then the contract might be terminated. This formalized process though leads to contract termination only exceptionally. For example, EcoVadis and Affectio Mutandi in their report find that from the studied contracts '[a]s much as 75 percent of clauses specify that a violation of the CSR clause can be a cause for an early termination, but only 12 percent have actually resorted to termination' (EcoVadis and Affectio Mutandi, 2018: 15). Legal enforcement through the courts is then very limited or practically non-existent due to legal hurdles as well as a lack of motivation (Mitkidis, 2019). Court proceedings are generally public, so companies would expose themselves to negative publicity, and retaining the business relationship with a supplier and thus securing uninterrupted delivery is often more important than pursuing sustainability goals.

As outlined above, the pharmaceutical industry is an atypical close-to-consumer industry, meaning that although it produces goods directly consumed by patients, it is not as sensitive to consumers' perception as ethical/unethical as other close-to-consumers industries. Yet the industry has been exposed to fierce ethical judgement, especially by investors (fearing the effects of any unethical behaviour on their investment), regulators (calling on large companies to take on their part of environmental responsibility), and the general public (not approving 'healing' pharmaceutical industry to gain profit by unethical practice). Finally, the business of pharmaceutical companies is about making peoples' health and life better (Alexandra, Countess of Frederiksborg, and Fort, 2014: 152). As Hank McKinnell, a former CEO of Pfizer, put it, '[b]ecause we have the ability to help in so many ways, we have a moral imperative to do so' (McKinnell and Hager, 2002). This dependence on the opinion of the general public, investors, and regulators is reflected in corporate sustainability procurement policies and practice. The PSCI finds that while the PiE stood at the top of the most important topics and trends for PSCI member companies in 2017–2018, it fell below supply chain resilience/business continuity and climate/emissions reduction in 2020 (PSCI, 2021: 11). The explanation of the drop stands out clearly. While in 2017–2018 the public discourse of PiE was intense in the expectation of the publication of the EU Strategic Approach (European Commission, 2019); 2020 was dominated by the COVID-19 crisis and its consequences as well as the climate discourse following the developments under the Paris Agreement, namely the re-entering of the United States, and the various extreme weather and climate events of 2020 (Yale Climate Connections, 2020). One of the COVID-19 crisis consequences was the increased fear of pharmaceutical supply chain disruptions, unequal access to medicines, and ethical questions in respect to vaccination. Environmental issues, and especially the invisible ones, such as the spread of AMR due to manufacturing discharges, were pushed into the background.

Finally, while possibly still ensuring that the PiE stands on the third place on the above-mentioned list, procurement policies of pharmaceutical companies and industry rarely address AMR expressly. For example, while the PSCI Principles speak of discharge controls, they do not make a specific link to the AMR hazard (PSCI Principles, 2019).

The potential of mutual reinforcing between public and private sustainable procurement practices in the fight against AMR

Following from the above, the interest in sustainable pharmaceutical procurement is detected in both the public and private sectors. Each of the sectors though presents only a part of the solution to the use of governance by contract to fight the global AMR challenge. Thus, governance by contract unfortunately remains largely ineffective, thus far. The shortcomings in each of the sectors individually are hard to overcome within the current business and regulatory framework.

One possibility of exploiting the full potential of procurement processes in this area is to facilitate mutual learning and reinforcement between the public and private procurement fields. As private procurement has been developing over several decades, it can contribute with experience, expertise, and knowledge of the market conditions regarding sustainability. For example, conducting sustainability audits of suppliers has become standard practice for most large close-to-consumer companies (Fraser et al., 2020), yet responsible private procurement is based on voluntary participation, lacking binding power and adequate enforcement. Furthermore, it has been criticized for aiming to postpone any EU regulatory action in respect of PiE in transnational supply chains by presenting itself as a viable alternative to hard regulation (Milmo, 2018). Public buyers, with more rigid administrative processes, may help to overcome these shortcomings of private procurement. They can stipulate sustainability criteria in a legally stronger manner, pool resources, and thus increase their influence over the private sphere; in other words, the market power and legitimacy of public buyers can cover the gap in the binding nature and enforcement of private regulation. Ultimately, the coordination of public and private procurement may help to bridge the regulatory gap while simultaneously avoiding the adoption of a rigid PiE legislation. The EU's Big Buyers initiative is an example of such pooling intending to deliver on the sustainability agenda (Big Buyers for Climate and Environment, n.d.).

The voices calling for public–private collaboration to fight AMR through procurement are getting louder (Schaaf, 2018). The AMR Industry Alliance, for example, says '[i]ndustry and governments must ... work together to ensure that supply chains are continuous, sustainable, and secure' (SustainAbility, 2020: 57). However, the drivers behind this call are preventing disruptions in pharmaceutical supply chains and medicines' shortages rather than addressing AMR (SustainAbility, 2020: 57). The Joint position paper on the Pharmaceutical Strategy for Europe makes a clearer link between green public procurement and the ability of pharmaceutical companies to 'reduce pharmaceutical pollution that contributes to AMR' throughout their supply chains (JPPPSE, 2020: 9). The background idea is that public procurement works as a natural driver for the development of private procurement. We can see this already in some suppliers in the developing countries, such as in India, who implement innovative solutions into their APIs' manufacturing processes to curb the spreading of AMR (SustainAbility, 2018: 82; see Chapter 17 for a further exploration of these initiatives).

This and other examples serve as evidence of the large potential hidden in the coordination between public and private procurement for global AMR governance.

But how can such coordination work? First, environmental requirements to suppliers need to be set and optimally harmonized. It is not an easy exercise to formulate such environmental criteria that would be measurable, be connected to the subject matter, and deliver on the AMR policy goals at the same time. European countries, particularly the Nordic ones, lead in the development of environmental criteria for pharmaceutical public procurement (Amgros, 2022; Lonaeus, 2016; Norwegian Hospital Procurement Trust, 2019). However, similar action takes also place at the global level under the auspices of the UN (Lindstrom and Coronado-Garcia, 2020: 18–19). Collaboration among public and private actors in preparing environmental criteria was identified as crucial, private parties coming in with information on the feasibility of any suggestions of public buyers (Lonaeus, 2016: 14). The EU legal framework, however, namely the requirement of the L2SM, may work as an obstacle rather than a facilitator of this exercise (Lonaeus, 2016: 16). This might be the reason why so-far formulated requirements are not specifically targeting AMR triggered by manufacturing effluents but rather the existence of corporate environmental management practices (Andhov et al., 2020: 10). A possible future direction for identifying concrete AMR-focused requirements could be the involvement of a new labelling scheme assuring the quality of wastewater treatment in suppliers' facilities. The requirement of environmental labels in EU public procurement is regulated in the Public Procurement Directive (Directive 2014/24/EU, recital 75 and Article 43). However, even such a label might still fail the L2SM test, providing a too general solution (Andhov et al., 2020: 38–9). To overcome this, it might be necessary to develop a methodology that would monitor the manufacturing discharges of a specific drug to such a wastewater treatment facility and, thus, connect clearly the subject matter of the contract to the label requirement.

After environmental requirements are identified, the contract execution, monitoring, and enforcement processes should be standardized for the suppliers to align expectations and avoid auditing fatigue (see e.g., Khalid et al., 2020). Audit results can be shared among public and private buyers to decrease audit-related costs. Achieving such a coordination will require engagement, will and trust on both sides. Already initiated collaborations, such as the RAMP (Stockholm International Water Institute (SIWI), 2020), bring hope and should be scaled up.

Optimally, public and private buyers should work in unison to influence future policy and regulation. While this would be optimal, it might take time to reconcile the profoundly different motivations of the public and private pharmaceutical buyers.

Finally, the public and private procurers could through collaboration minimize double work and, thus, expenses. While public procurement focuses on articulating sustainability requirements primarily in the initial phases of the procurement process (pre-tender and tender), private procurement does the opposite and focuses on contract language and contract execution. The sharing of experience and combining best practice from both is desirable.

Conclusion

Production discharges from pharmaceutical manufacturing have been standing at the outskirts of the EU AMR policy and governance. With the increasing scientific knowledge of the scope of those discharges to the environment and their detrimental effects, the regulatory eyes are turning to this issue. The complexity of transnational supply chains and the need of extraterritorial regulation combined with the prevailing opposition of the private sphere to any new EU legislation on PiE have, however, been hindering further regulatory development. The coordination of public and private procurement can help us to move away from this regulatory stalemate and present a valuable piece in the global AMR governance puzzle. This will require the will, trust, and engagement among the involved subjects.

Several policy implications and recommendations can be identified. First, a development of platforms facilitating an open discussion among all involved subjects, public and private buyers as well as suppliers, scientists, and engineers, is a necessary initial step (SIWI, 2020). Secondly, such platforms should help to formulate public procurers' requirements that are feasible and legal, benefitting from the experience and knowledge from other spheres, such as product labelling. Finally, the ultimate target for using governance by contract to fight global AMR is to exploit all stages of the procurement process and avoid 'reinventing the wheel' while scaling up the leverage of the stricter environmental standards of developed countries over the pharmaceutical production processes in developing countries. Optimally, this all can happen without the necessity to adopt new legislation.

The EU regulator might facilitate the above through a revision of the current public procurement rules. In particular, the L2SM requirement should be reconsidered and possibly replaced. Moreover, the possibility to include environmental criteria into the good manufacturing practice rules should be considered (EMA, n.d.). Overall, the current legal framework should be reviewed to ensure that it enables rather than hinders the use of governance by contract to fight global AMR. By mounting procurement processes as a global AMR governance tool, the EU can exercise both directional and structural leadership (Elgström, 2011) globally and motivate similar developments in other jurisdictions.

Acknowledgement

The author thanks research assistant Adriana Šefčíková for excellent support during the writing of this chapter. The work on this chapter was conducted within the framework of the research project Regulating emerging pollutants: Designing law amidst constant scientific knowledge development, funded by the Carlsberg Foundation, grant no. CF19-0170.

References

Affolder, N. (2018). 'Looking for Law in Unusual Places: Cross-Border Diffusion of Environmental Norms'. *Transnational Environmental Law*, 7/3, 425–49. <https://doi.org/10.1017/s2047102518000080>.

Alexandra, Countess of Frederiksborg, and Fort, T. L. (2014). 'The Paradox of Pharmaceutical CSR: The Sincerity Nexus'. *Business Horizons*, 57/2, 151–60. <https://doi.org/10.1016/j.bushor.2013.10.006>.

Amgros. (2022). *European Award for Joint Nordic Environmental Criteria*. <https://amgros.dk/en/knowledge-and-analyses/articles/european-award-for-joint-nordic-environmental-criteria/> accessed 3 February 2023.

SustainAbility (2018). *Tracking Progress to Address AMR*. AMR Industry Alliance. Geneva, Switzerland. <https://www.amrindustryalliance.org/wp-content/uploads/2018/01/AMR_Industry_Alliance_Progress_Report_January2018.pdf>.

AMR Industry Alliance. (2019). *Making Antibiotics Responsibly a Common Manufacturing Framework to Tackle Antimicrobial Resistance*. <https://www.amrindustryalliance.org/wp-content/uploads/2019/11/Making-antibiotics-responsibly_A-common-manufacturing-framework-to-tackle-AMR.pdf>.

SustainAbility. (2020). *AMR Industry Alliance 2020 Progress Report*. AMR Industry Alliance. Geneva, Switzerland. <https://www.amrindustryalliance.org/wp-content/uploads/2020/01/AMR-2020-Progress-Report.pdf>.

Andhov, M. et al. (2020). *Sustainability through Public Procurement: The Way Forward—Reform Proposals*.

Andrecka, M., and Mitkidis, K. P. (2017). 'Sustainability Requirements in EU Public and Private Procurement—a Right or an Obligation?', *Nordic Journal of Commercial Law*, 1, 55–89. <https://doi.org/10.5278/ojs.njcl.v0i1.1982>.

Big Buyers for Climate and Environment. (n.d.). <https://bigbuyers.eu> accessed 3 August 2021.

Cafaggi, F. (2016). 'Regulation through Contracts: Supply-chain Contracting and Sustainability Standards'. *European Review of Contract Law*, 12/3, 218–58. <https://doi.org/10.1515/ercl-2016-0013>.

Cassini, A., Högberg, L. D., Plachouras, D., Quattrocchi, A., Hoxha, A., Simonsen, G. S., et al. (2019). 'Attributable Deaths and Disability-Adjusted Life-Years Caused by Infections with Antibiotic-Resistant Bacteria in the EU and the European Economic Area in 2015: A Population-Level Modelling Analysis'. *The Lancet Infectious Diseases*, 19/1, 56–66. <https://doi.org/10.1016/S1473-3099(18)30605-4>.

Committee on Antimicrobial Resistance. (2018). *Today's Actions for a Healthier Tomorrow 2017-2018*. European Health Parliament. <https://www.healthparliament.eu/wp-content/uploads/2018/04/Walking-the-Talk-on-Antimicrobial-Resistance.pdf>.

Deva, S. (2006). 'Global Compact: A Critique of The U.N.'s "Public-Private" Partnership For Promoting Corporate Citizenship'. *Syracuse Journal of International Law and Commerce*, 34/1, 107–151.

Directive 2014/24/EU of The European Parliament and of The Council of 26 February 2014 on public procurement and repealing Directive 2004/18/EC.

EcoVadis and Affectio Mutandi. (2018). *Sustainability Clauses in Commercial Contracts: The Key to Corporate Responsibility 2018 Study of CSR Contractual Practices Among Buyers and Suppliers*. <https://www.eticanews.it/wp-content/uploads/2018/07/ecovadis_contrat_clauses_RSE__20.06.2018_eng_v5-1.pdf>.

Elgström, O. (2011). 'EU Leadership in an Emerging New World Order', in C. G. Alvstam, B. Jännebring, and D. Naurin, eds, *I Europamissionens tjänst. Vänbok till Rutger Lindahl* (Göteborg: Centrum för Europaforskning vid Göteborgs universitet), 311–21.

EMA (European Medicines Agency) (n.d.). *Good Manufacturing Practice*. <https://www.ema.europa.eu/en/human-regulatory/research-development/compliance/good-manufacturing-practice>.

European Centre for Disease Prevention and Control. (2021). *Geographical Distribution of Antimicrobial Consumption.* <https://www.ecdc.europa.eu/en/antimicrobial-consumption/datab ase/geographical-distribution> accessed 3 August 2021.

European Commission. (2017a). *AMR: A Major European and Global Challenge* [Fact sheet]. <https://ec.europa.eu/health/sites/default/files/antimicrobial_resistance/docs/amr_2017_fa ctsheet.pdf>.

European Commission. (2017b). *Communication from the Commission to the European Parliament, the Council, the European Economic and Social Committee and the Committee of the Regions. Making Public Procurement Work in and for Europe.* Strasbourg. COM(2017)572 Final.

European Commission. (2017c). *A European One Health Action Plan against Antimicrobial Resistance (AMR).* <https://ec.europa.eu/health/sites/default/files/antimicrobial_resistance/docs/amr_2017 _action-plan.pdf>.

European Commission. (2019). *Communication from The Commission to The European Parliament, The Council and The European Economic and Social Committee. European Union Strategic Approach to Pharmaceuticals in the Environment.* Brussels. COM(2019) 128 final (EU Strategic Approach to PiE).

European Commission. (2020). *Communication from The Commission to The European Parliament, The Council, The European Economic and Social Committee and The Committee of The Regions. Pharmaceutical Strategy for Europe.* Brussels. COM(2020) 761 final, SWD(2020) 286 Final (Pharmaceutical Strategy for Europe).

European Court of Justice, Case C-368/10 *Commission v. Kingdom of the Netherlands* [2012] ECR I-284.

European Court of Justice, Case C-513/99, *Concordia Bus* [2002] ECR I-7213; Case C-448/01, *EVN and Wienstrom* [2003] ECR I-14527.

Fraser, I. J., Schwarzkopf, J., and Müller, M. (2020). 'Exploring Supplier Sustainability Audit Standards: Potential for and Barriers to Standardization'. *Sustainability*, 12, 8223. <https://doi.org/ 10.3390/su12198223>.

Grundmann, S., Möslein, F., and Riesenhuber, K. (2015). *Contract Governance: Dimensions in Law and Interdisciplinary Research* (1st edn, Oxford: Oxford University Press).

Guiu Segura, J. M., Gilabert Perramon, A., Sans Calle, V., and Hors Comadira, P. (2019). 'Introducing Concepts of Circular Economy into the Public Procurement of Medicines in Europe'. *European Journal of Hospital Pharmacy. Science and Practice*, 26(4), 238–40. <https://doi.org/10.1136/ejhph arm-2018-001717>.

Haddock-Fraser, J., and Fraser, I. (2008). 'Assessing Corporate Environmental Reporting Motivations: Differences Between "Close-to-Market" and "Business-to-Business" Companies'. *Corporate Social Responsibility and Environmental Management*, 15/3, 140–15. <https://doi.org/ 10.1002/csr.147>.

HCWH. (2019, September). *Tackling AMR in Europe's Healthcare Facilities: Best Practice to Prevent the Development and Spread of Drug-Resistant Bacteria.* Brussels. <https://noharm-europe. org/sites/default/files/documents-files/5994/2019_09_24_HCWH_AMR_European_Hospit als_WEB.pdf>.

JPPPSE (Joint position paper on the Pharmaceutical Strategy for Europe). (2020). *Improving Transparency and Access to Affordable, Quality, and Sustainable Medicines in Europe.* <https://me-dicinesalliance.eu/wp-content/uploads/2020/07/Joint-position-pharma-strat_200713.pdf>.

Khalid, M. K., Agha, M. H., Shah, S. T. H., and Akhtar, M. N. (2020). 'Conceptualizing Audit Fatigue in the Context of Sustainable Supply Chains'. *Sustainability*, 12/21, 9135. <http://dx.doi.org/10.3390/ su12219135>.

Kurucz, E. C., Colbert, B. A., and Wheeler, D. (2008). 'The Business Case for Corporate Social Responsibility', in A. Crane, D. Matten, A. McWilliams, J. Moon, and D. S. Siegel, eds, *The Oxford Handbook of Corporate Social Responsibility* (1st edn, Oxford: Oxford University Press), 83–112. <https://doi.org/10.1093/oxfordhb/9780199211593.003.0004>.

Larsson, D. G. J. (2014). 'Pollution from Drug Manufacturing: Review and Perspectives'. *Philosophical Transactions of the Royal Society B: Biological Sciences*, 369/1656, 20130571, 1–7. <https://doi.org/ 10.1098/rstb.2013.0571>.

Larsson, D. G. J., de Pedro, C., and Paxeus, N. (2007). 'Effluent from Drug Manufactures Contains Extremely High Levels of Pharmaceuticals'. *Journal of Hazardous Materials*, 148/3, 751–5. <https://doi.org/10.1016/j.jhazmat.2007.07.008>.

Lee, M., and Kohler, J. (2010). 'Benchmarking and Transparency: Incentives for the Pharmaceutical Industry's Corporate Social Responsibility'. *Journal of Business Ethics*, 95/4, 641–58. <https://doi.org/10.1007/s10551-010-0444-y>.

Leisinger, K. M. (2005). 'The Corporate Social Responsibility of the Pharmaceutical Industry: Idealism without Illusion and Realism without Resignation'. *Business Ethics Quarterly*, 15(4), 577–94. <https://doi.org/10.5840/beq200515440>.

Lindstrom, A., and Coronado-Garcia, L. (2020). *Sustainable Health Procurement Guidance Note*, UN Development Programme.

Lonaeus, K. (2016). *Sustainable Pharmaceuticals—Public procurement as a Political Tool* (Stockholm: SIWI).

Marschang, S. (2017). *AMR and Antibiotic Production: A Vicious Cycle* (European Public Health Alliance). <https://epha.org/amr-and-antibiotic-production-a-vicious-cycle/>.

McKinnell, H., and Hager, M. (2002). 'We Are Not the Problem'. *Chief Executive*, 180, 20.

Medicines for Europe. (2021). *Medicines for Europe Factsheets on Market and regulatory reforms to ensure availability and resilience of the supply chain* [Fact sheet]. Brussels. <https://www.medicinesforeurope.com/wp-content/uploads/2021/05/Medicines-for-Europe-Factsheets-on-Market-and-regulatory-reforms-to-ensure-availability-and-resilience-of-the-supply-chain.pdf>.

Milmo, S. (2018). 'Pharmaceuticals in the Environment'. *Pharmaceutical Technology Europe*, 30/8, 6–7.

Mitkidis, K. P. (2015). *Sustainability Clauses in International Business Contracts*. Eleven International Publishing.

Mitkidis, K. (2019). 'Enforcement of Sustainability Contractual Clauses in Supply Chains by Third Parties', in V. Ulfbeck, A. Andhov and K. Mitkidis, eds, *Law and Responsible Supply Chain Management: Contract and Tort Interplay and Overlap* (London: Routledge), 65–87. <https://doi.org/10.4324/9780429461231-4>.

Mitkidis, K., Walter, S. E., and Obolevich, V. (2018). 'Towards Responsible Management of Pharmaceutical Waste in the EU', in H. T. Anker and B. E. Olsen, eds, *Sustainable Management of Natural Resources: Legal Instruments and Approaches* (Cambridge: Intersentia), 63–80.

Norwegian Hospital Procurement Trust (Sykehusinnkjøp HF). (2019). *New Environmental Criteria for the Procurement of Pharmaceuticals*. <https://sykehusinnkjop.no/nyheter/new-environmental-criteria-for-the-procurement-of-pharmaceuticals> accessed 3 August 2021.

Peterkova, K. (2014). 'General or Specific? Wording Matters in a Supplier's Code of Conduct'. *Contracting Excellence Journal*, November/December 2014.

Polianciuc, S. I., Gurzău, A. E., Kiss, B., Ştefan, M. G., and Loghin, F. (2020). 'Antibiotics in the Environment: Causes and Consequences'. *Medicine and Pharmacy Reports*, 93/3, 231–40. <https://doi.org/10.15386/mpr-1742>.

PSCI. (2021). *Benchmarking Report: Responsible Procurement and PSCI's Impact*. London. <https://pscinitiative.org/resource?resource=943>.

PSCI Principles, v2.0. (2019). <https://pscinitiative.org/resource?resource=1>.

Schaaf, N. (2018). 'It Takes Two to Tango'. *Waterfront*, 3–4, 22–3. <https://www.yumpu.com/en/document/read/62284259/water-front-3-4-2018/23>.

Schaaf, N. (2020). *AMR driven by manufacturing our next big challenge*. DownToEarth. <https://www.downtoearth.org.in/blog/health/amr-driven-by-manufacturing-our-next-big-challenge-74259>.

Semple, A. (2015). 'The Link to the Subject Matter: A Glass Ceiling for Sustainable Public Contracts?', in B. Sjåfjell and A. Wiesbrock, eds, *Sustainable Public Procurement under EU Law* (Cambridge: Cambridge University Press), 50–74. <https://doi.org/10.1017/CBO9781316423288.005>.

Stevens, H., and Huys, I. (2017). 'Innovative Approaches to Increase Access to Medicines in Developing Countries'. *Frontiers in Medicine*, 4, 218. <https://doi.org/10.3389/fmed.2017.00218>.

Stockhom International Water Institute. (2020). *Responsible Antibiotics Manufacturing Platform (RAMP)*. <https://siwi.org/amr-ramp/>.

SumOfUs (based on research by Changing Markets and Profundo). (2015). *Bad medicine: How the Pharmaceutical Industry is Contributing to the Global Rise of Antibiotic-Resistant Superbugs.* New York. <https://changingmarket.wpengine.com/wp-content/uploads/2016/12/BAD-MEDIC INE-Report-FINAL.pdf>.

VIVE, Wadmann, S., and Kjellberg J. (2018). *Value-based Procurement of Hospital Medicines— Denmark.* <https://www.vive.dk/media/pure/10767/2302250>.

WHO. (2020). *Antimicrobial Resistance.* <https://www.who.int/news-room/fact-sheets/detail/antimi crobial-resistance>.

Yale Climate Connections. (2020). *The Top 10 Extreme Weather and Climate Events of 2020.* <https:// www.ecowatch.com/extreme-weather-climate-2020-2649628910.html>.

19

International Law and Antimicrobial Resistance

Learning from Fifteen Years Implementing the International Health Regulations

Louise Munkholm and Susan Rogers Van Katwyk

Introduction

Antimicrobial resistance (AMR) constitutes a creeping crisis for global health (Baekkeskov et al., 2020). Caused by the production and use of antimicrobial agents that we depend on to treat infectious diseases, AMR is a 'super wicked problem' and extremely difficult to mitigate (Baekkeskov et al., 2020). As resistant micro-organisms do not respect national borders, tackling the root causes and transmission of AMR necessitates substantial global cooperation. Achieving the necessary level of global cooperation requires a strong global governance regime, and there has been widespread discussion concerning the need for an international legal instrument to boost global collective action on AMR (Behdinan et al., 2015; Hoffman, et al., 2015; Rogers Van Katwyk, Giubilini, et al., 2020; Rogers Van Katwyk, Weldon, et al., 2020). In general, international legal agreements are the strongest mechanisms through which states can make commitments to each other, and thus constitute a valuable tool for coordinating responses to problems with substantial global reach or the potential to cross international borders (Hoffman et al., 2015). Research suggests that a global health treaty has a reasonable chance of being impactful if the health challenge has a significant transnational dimension, if the treaty addresses multilateral challenges that cannot be addressed by a single country, and if the treaty incentivizes action, institutionalizes accountability, and activates interest groups (Hoffman et al., 2015). Yet, the slow pace of developing new international laws is a barrier to achieving global AMR goals, and when contrasted against the need for timely AMR action (Rogers Van Katwyk, Weldon, et al., 2020), it provides a strong incentive to use established legal mechanisms rather than creating entirely new systems. As the primary mechanism for coordinating global health emergency responses, the International Health Regulations (2005) (IHRs) are often cited as the most likely existing option for governing the global AMR response. While previous iterations of the IHRs focused on a few specified infectious disease threats, the 2005 revision defines Member States' rights and obligations in handling health emergencies with the potential to cross borders, including but not limited to infectious diseases. In particular, the IHRs require the World Health Organization

Louise Munkholm and Susan Rogers Van Katwyk, *International Law and Antimicrobial Resistance* In: *Steering against Superbugs*. Edited by: Olivier Rubin, Erik Baekkeskov, and Louise Munkholm, Oxford University Press. © Oxford University Press 2023. DOI: 10.1093/oso/9780192899477.003.0019

(WHO) and its Member States to implement a coordinated global system of prepared-ness, surveillance, alerts, and response for any health threat that puts humans at risk (World Health Organization, 2005a). This focus on preparedness and surveillance in the revised IHRs creates the opportunity to see the Regulations as a tool for tackling the global spread of AMR (Wernli et al., 2011).

In this chapter, we discuss the potential and pitfalls of using the IHRs as a legal frame-work for global AMR governance. We base the discussion on our analysis of the experi-ences of the WHO in IHR implementation with focus on global, regional, and national capacity scores from the period 2010–2020,[1] and a document analysis of sixty reports on IHR implementation presented to the World Health Assembly (WHA), covering the years 2006–2021.[2] Building on the criteria for an effective international legal in-strument outlined by Hoffman, Røttingen, and Frenk (2015), attention is paid to the extent to which the IHRs incentivize action, institutionalize accountability, and acti-vate interest groups. Our analysis shows that IHR implementation suffers from lack of sustained action, lack of enforcement mechanisms and lack of activation of all interest groups. This in turn makes the IHRs less suitable as an international legal framework for dealing with AMR. The chapter concludes by suggesting how to draw from this knowledge when designing future global AMR responses.

Background

The IHRs date back to the Sanitary Conference in 1851 (Gostin and Katz, 2016). At that time, cholera, plague, and yellow fever entered Europe from Asia, causing European leaders call for international agreements to curb the ongoing spread of infectious dis-eases (Howard-Jones, 1975). The first legally binding agreement, the International Sanitary Convention (ISC), was adopted in 1892 to mitigate the spread of cholera. By 1926, the ISC also covered plague and yellow fever. Those earliest agreements grew out of concern from European governments who wanted 'self-protection against ex-ternal threats, rather than safeguarding the public's health in every region of the world' (Gostin and Katz, 2016: 266). Upon its creation in 1948, the WHO assumed the over-sight of the ISC, and the WHO Constitution gave the WHO the mandate to adopt regu-lations to prevent the international spread of disease (see World Health Organization, 1948, Articles 21–22), regulations that are binding on WHO Member States unless they affirmatively opt out. In 1951, the WHA used this mandate to replace the ISC with the International Sanitary Regulations, now covering six diseases. A 1969 revision changed the name of the regulations to the IHRs and removed typhus and relapsing fever from

---

[1] Data have been derived from the e-Spar Repository of the WHO: <https://extranet.who.int/e-spar>. 31 January 2022 (last accessed).
[2] The World Health Assembly archive can be accessed here: <https://apps.who.int/gb/index.html>. Documents from the latest WHA in May 2021 were found here: <https://apps.who.int/gb/e/e_wha74.html>. 31 January 2022 (last accessed).

the covered diseases, and a later revision also removed smallpox, resulting in an IHR that covered the original diseases from the ISC: cholera, plague, and yellow fever.

In 1995, the WHA called for fundamental revision of the IHRs as they proved insufficiently flexible to respond to new infectious disease threats (Gostin and Katz, 2016). A ten-year revision process resulted in the adoption of the revised IHRs in 2005. According to the WHO, the revised Regulations

> contain a range of innovations, including: (a) a scope not limited to any specific disease or manner of transmission, but covering 'illness or medical condition, irrespective of origin or source, that presents or could present significant harm to humans'; (b) State Party obligations to develop certain minimum core public health capacities; (c) obligations on States Parties to notify WHO of events that may constitute a public health emergency of international concern according to defined criteria; (d) provisions authorizing WHO to take into consideration unofficial reports of public health events and to obtain verification from States Parties concerning such events; (e) procedures for the determination by the Director-General of a 'public health emergency of international concern' and issuance of corresponding temporary recommendations, after taking into account the views of an Emergency Committee; (f) protection of the human rights of persons and travellers; and (g) the establishment of National IHR Focal Points and WHO IHR Contact Points for urgent communications between States Parties and WHO. (World Health Organization, 2005a: 1–2)

In short, the IHRs require WHO and its Member States to implement a coordinated global system of preparedness, surveillance, alerts, and response for any health threat that puts humans at risk. AMR is indisputably a health threat that puts humans at risk (O'Neill, 2016), and building capacity for preparedness, surveillance, alerts, and health risk response are at the core of existing action plans and non-binding international agreements, including the Global Action Plan endorsed by the WHA in 2015 and the 2016 Political Declaration on Antimicrobial Resistance adopted by the UN General Assembly. This suggests good reasons for using the IHRs as framework for governing AMR. However, careful analysis is needed to determine the extent to which the existing IHR structure supports specific AMR governance needs.

Analysis of IHR implementation

Our analysis is divided into three sections. Section 1 focuses on the extent to which the IHRs incentivize action. Sections 2 and 3 investigate the extent to which the IHRs institutionalize accountability and activate interest groups, respectively.

1. Incentivizing action

The IHRs seek to improve Member States' capacities to detect, assess, notify, and report events that may constitute a public health risk of international concern. With June 2012 set as the initial target date for establishment of these capacities (World Health Organization, 2005a), WHO has conducted an annual self-assessment survey at the country level since 2010. This assessment focuses on thirteen areas: legislation, coordination, surveillance, response, preparedness, risk communication, human resources, laboratory, points of entry, zoonotic events, food safety, chemical events, and radionuclear accidents.[3] Based on the self-assessments, each country gets a capacity score calculated as a percentage (from 0 to 100) for each of the thirteen areas. These data provide a useful starting point for evaluating the extent to which the IHRs incentivize Member States to develop and maintain their capacities to deal with public health risks of international concern. Analysing global average capacity scores over time, it becomes clear that implementation falls short in many areas. For example, the global average score on human resources, which concerns '[s]trategies … to ensure that a multisectoral workforce is available and trained to enable early detection, prevention, preparedness and response to potential events of international concern at all levels of health systems' (World Health Organization, 2018a: 19), only grows from forty-two in 2010 to sixty-four in 2020 (World Health Organization, 2021a), suggesting ongoing challenges in recruiting and training personnel on how to translate the IHRs effectively from paper into practice. In comparison, progress has happened to a larger degree in the areas of surveillance, outbreak response, and laboratory capacities where the global average scores are generally high (91, 79, and 81 in 2017, respectively, compared to 63, 69, and 66 in 2010, respectively) (World Health Organization, 2021a).

Both regionally and nationally, there is great variation as to the extent to which the core capacities have been developed and maintained. The African region scores lowest in all capacity categories in all years whereas the European region tend to score significantly higher than the global average in all capacity categories (World Health Organization, 2021a). This indicates that the IHRs' ability to incentivize action depends on income levels and regional efforts: rich Member States in regions with high levels of regional coordination and collaboration have higher capacity scores than poorer Member States in regions with lower levels of regional coordination and collaboration—a finding that resonates with other studies, showing that high-income countries (HICs) in Europe are frontrunners when it comes to AMR mitigation whereas low- and middle-income countries (LMICs) are often left behind (e.g., Munkholm and

---

[3] From 2018, implementation efforts have been assessed based on a revised self-assessment questionnaire that merges response and preparedness under a new category termed 'National Health Emergency Framework' and introduces a new capacity named 'Health service provision'. Also the former 'Yes/no/not known' responses are replaced by five progressive levels of capacity. This change in how capacity scores are accessed makes it difficult to compare the exact capacity scores over time. Nevertheless, the exercise remains relevant as a means to establish a baseline for analysing progress and lack thereof when it comes to IHR implementation.

Rubin, 2021; see also Chapters 5, 6, and 7). In 2020, almost all countries with capacity scores below the global average (65) are LMICs, and the pattern of big differences in capacity scores between LMICs and HICs is particularly profound in the case of the African region, the South-East Asian region, the Eastern Mediterranean region, as well as the Western Pacific region (World Health Organization, 2021a). The capacity scores must, of course, be treated with caution as they result from self-assessments with only sporadic participation. As noted by the WHO: '100% of States Parties have reported on IHR indicators at least once in past 9 years' (World Health Organization, n.d.). While the findings from an analysis of self-assessed capacity scores should not be overstated, these scores nevertheless suggest that capacity building happens slowly, raising the issue of whether the IHRs can be used as a tool to boost action when it comes to global health threats such as AMR.

In their annual reports to the WHA, the WHO Director-General explicitly considers the lack of progress in Member States' capacity scores and outlines different types of hurdles and barriers to overcome. Recurrent themes include lack of technical and financial resources; lack of governmental commitment and political leadership; lack of time and personnel at national level; and lack of awareness of the Regulations (see, e.g., World Health Organization, 2012b). The Director-General also highlights uneven levels of support by various stakeholders and a lack of alignment between priorities of donors, the WHO itself, and the needs of the most vulnerable member states (World Health Organization, 2014), as well as lack of intersectoral collaboration, public–private partnerships, and community involvement (World Health Organization, 2017). While these challenges are clearly identified, and repeated throughout the years, the WHO seems to have struggled to overcome them. In the implementation reports and their supplementary material (such as resolutions to be adopted by the WHA), the most often proposed solution to these capacity deficits entails training through workshops, toolkits, simulation exercises, and new/improved online information sites (see, e.g., World Health Organization, 2008, 2012a, 2013, 2020). In summary, although the IHRs are legally binding upon Member States, WHO addresses challenges to the implementation of IHRs through soft law tools rather than advocating for more hard law approaches, such as developing mechanisms for sanctioning non-compliance or low performance. Action is thus incentivized through soft law methods, however, with different degrees of success as indicated by the great variance in capacity scores over time and within specific areas. As AMR mitigation requires timely and sustained action from all stakeholders, this soft approach to incentives makes the IHRs less useful as legal framework for AMR governance.

2. Institutionalizing accountability

Apart from being a means to incentivize action, the collection and public sharing of capacity scores can also be seen as one way in which accountability is institutionalized under the IHRs: Using capacity scores, WHO seeks to hold member states accountable for their actions under the IHRs.

The IHRs also establish two other paths for institutionalized accountability. First, Article 5 of the Regulations establishes the right of Member States to apply for an extension of two years to fulfil their obligations 'on basis of a justified need and an implementation plan', and Article 13 establishes that in 'exceptional circumstances . . . the State Party may request a further extension not exceeding two years' (World Health Organization, 2005a). These provisions provide the WHO with a mechanism to monitor the implementation process and push Member States to prepare realistic implementation plans, thereby holding them accountable through institutionalized means. More than half of the Member States (118 out of 194) requested and were granted a two-year extension in 2012 (World Health Organization, 2015a), and in 2014, eighty-one Member States were granted an additional extension (World Health Organization, 2015b).

The other path for institutionalized accountability in the IHRs relates to Article 43, which allows Member States to implement additional health measures in response to public health risks or public health emergencies of international concern, as long as these are not 'more restrictive of international traffic and not more invasive or intrusive to persons than reasonably available alternatives that would achieve the appropriate level of health protection' (World Health Organization, 2005a). Article 43 obliges Member States that implement additional health measures to 'inform WHO, within 48 hours of implementation, of such measures and their health rationale' (unless these are covered by a temporary or standing recommendation issued by the WHO) (World Health Organization, 2005a). On the basis of the information received, the WHO 'may request that the member state concerned reconsider the application of the measures' (World Health Organization, 2005a). This provision not only provides the WHO with the mandate to request that Member States justify their adoption of additional measures but also with the mandate to ask Member States to withdraw measures interpreted by the WHO to be counterproductive.

While these three mechanisms (self-assessments, extension procedures, and review of health measures) serve to institutionalize accountability, they suffer from a lack of enforcement mechanisms. There are no legal consequences if Member States do not submit annual self-assessment questionnaires, do not apply for extensions when failing to meet deadlines, or who do not follow WHO recommendations regarding withdrawing health measures that interfere unnecessarily with international traffic and trade. As emphasized by the Review Committee in 2011, 'The most important structural shortcoming of the IHR is the lack of enforceable sanctions" (World Health Organization, 2011: 13). In its 2015 report, the Review Committee flagged unresolved problems with the extension process, noting that by June 2014, forty-two Member States had not communicated their intentions and 'should be reminded of the importance of transparency in relation to both the letter and the spirit of the IHR' (World Health Organization, 2015a: 8). Thus, while the extension option institutionalizes accountability, it also acts as a loophole for Member States to postpone the fulfilment of their obligations. In 2016, in reference to the fact that several Member States simply ignored reprimands from the WHO, the Review Committee report concluded that there is 'an unacceptable disregard for their obligations under the IHR' (World Health Organization, 2016: 32). In a similar vein, the Review Committee report presented in May 2021 in the midst of the COVID-19 pandemic notes:

> As we reviewed the IHR article by article, we found that much of what is in the Regulations is well considered, appropriate and meaningful in any public health emergency of international concern. However, ... in the context of a pandemic, countries that in 2005 approved the IHR, in 2020 only applied the Regulations in part, were not sufficiently aware of them, or deliberately ignored them. (World Health Organization, 2021b: 7)

The IHRs do not establish any enforceable sanctions, and creating these enforcement tools would require renegotiation of the IHR. This renegotiation is unlikely as recent moves suggest that the WHO no longer expects strict compliance with the IHRs. In the first years after its adoption, WHO monitored implementation with an emphasis on meeting specific deadlines, such as the entry into force of the Regulations in June 2012 (see e.g., World Health Organization, 2005b), and the deadlines for seeking extensions (see e.g., World Health Organization, 2012a). In 2015, WHO shifted its approach, emphasizing that, going forward, implementation should be seen as a continuous process based on a 'progressive realization of rights and obligations' as opposed to 'one that comes to an end at any particular date' (World Health Organization, 2015c: 6). In 2018, the WHO suggested the use of a five-year global strategic plan that 'does not create any legally binding obligations for Member States' to improve IHR implementation (World Health Organization, 2018b: 39). Thus, WHO has moved away from requiring strict compliance with the commitments under the Regulations. This suggests a view that when enforceable sanctions are non-existent, and there is no will for developing them, non-binding measures seem to be the only viable way for improving IHR implementation.

In contrast to Member State accountability, it is less clear what mechanisms exist to hold WHO itself accountable for its responsibilities under the IHRs. The IHR s(2005) place a number of obligations on the Director-General, including (i) having to co-operate with other intergovernmental organizations 'to coordinate with them the activities of WHO ... with a view to ensuring application of adequate measures for the protection of public health and strengthening of the global public health response to the international spread of disease', (ii) to build and strengthen the capacities of WHO to 'perform fully and effectively the functions entrusted to it', and (iii) provide support to developing countries in building, strengthening, and maintaining the capacities required under the IHRs (World Health Organization, 2005a: 4). From the information available, it seems that the accountability of WHO bodies is only assessed by the external Review Committees who may raise issues and make recommendations but who have no mandate to sanction non-compliance.

In summary, the IHRs establish clear procedures for how to measure and assess accountability but lack concrete tools for sanctioning Member States who do not participate in these procedures and WHO bodies who do not perform in accordance with the Regulations. This partial institutionalization of accountability in turn hampers the effectiveness of the IHRs to meet their objectives. It also makes the IHRs ill-equipped as a global framework for mitigating AMR, only adding another layer of self-assessments and voluntary alignment to the existing governance regime.

3. Activating interest groups

Our analysis of IHR implementation reports from 2006 to 2021 shows that the Regulations have activated some interest groups more than others. While serving public health interests in general and being sensitive to the interests of international traffic and trade (World Health Organization, 2005a: Article 2), the IHRs are primarily designed to serve member states' interests. The Regulations emphasize the sovereign right of states to legislate and implement health legislation and policies and highlight that '[i]n doing so they should uphold the purpose of these Regulations' (World Health Organization, 2005a: Article 3.4). If reports about potential public health risks come from non-state sources, the WHO is obliged to 'consult and obtain verification from the State Party in whose territory the event is allegedly occurring' (World Health Organization, 2005a: Article 9.1). At the same time, several Member States have obtained different types of reservations with the IHRs, illustrating how public health needs are constantly balance against interests of Member States (World Health Organization, 2005a: 60–8). By contrast, the activation of other interest groups receives much less attention in the legal document. The Regulations only emphasize a small number of international bodies as relevant partners (e.g., the United Nations (UN), International Labour Organization (ILO), Food and Agriculture Association (FAO), World Organisation for Animal Health (OIE), International Atomic Energy Association (IAEA), International Civil Aviation Authority (ICAO), International Maritime Organization (IMO), International Committee of the Red Cross (ICRC), International Air Transport Association (IATA), International Shipping Federation (ISF)) (World Health Organization, 2005a: 3–4) while the interests of ordinary people are considered only briefly, for example in Article 3 which highlights that the 'implementation of these Regulations shall be with full respect for the dignity, human rights and fundamental freedoms of persons', and in Article 32 which establishes that Member States must 'treat travellers with respect for their dignity, human rights and fundamental freedoms' (World Health Organization, 2005a: 10). While WHO reports an increase in the involvement of stakeholders in IHR implementation, there is little or no reference to international donors, the development community, or interest groups from the environmental or pharmaceutical sectors, or human rights organizations.

By contrast, other interest groups seem to be activated consistently including those in international transport sectors (e.g., ICAO), those who work with food safety and animal health (e.g., FAO, OIE, and the International Food Safety Authorities Network (INFOSAN)), and those who work with nuclear emergencies (e.g., IAEA).

The lack of activation of all relevant interest groups hampers the effectiveness of the IHRs in several ways. For example, in assessing the functioning of the IHRs in relation to the H1N1 pandemic in 2009, the Review Committee concludes that WHO suffers from 'systemic difficulties' and highlights 'WHO's dual role as moral voice for health in the world and as a servant of its member states' as particularly problematic (World Health Organization, 2011: 10). The statement is elaborated with the observation that 'WHO's scientific and technical aspirations for global health are constantly conditioned by the multiplicity of views, needs and preferences of its Member States' (World Health Organization, 2011: 27). Put differently, the IHRs are implemented in ways that privilege the interests of national authorities at the expense of other important and relevant stakeholders whose voices and potential for acting are, as a consequence, overlooked or ignored. From the perspective of AMR, the lack of ability of the IHRs to activate all relevant interest groups is problematic. While the IHRs activate important actors for AMR mitigation, such as FAO, OIE, and INFOSAN, the failure to engage with groups in the development community, environmental sectors, and pharmaceutical manufacturers, limits opportunities to develop a coherent AMR response that includes disease prevention, access to antimicrobials, and pharmaceutical innovation.

Challenges for AMR

Despite having been adopted more than fifteen years ago, and giving Member States five years to implement, it is clear that the Regulations are not fully functional as a mechanism to mitigate threats to human health. Our analysis of the IHR implementation reports reveals several issues that appear difficult to correct within the existing system, including the inherent tension between WHO's role as a moral voice for public health and a servant for Member States, and the lack of mechanisms to enforce action on IHR obligations. Thus, the IHRs fail to incentivize action, institutionalize accountability, and activate interest groups sufficiently, thereby failing to give WHO the necessary mechanisms and influence to create action on urgent global health threats, including AMR.

On this basis, several lessons can be drawn from fifteen years implementing the IHRs. First, without compliance mechanisms an international legal instrument works poorly, resulting in a lack of incentives to deliver on developing core capacities as required by the instrument, and on participating in the institutionalized accountability frameworks. A lack of incentives and enforcement mechanisms in the IHRs may also prevent Member States from reporting global health threats. For example, LMICs may benefit little from reporting threats while they serve as an early warning system for HICs with more capacity (Wilson et al., 2008). To combat AMR, it is vital to develop a global framework that provides strong incentives for all stakeholders to act. It is crucial to activate all relevant interest groups at all stages, from design to implementation of the international legal instrument. This is a key impediment to applying the IHRs to AMR and other emerging One Health threats that require collaborative action between sectors. Secondly, as a reactive tool for dealing with public health emergencies, the IHRs take an event-based approach, responding to outbreak notifications from Member States. While the development and spread of new antimicrobial resistance strains meets the criteria constituting a Public Health Emergency of International Concern (PHEIC) both in terms of serious public health impact and potential for international spread (Wernli et al., 2011), resistance is often seen as a single phenomenon rather than as a series of discrete acute outbreak events (Kamradt-Scott, 2011). It is therefore unlikely that many discrete outbreaks of a resistant pathogen would be deemed a PHEIC. Furthermore, as IHR implementation suffers from lack of capacity in many member states to detect and report on public health risks and emergencies, it is unlikely the IHR National Focal Points would use their reporting mechanisms for repeated AMR events (Kamradt-Scott, 2011). Even if the IHR National Focal Point frequently reported AMR outbreaks, there is a risk that without similarly frequent declarations of PHEIC, the importance of AMR would be minimized, giving rise to the impression that AMR is not a serious public health threat and detracting from efforts to rally collaboration through other international mechanisms.

Another crucial challenge is that while individual outbreaks could rise to the level of PHEIC, overall, the IHRs lack mechanisms to address the underlying drivers of resistance development. As an evolutionary process rather than a single infectious agent, AMR requires a substantial focus on investments that address the root causes of infection, and the collaborative global response must include coordination on the processes that accelerate AMR. Attempting to use the event-based tools under the IHRs as the primary mechanism for coordinated and collaborative response to global AMR also risks shifting global focus away from the current approach, which emphasizes multisectoral coordination across access, conservation and innovation challenges, and towards a reactionary approach that prioritizes AMR action only when an outbreak becomes severe enough to be a PHEIC. While the IHRs do provide a mechanism for strengthening surveillance, they do not provide a mechanism for strengthening action on access, conservation, or innovation.

Conclusion

The creeping AMR crisis requires immediate and sustained action, yet substantial financial and time investments would be needed to develop a new AMR-focused treaty. Previous research has recommended a number of revisions to the IHRs that would promote appropriate antibiotic use, including creating and financing a global fund to improve access, stewardship, healthcare, food security, and WASH systems; strengthening health systems to improve infection prevention and control and reduce the need for antimicrobials; strengthening the surveillance of antimicrobial use and AMR in humans, animals, and the environment through setting international standards for laboratory testing and data harmonization; or safeguarding the effectiveness of new antimicrobials through the creation of expert committee to monitor resistance and, as needed, designating and reserving particular antimicrobials for human-only use (Rogers Van Katwyk, Weldon, et al., 2020). However, based on our analysis, we argue there are too many pitfalls with using the IHRs as an international legal framework for governing the antimicrobial commons: it is too vulnerable to Member States interests, it fails to incentivize action, institutionalize accountability, and activate all relevant interest groups.

On this basis, we suggest three policy recommendations for international legally binding AMR agreements. First, given the limitations of the IHRs, there is a need to develop a new standalone AMR treaty with the necessary reach and sanctions to ensure One Health action. Such a treaty would need to prioritise preparedness over reactive event-based responsiveness and enhance stakeholders' compliance with obligations. Second, there is a need to establish new One Health AMR leadership (for a contrary view, see Chapter 11). The IHRs do not provide the WHO with sufficient mandate or resources to address AMR as a One Health challenge. To ensure engagement with all relevant interest groups, a new AMR governance regime should be lead either by the UN or by a new multisectoral body. Finally, given the identified challenges in using global health focused legal structures like the IHRs to incentivize action, we suggest that a new AMR treaty draws inspiration from other governance sectors than public health, such as international trade law. Here, a 'predictable legal framework' is seen as 'the precondition for efficient international commerce' (Mitkidis, 2019: 97) as predictability creates stability and sustained action through the use of contractual standards which outline both the responsibilities of each party and the procedures for resolving non-compliance (Mitkidis, 2019: 105–6). Put differently, clear and well-defined responsibilities and enforcement procedures provide strong incentives to act in accordance with the agreed upon rules. Thus, apart from drawing on the lessons learnt from fifteen years implementing the IHRs, it also makes sense to look to trade and other regimes to identify the building blocks of a new and strong AMR global governance regime.

References

Behdinan, A., Hoffman, S. J., and Pearcey, M. (2015). 'Some Global Policies for Antibiotic Resistance Depend on Legally Binding and Enforceable Commitments', *Journal of Law, Medicine & Ethics*, 43/ S3, 68–73. <https://doi.org/10.1111/jlme.12277>.

Bækkeskov, E., Rubin, O., Munkholm, L., and Zaman, W. (2020). 'Antimicrobial Resistance as a Global Health Crisis', in E. Stern, ed., *Oxford Encyclopaedia of Crisis Analysis* (Oxford: Oxford University Press). Retrieved 27 January 2023, from <https://oxfordre.com/politics/view/10.1093/acrefore/9780190228637.001.0001/acrefore-9780190228637-e-1626>.

Gostin, L. O., and Katz, R. (2016). 'The International Health Regulations: The Governing Framework for Global Health Security', *The Milbank Quarterly*, 94/2, 264–313.

Hoffman, S. J., Outterson, K., Røttingen, J.-A., Cars, O., Clift, C., Rizvi, Z., Rotberg, F., Tomson, G., and Zorzet, A. (2015). 'An International Legal Framework to Address Antimicrobial Resistance', *Bulletin of the World Health Organization*, 93/2, 66. <http://dx.doi.org/10.2471/BLT.15.152710>.

Hoffman, S. J., Røttingen, J.-A., and Frenk, J. (2015). 'Assessing Proposals for New Global Health Treaties: An Analytic Framework', *American Journal of Public Health*, 105/8, 1523–30. <https://doi.org/10.2105/AJPH.2015.302726>.

Howard-Jones, N. (1975). The Scientific Background of the International Sanitary Conferences 1851–1938 (Geneva: World Health Organization).

Kamradt-Scott, A. (2011). 'A Public Health Emergency of International Concern? Response to a Proposal to Apply the International Health Regulations to Antimicrobial Resistance', *PLoS Medicine*, 8/4, e1001021.< https://doi.org/10.1371/journal.pmed.1001021>.

Mitkidis, K. (2019). 'Development of Transnational Contract Law?', in B. L. Kristiansen, K. Mitkidis, L. Munkholm, L. Neumann, and Cécile Pelaudeix, eds, *Transnationalisation and Legal Actors: Legitimacy in Question* (London: Routledge), 97–111.

Munkholm, L., and Rubin, O. (2021). 'The Global Governance of Antimicrobial Resistance: A Cross-Country Study of Alignment Between the Global Action Plan and National Action Plans', *Globalization and Health*, 16, 109. doi:10.1186/s12992-020-00639-3.

O'Neill, J. (2016). *Tackling Drug-resistant infections Globally: Final Report and Recommendations* (Wellcome Trust and HM Government).

Rogers Van Katwyk, S., Giubilini, A., Kirchhelle, C., Weldon, I., Harrison, M., McLean, A., Savulescu, J., and Hoffman, S. J. (2020). 'Exploring Models for an International Legal Agreement on the Global Antimicrobial Commons: Lessons from Climate Agreements'. *Health Care Analysis*. <https://doi.org/10.1007/s10728-019-00389-3>.

Rogers van Katwyk, S., Weldon, I., Giubilini, A., Kirchhelle, C., Harrison, M., McLean, A., et al. (2020). 'Making Use of Existing International Legal Mechanisms to Manage the Global Antimicrobial Commons: Identifying Legal Hooks and Institutional Mandates', *Health Care Analysis*. <https://doi.org/10.1007/s10728-020-00393-y>.

Wernli, D., Haustein, T., Conly, J., Carmeli, Y., Kickbusch, I., and Harbarth, S. (2011). 'A Call for Action: The Application of the International Health Regulations to the Global Threat of Antimicrobial Resistance', *PLoS Medicine*, 8/4, e1001022. <https://doi.org/10.1371/journal.pmed.1001022>.

Wilson, K., von Tigerstrom, B., and McDougall, C. (2008). 'Protecting Global Health Security through the International Health Regulations: Requirements and Challenges', *Canadian Medical Association Journal*, 179/1, 44–8. <https://doi.org/10.1503/cmaj.080516>.

World Health Assembly archives. (n.d.). <https://apps.who.int/gb/index.html>. Documents from the latest WHA in May 2021 were found here: <https://apps.who.int/gb/e/e_wha74.html>.

World Health Organization. (n.d.). *International Health Regulations: Overview*. <https://www.who.int/health-topics/international-health-regulations#tab=tab_2> (last accessed: 31 January 2022).

World Health Organization. (1948). *Constitution of the World Health Organization* (Geneva: World Health Organization).

World Health Organization. (2005a). *International Health Regulations (2005)* (Geneva: World Health Organization).

World Health Organization. (2005b). *Revision of the International Health Regulations. Note by the Secretariat.* (Document No. A58/4) (Geneva: World Health Organization).

World Health Organization. (2008). *Implementation of the International Health Regulations (2005). Report by the Secretariat* (Document No. A61/7) (Geneva: World Health Organization).

World Health Organization. (2011). *Implementation of the International Health Regulations (2005). Report of the Review Committee on the Functioning of the International Health Regulations (2005) in relation to Pandemic (H1N1) 2009. Report by the Director-General* (Document No. A64/10) (Geneva: World Health Organization).

World Health Organization. (2012a). *Implementation of the International Health Regulations (2005). Report by the Director-General* (Document No. A65/17) (Geneva: World Health Organization).

World Health Organization. (2012b). *Implementation of the International Health Regulations (2005). Report on development of national core capacities required under the Regulations. Report by the Secretariat* (Document No. A65/17 Add.1) (Geneva: World Health Organization).

World Health Organization. (2013). *Implementation of the International Health Regulations (2005). Report by the Director-General* (Document No. A66/16) (Geneva: World Health Organization).

World Health Organization. (2014). *Implementation of the International Health Regulations (2005). Report by the Director-General* (Document No. A67/35) (Geneva: World Health Organization).

World Health Organization. (2015a). *Implementation of the International Health Regulations (2005). Report of the Review Committee on Second Extensions for Establishing National Public Health Capacities and on IHR Implementation. Report by the Director-General* (Document No. A68/22 Add.1) (Geneva: World Health Organization).

World Health Organization. (2015b). *Resolutions and Decisions Annexes* (Document No. WHA68/2015/REC/1) (Geneva: World Health Organization).

World Health Organization. (2015c). *Implementation of the International Health Regulations (2005). Responding to Public Health Emergencies. Report by the Director-General* (Document No. A68/22) (Geneva: World Health Organization).

World Health Organization. (2016). *Implementation of the International Health Regulations (2005). Report of the Review Committee on the Role of the International Health Regulations (2005) in the Ebola Outbreak and Response. Report by the Director-General* (Document No. A69/21) (Geneva: World Health Organization).

World Health Organization. (2017). *Implementation of the International Health Regulations (2005). Annual Report on the Implementation of the International Health Regulations (2005). Report by the Director-General* (Document No. A70/15) (Geneva: World Health Organization).

World Health Organization (2018a), *International Health Regulations (2005). State Party Self-Assessment Annual Reporting Tool* (Geneva: World Health Organization).

World Health Organization. (2018b). *Resolutions and Decisions Annexes* (Document No. WHA71/2018/REC/1) (Geneva: World Health Organization).

World Health Organization. (2020). *International Health Regulations (2005). Annual Report on the Implementation of the International Health Regulations (2005). Report by the Director-General* (Document No. A73/14) (Geneva: World Health Organization).

World Health Organization. (2021a). *e-Spar State Party Annual Report.* <https://extranet.who.int/e-spar>. Geneva: World Health Organization.

World Health Organization. (2021b). *WHO's Work in Health Emergencies. Strengthening Preparedness for Health Emergencies: Implementation of the International Health Regulations (2005)* (Document A74/9 Add1) (Geneva: World Health Organization).

Index

For the benefit of digital users, indexed terms that span two pages (e.g., 52–53) may, on occasion, appear on only one of those pages.